HYPNOTISM

First Edition (Grant Richards), 1903
Second Edition (Alexander Moring, Ltd.), 1906

HYPNOTISM

ITS HISTORY, PRACTICE
AND THEORY

BY

J. MILNE BRAMWELL, M.B., C.M.

AUTHOR OF NUMEROUS ARTICLES ON
THE PRACTICE AND THEORY OF HYPNOTISM

SECOND EDITION

London

ALEXANDER MORING, Limited

DE LA MORE PRESS

32 GEORGE STREET, HANOVER SQUARE, W.

1906

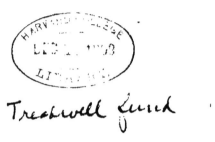

PREFACE TO THE SECOND EDITION

THE First Edition of the above work was practically exhausted in ten months, and has now, for some time, been entirely out of print.

Since it appeared, little of importance has been added to the literature of hypnotism, and nothing which has caused me to alter the views I have already expressed.

Under these circumstances, I feel justified in making the Second Edition a practically unaltered reproduction of the First.

J. MILNE BRAMWELL.

33 WIMPOLE STREET,
    LONDON, W.

CONTENTS.

CHAPTER I.

CHAPTER II.

CHAPTER III

CHAPTER IV.

CHAPTER V.

CHAPTER VI.

CHAPTER VII.

CHAPTER VIII.

CHAPTER XI.

CHAPTER XII.

CHAPTER XIII.

X's views, 429. Cases of harm reported by X, 430. Objections to his
statements, 430. Instances of alleged evil results of hypnotic practice
generally nothing but cases of delusional insanity, 431.

CHAPTER I.

ALTHOUGH of late years hundreds of books have been written on hypnotism, nearly all have been contributed by foreign workers, and few have been translated. Apparently the latter do not fulfil the requirements of English students, as I am frequently asked for information which they do not contain. I propose, therefore, not only to refer to my twelve years' hypnotic practice and research, but also to give such a general account of the subject as can be brought within reasonable compass.

In the chapter on history, much is purposely omitted that has already been given by Moll, Liégeois, and others, regarding Mesmer, his predecessors and immediate followers. On the other hand, I have drawn particular attention to the work of Elliotson, Esdaile, and Braid, as what was done, especially by the two former, is apparently almost entirely forgotten.

I hope the description of the different methods may prove useful to those who wish to begin hypnotic work.

It is impossible to give anything like a full account of the medical and surgical cases that have been recorded. I have therefore (1) selected some from my own practice, and (2) chosen others, most of which have neither been previously translated into English nor published abroad in easily accessible form— the majority being taken from foreign medical journals, etc.

I have found it equally difficult to condense the experimental phenomena of hypnosis, and have been compelled to give a short account of most of them; but post-hypnotic appreciation of time, which apparently has an important bearing on hypnotic theory, is dealt with in greater detail.

The chapter on stages occupies little space. I have given,

however, more fully the causes which influence susceptibility to hypnosis, as these are of great practical importance.

I have drawn attention to the importance of care in the management of medical and particularly experimental cases, as it is to want of caution in the conduct of the latter that we owe most of our fallacies.

Hypnotic theories are too numerous and complicated to be described at length, but the principal ones have been outlined and discussed.

Finally, I have endeavoured to show what awaits those who embark on hypnotic practice—to picture its successes and failures, and the dangers, mainly theoretical, which are said to be associated with it.

CHAPTER II.

(A) THE EARLY HISTORY OF HYPNOTISM.

JUST as chemistry arose from alchemy, astronomy from astrology, and the therapeutics of to-day were formerly represented by disgusting compounds, largely drawn from the living or dead human body, so Hypnotism had its origin in Mesmerism. Hence, amongst hypnotic phenomena are to be found those mesmeric ones which have stood the test of a rigorous investigation, and are now explained in a more scientific way. Phenomena, such as Mesmer (b. 1734, d. 1815) described, had been observed from an early date in human history; but after his day they were usually called by his name and explained by his theory, i.e. by the action of a mysterious force or fluid, supposed to emanate from the operator.

The phenomena themselves, the methods supposed to evoke them, and their theoretical explanation, will be again referred to more fully. For the present it is only necessary to remember that the mesmerists believed that they excited the phenomena by various physical means, such as fixed gazing and passes with contact. The subjects then passed either into a condition resembling lethargy, in which anæsthesia and other symptoms of decreased sensibility occurred, or into what was termed " lucid trance," characterised by hyperæsthesia of the special senses. The mysterious force or fluid just referred to was held to explain everything.

In 1814, the Abbé Faria suggested that the phenomena were subjective in origin, but his views made little impression and were soon forgotten. On the other hand, the influence of Mesmer continued to be widely felt: numerous observers in different

3

Ones author's explanation about the differences
between Salpetriere & Nacy schools False because at
least The people of Nancy knew, what was occurring at
Salpetrier

countries produced phenomena resembling those he had shown,
and explained them in much the same way.

It is only by studying the work of the later mesmerists,
and contrasting it with that of Braid, that we are able to understand how hypnotism arose, shook itself free from the fallacies
and misconceptions which preceded its birth, and finally established itself among the sciences. Ignorance of what was done
by the rival schools of Mesmerism and Hypnotism probably
accounted in some measure, at all events, for the reproduction
of mesmeric errors at the Salpêtrière, and for the claims of
the Nancy school to be the discoverers of much that had
already been demonstrated by Braid.

John Elliotson was the leader of a great mesmeric movement which began in England in 1837. This I propose to
sketch, as well as the antagonism between Braid and the
mesmerists, and possibly can do so best by presenting short
histories of Elliotson, Esdaile, and Braid.

JOHN ELLIOTSON.

John Elliotson, the son of a Southwark chemist, was born
in 1791. He received a sound classical education, then went
to Edinburgh and graduated as M.D. He next visited the
most important Continental medical schools, and, on his return
to England, continued his studies at Cambridge and St. Thomas
and Guy's Hospitals.

In 1817, he was appointed assistant physician to St.
Thomas's Hospital, and physician six years later, but only
obtained the privilege of giving clinical lectures with great
difficulty. These were at once successful, and I can best
describe them by giving, almost in his own words, the account
published by a contemporary writer in the *Medical Times*, vol.
xi. 1844–45. They were telling things, he said, full of
learning, acuteness, careful discrimination, philosophic liberality
and daring, and often wonderfully accurate decisiveness. Their
interest was quite peculiar. The cases were carefully selected,
each stage marked with the greatest nicety, and the principles,
whatever they were, on which the patient was treated, recklessly
bared to the world. In addition, there was a large dash of
novelty, either in the treatment or in its explanation. Elliot-

son's motto was everlastingly "Onward!" If he did not look with hate, he did with distrust, on all that was old—the past seemed nothing to him, the future boundless. Beyond the mere narrative description of disease, he thought that nothing had been done before his time—that the medical edifice had yet to be erected, and he was determined to have his full share of the labour. The spirit of progress had permeated his whole being. With so much of art unexplored before him, and so little of life for the task, his genius strove to reach the goal in leaps, and sought distinction in medicine like a youthful Napoleon in war. . . . We owe to him the employment of quinine in heroic doses, the recognition of the value of iodide of potassium, the use of prussic acid in vomiting, iron in chorea, sulphate of copper in diarrhœa, the employment of creosote, etc.

The *Lancet* also pointed out that Elliotson had shown how the heart sounds were influenced by posture, and had also drawn attention to many other hitherto unnoticed phenomena connected with auscultation. Elliotson, in fact, was the earliest to use the stethoscope in England, and began to do so immediately after the publication of Laennec's work. At first he made his observations quietly in his hospital wards, but, as soon as he drew attention to them, he was ridiculed and abused. The stethoscope, as well as the facts of percussion and auscultation as described by Avenbrugger, were condemned as fallacies by the foremost teachers of medicine in London, while, even at a much later date, they were treated at St. Thomas's with indignation or silent contempt. At the College of Physicians a senior fellow, in a Croonian Lecture, denounced the folly of carrying a piece of wood into a sick-room. Another condemned the stethoscope as worse than nonsense, and said: "Oh! It's just the thing for Elliotson to rave about." While a third, on seeing one on Elliotson's table, said: "Ah! Do you use that hocus pocus?" On Elliotson replying that it was highly important, he added: "You will learn nothing by it, and, if you do, you cannot treat disease the better."

In 1831, Elliotson was appointed Professor of the Practice of Medicine at University College. His connection with that institution and the commencement of his mesmeric researches were described in the *Medical Times* by the writer already referred to, and I again quote the latter almost in his own words.

Thus, he said, on the establishment of the University of London, or, as it is now called, University College, Elliotson moved there, as to a temple after his own heart, and devoted himself enthusiastically to its interests. He was all for the College, was its great impelling force, and worked for it with an alacrity and energy that explains much of its early progress. The Hospital may be said to have been mainly his erection. Yet here, in the home of his labours, the scene of his triumphs, he received his greatest check. Dupotet's visit to this country attracted much attention to mesmerism, and led Elliotson to investigate the subject. His experiments were successful, and, believing that he had found an opening into an unexplored science, he pursued them with zeal and daring enthusiasm. His reckless independence made many enemies, and official opposition to mesmerism led him to resign his Hospital appointments. Notwithstanding this, Elliotson adhered to mesmerism, and sacrificed to it friends, position, and practice, but still looked sanguinely forward to the hour when the profession would say of it as of creosote, iodide of potash, prussic acid, auscultation, etc.: " Useful novelties if properly employed."

This account understates both the amount of mesmeric work done at University College and the opposition it received. The demonstrations of Chenevix, in 1829, first drew Elliotson's attention to the subject, but it was only after seeing Dupotet, in 1837, that he commenced his own researches. In conjunction with his clinical clerk, Mr. Wood, he regularly mesmerised some of the patients, and obtained important therapeutic results. His students, as well as those of other hospitals, soon became greatly interested, and attended in such numbers that Elliotson was obliged to mesmerise in the theatre, instead of in the wards. His colleagues, while boasting of their refusal to witness his demonstrations, persecuted and annoyed him in many petty and disgraceful ways. The Dean, in advising him to desist, urged that the interests of the School ought to be considered, rather than those of science and humanity, and that the risk of the loss of public favour was of more importance than the truth of the wonderful facts alleged, or of their benefit in the treatment of disease. To this Elliotson replied " that the institution was established for the discovery and dissemination of truth; all other considerations were secondary, and we should lead the public, not the public us.

The sole question was whether the matter were the truth or not."

In 1838, the Council of University College passed the following resolution : " That the Hospital Committee be instructed to take such steps as they shall deem most advisable to prevent the practice of mesmerism or animal magnetism in future within the Hospital." Elliotson was therefore ordered to cease mesmerising his patients, and immediately resigned his appointments, never afterwards entering either College or Hospital. He felt the insult keenly, especially as he was senior physician, and had done much to increase the reputation and prosperity of the School. In addition, the Hospital owed its origin to him, and he had made enemies amongst his colleagues by insisting that the Medical School was inefficient without one. Further, he asserted that the action of the Council was unreasonable, as the majority of its members had refused to witness his experiments or even to discuss the subject with him.

In 1846, Elliotson's turn came to deliver the Harveian Oration, but, as soon as it was known that he had accepted the office, he was attacked in the most savage manner, in order to prevent his appearing. For example, the *Lancet* called him a professional pariah, stated that his oration would strike a vital blow at legitimate medicine, and would be a black infamy degrading the arms of the College.

Undeterred by this, Elliotson made mesmerism the subject of his address. Without referring to the attacks which had been made upon him, he simply stated the result of his researches, and respectfully invited the College to examine alleged facts of overwhelming interest and importance. He exhorted his hearers to study mesmerism calmly and dispassionately, and reminded them, with more truth than tact, that all the greatest discoveries in medical science, and the most important improvements in its practice, had been opposed by the profession in the most violent and unprincipled manner. As examples of scientific discoveries which had been received in this way, he cited those of the lacteal vessels, the thoracic duct, the sexual system of plants, the circulation of the blood, the sounds of the chest and their relation to the diseases of the heart and lungs and their coverings, etc. As instances of improvement in practice which had been treated in like manner, he referred to the employment of Peruvian bark,

In the Early 19 century, after mesmerism had been in
decline, people still believed the claims of the early
mesmerists.

8   *HYPNOTISM*

inoculation and vaccination for small-pox, the use of mild
dressings, instead of boiling oil, in gun-shot wounds, the ligature
of the bleeding vessels after operation, instead of the application
of burning pitch or red-hot irons, etc. We should, Elliotson said,
never forget these things, nor allow authority, conceit, habit, or
the fear of ridicule to make us hostile to truth. We should
always have before our eyes that memorable passage in Harvey's
works : "True philosophers, compelled by the love of truth and
wisdom, never fancy themselves so wise and full of sense as not
to yield to truth from any source and at all times : nor are they
so narrow-minded as to believe any art or science has been
handed down in such a state of perfection to us by our predecessors
that nothing remains for future industry." All this, Elliotson said,
should be borne in mind when considering the alleged facts of
mesmerism. In his opinion many of these were indisputable ;
for ten years he had shown how mesmerism could prevent pain
during surgical operation, produce sleep and ease in sickness, and
even cure many diseases which had been unrelieved by ordinary
methods. It was the imperative and solemn duty of the profession
to carefully and dispassionately examine the subject. He therefore earnestly implored them to do so, if they cared for truth,
their own dignity, and the good of mankind.

In 1843, Elliotson and his sympathisers started the *Zoist*, a
journal for the collection and diffusion of information connected
with cerebral physiology and mesmerism. It appeared quarterly,
from April, 1843, until it was discontinued on December 31st,
1855. Its writers then claimed that its object had been fulfilled
—their views had been made public for thirteen years. The whole
work comprises thirteen volumes, averaging about 500 pages each.

Elliotson was a constant writer in the *Zoist*, and contributed many medical and surgical cases observed by himself
or others. These comprised amputations of the thigh, leg, arm,
breast, etc., which had been performed painlessly during mesmeric
trance in England and Scotland, as well as on the Continent and
in America. The most important operations, however, were those
recorded by Esdaile in India, and published in the *Zoist* from
time to time. Cure or improvement was alleged to have followed
mesmeric treatment in insanity, epilepsy, hystero-epilepsy,
hysteria, stammering, neuralgia, asthma, torticollis, headache,
functional affections of the heart, rheumatism, and other diseases,

Elliotson asserted that mesmerism was especially useful in hysteria and other functional nervous disorders. These diseases, he said, were generally misunderstood, and treated in a worse than useless manner by blistering, bleeding, and salivation. Marriage, with disastrous results, was sometimes suggested as a remedy for hysterical women, on the supposition that the disease was essentially of a sexual character. It was not, however, necessarily connected with the uterus, nor confined to the female sex, but occurred frequently both in boys and men. Mesmerism, not medicine, was the appropriate treatment for hysteria.

In addition to mesmerism, sanitation, education, the undue harshness of the criminal code, and the insufficient attention paid to the mental condition of criminals, were subjects which occupied prominent places in the *Zoist*, and views were expressed which, though long since accepted, were doubtless at that time regarded as extremely revolutionary.

In an essay entitled "*Physical Well-being, a Necessary Preliminary to Moral and Intellectual Progression*," attention was forcibly drawn to the evils arising from the overcrowded and insanitary conditions of the houses of the poor.

The crying necessity for national education was insisted upon, and the injustice of a Government scheme, afterwards given up, was thus referred to: "Dissenters are to be compelled to pay towards the support of schools where religious doctrines are taught of which they disapprove, and the schools are to be under the absolute control of the clergy. Not only must they pay for exclusive Church schools and send their children to them, but they are themselves debarred from receiving one farthing from the poor-rates towards their own schools. . . . Education is the proper remedy for crime, and there ought to be a national system of education, apart from religious belief and sectarian influence."

As the result of the influence of the *Zoist*, a Mesmeric Infirmary was opened in London, and Mesmeric Institutions were formed in Edinburgh, Dublin, and elsewhere. At one of these, in Exeter, Mr. Parker, surgeon, claimed to have mesmerised 1200 persons, and to have performed 200 painless surgical operations. The medical journals almost entirely ignored the surgical and therapeutic claims of mesmerism, and usually only referred to it in order to assail its followers with the most violent abuse. In the *Lancet* of July 31st, 1847, for example, the following editorial statement appeared: "Of course the parties concerned in the infamous publication (the *Zoist*) are in a state of perpetual mortification at their fallen and degraded position, and therefore they bite and rail; the leper [*sic*] must be taken with his spots."

The subjects of the various surgical operations were universally regarded either as impostors or as persons insensible to pain. In Nottinghamshire, in 1842, Mr. Ward, surgeon, amputated a thigh during mesmeric trance; the patient lay perfectly calm during the whole operation, and not a muscle was seen to twitch. The case, reported to the Royal Medical and Chirurgical Society, was badly received; and it was even asserted that the patient had been trained not to express pain. Dr. Marshall Hall suggested that the man was an impostor, because he had been absolutely quiet during the operation; if he had not been simulating insensibility, he would have had reflex movements in the other leg. Dr. Copland proposed that no account of such a paper having been read before the Society should be entered in its minutes. He asserted that "if the history of the man experiencing no agony during the operation were true, the fact was unworthy of their consideration, because pain was a wise provision of nature, and patients ought to suffer pain while their surgeons were operating; they were all the better for it and recovered better." Eight years afterwards, Dr. Marshall Hall publicly stated at a meeting of the Society that the patient had confessed that he had suffered during the operation. The doctor was promptly challenged to give his authority, and replied that he had received the information from a personal acquaintance, who, in his turn, had received it from a third party, but that he was not permitted to divulge their names, and would not give any further information on the subject. The man was still living, and signed a solemn declaration to the effect that the operation had been absolutely painless. Dr. Ashburner attended the next meeting, and asked permission to read this statement in opposition to Dr. Marshall Hall's, but the Society would not hear him.

Elliotson opposed and constantly attacked spiritualism, but, on the other hand, shared the mesmeric errors of his day; he believed in clairvoyance, phrenology, and odylic force, and translated Burq's *Metallo-Therapia*.

Elliotson's fallacies, especially as to clairvoyance, were eagerly seized upon by his opponents, and made the subject of constant and virulent attack. He, in his turn, assailed what he regarded as medical errors. Thus, in referring to the treatment of a case of nervous exhaustion by blood-letting, he said ammonia and not the lancet was required. He asserted that the indiscriminate use of blood-letting, and other debilitating measures, had caused the death of thousands of human beings, and had left a still greater number enfeebled for the rest of their lives. Formerly, the surgeries of country practitioners were crowded at spring and fall with healthy persons waiting to be bled. He had protested against this practice thirty years ago, but now medical men had run into the other extreme, and had entirely abandoned depletion, which, in properly selected cases, was a valuable remedy.

As to the administration of medicines, Elliotson said, our aim should be to benefit the patient with the smallest number of grains or drops, but the dose ought to be steadily increased until the system had felt its power. Some practitioners had actually a fixed dose for each medicine; others changed their prescriptions incessantly, and the patient believed he had tried everything, whereas time had simply been wasted. Thus, one of the physicians at University College Hospital made a clean sweep at every visit of all the drugs he had prescribed at the previous one. The public had no conception of the absurd mode in which medicines were administered; for example, when iodide of potassium was first introduced Sir —— began by opposing it, then prescribed it in the invariable dose of two grains, never giving more, even if it produced no effect.

Elliotson also complained of the rôle played by fashion in medicine. For thirty years, he said, the liver was the favourite organ; all diseases were referred to it, all treatment directed to it. Of late the kidneys had had an equal run; but he was sick of hearing about renal diseases, and twenty years previously had steadily opposed the doctrine that albumen in the urine necessarily indicated structural disease of the kidneys.

Elliotson found children easy to mesmerise, and stated that he could thus cure or relieve many of their diseases; at the same time he insisted upon the injury done to them by the ordinary medical treatment of his time. His views on the management of children were remarkable, and he drew a vivid picture of their sufferings from the cruelty of parents, medical men, and teachers.

What he said about corporal punishment might be read with profit by those who are still advocating its retention in girls' schools. Children suffering from nervous diseases were made worse, he said, by being needlessly tortured with blisters and other external irritants. Yet the little creatures were far more sensitive than we were, and felt more pain from an equal cause. When he thought of medical men's cruelty to innocent little children, he often wished their complaints had been left to nature.

If well treated and managed, children were positively heavenly beings, far superior to their elders in moral excellence. They were affectionate, confiding, and disposed to truth, and yet, at home, at school, and elsewhere, they were the most persecuted of all human beings. Their faults resulted from bad management, and could be corrected by good example and advice. Dulness and crossness were often the result of over-fatigue, and the poor child was punished when he ought really to have been sent to bed. Many little things made *us* cross, but no allowance was made for the young. Convulsions sometimes arose from over-work, and terror was no uncommon cause of nervous affections. Such maladies were often not recognised, and punished as obstinate faults. St. Vitus' dance, local twitchings and the like were often supposed to be due to bad habits or obstinacy. Momentary fits of epileptic unconsciousness, little paroxysms of insanity, causing absurdity or anger for a few minutes, were frequently mistaken for bad conduct, and the child punished accordingly.

As far as I can learn, Elliotson, up to the time of his death, continued to believe in clairvoyance and other alleged mesmeric phenomena of a similar nature. The following statement, however, at the conclusion of the last volume of the *Zoist*, indicated that these beliefs were losing ground among its writers: "Examples of clairvoyance abound in all the volumes, but, though this phenomenon appears unquestionable, we all know that gross imposition is hourly practised in regard to it, both by professional clairvoyants and private individuals considered to be trustworthy, but influenced by vanity and wickedness. The assertions of a clairvoyant are to be believed in scarcely one instance out of a hundred, and only then when they are free from the possibility of lucky guess or trickery, and the facts otherwise verified. A host of clairvoyants are impostors."

One of the contributors to the *Zoist* has certainly changed his views on the subject of phrenology. I refer to Herbert Spencer, who appears there as the author of the following essays : "*A New View of the Functions of Imitation and Benevolence,*" "*On the Situation of the Organ of Amativeness,*" "*A Theory concerning the Organ of Wonder*"!

Although Elliotson was firmly convinced of the value of mesmerism as a remedial agent, he contented himself with urging its claims in the *Zoist*. He did not consider it universally applicable, and only suggested it in cases which he thought specially suitable, and where, in addition, there existed no prejudice concerning it. In all other instances he treated his patients by ordinary methods, and still displayed the same high diagnostic and therapeutic powers for which he had been so justly celebrated. Despite this, he was constantly abused and attacked in the grossest manner possible, the term madman being one of the mildest that was applied to him. Of this he complained at last in strong and pathetic terms. For fifteen years, he said, he had supported the unprovoked persecution of his professional brethren. He had been ridiculed and abused by them in their daily conversations among themselves and their patients, and in all the medical journals. Those who had formerly called him in consultation had now not only ceased to do so, but were untiring in their efforts to prevent his being employed by others, and thus his professional income had been reduced two-thirds. This, however, was not his greatest affliction; one, in whose judgment he had confided, had caused him losses equal to his professional ones, and, what was worse than all, those whom he had loved from infancy had unexpectedly turned upon him without provocation, and conducted themselves in such a way as nothing but mental aberration could explain.

In 1829, Elliotson delivered the Lumley Lectures, his subject being "*The Recent Improvement in the Art of distinguishing various Diseases of the Heart.*" These he published in 1830. He also contributed many papers on different subjects to the medical journals, translated Blumenbach's *Physiology*, and, at a later date, brought out an independent work on the same subject, as well as on the *Principles and Practice of Medicine*. He was Censor of the Royal College of Physicians, and President of the Royal Medical and Chirurgical Society of London.

Elliotson, who had never married, died, after a lingering

illness, on July 29th, 1868, in Davies Street, Berkeley Square, in the house of his friend, Dr. Symes, a former pupil who had always been devoted to him.

JAMES ESDAILE.

James Esdaile, son of the Rev. Dr. Esdaile of Perth, was born on February 6th, 1808. He graduated at Edinburgh in 1830, and then obtained an appointment in the East India Company.

On April 4th, 1845, when in charge of the Native Hospital at Hooghly, Esdaile made his first mesmeric experiment, his subject being a Hindoo convict with double hydrocele. As the usual injection had produced severe pain, Esdaile tried to mesmerise the patient, but did not expect to succeed, as he knew nothing about mesmerism except what he had read of Elliotson's doings. The man, however, fell into a deep trance, and became profoundly analgesic. Encouraged by this, and a still more striking success with the same patient, Esdaile continued his experiments, and soon reported seventy-five mesmeric operations to the Medical Board. His letter was not even acknowledged. At the end of the year, when his operations amounted to over a hundred, he placed the results before the Government. The Deputy-Governor of Bengal, Sir Herbert Maddock, at once appointed a Committee of Investigation, mainly composed of medical men. Their report was an extremely favourable one. On receiving it, the Government sent the following official communication to the President of the Committee :—

"The Committee's report has been ordered to be published, and the Deputy-Governor entirely concurs with the remark of the President in Council, that it is sufficient for the present that it should be allowed to work its own way towards producing conviction among the profession and the public, and, at this stage, any more direct encouragement on the part of the Government to the general introduction of mesmeric practice would be premature. But so far has the possibility of rendering the most serious operations painless to the subject of them been, in his Honour's opinion, established by the late experiments performed under the eye of the Committee appointed for that purpose, as to render it incumbent on the Government to afford to the meritorious and zealous officer by whom the subject was first brought to its notice, such assistance as may facilitate his investigations, and enable him to prosecute his interesting experiments under the most favourable and promising circumstances.

"With this view his Honour has determined, with the sanction of the

Supreme Government, to place Dr. Esdaile for a year in charge of a small experimental hospital, in some favourable situation in Calcutta, in order that he may, as recommended by the Committee, extend his investigations to the applicability of this alleged agency to all descriptions of cases, medical as well as surgical, and all classes of patients, European as well as Native. Dr. Esdaile will be directed to encourage the resort to his hospital of all respectable persons, especially medical and scientific, whether in or out of the service, who may be desirous of satisfying themselves of the nature and effect of his experiments, and his Honour will nominate, from among the medical officers of the Presidency, "Visitors," whose duty it will be to visit the hospital from time to time, inspect Dr. Esdaile's proceedings, without exercising any interference, and occasionally, or when called upon, report upon them, through the Medical Board, for the information of the Government. On these reports will mainly depend what future steps the Government may deem it expedient to take in the matter.— I have the honour to be, Gentlemen, your most obedient servant,

FRED. JAS. HALLIDAY,

Secretary to the Government of Bengal."

In accordance with this, a small hospital in Calcutta was placed at Esdaile's disposal by the Government in November, — 1846, and the following official visitors appointed : R. Thompson, M.D.; D. Stewart, M.D.; J. Jackson, F.R.C.S.; F. Mouatt, M.D.; and R. O'Shaughnessy, F.R.C.S. Esdaile was as successful here as he had been at Hooghly, the class of cases and the character of the operations being very similar. At the end of the year (December, 1847), the medical officers reported that complete insensibility to pain was obtained by mesmerism in the most severe operations, and that its influence in reducing shock was decidedly favourable.

In June, 1847, Esdaile wrote to the Government of Bengal as follows :—

"Since his Honour the Deputy-Governor has determined upon printing the Report of the Mesmeric Hospital for the last six months, I hope that I may be permitted to take this opportunity to make a few remarks on the working and prospects of the experimental hospital so liberally and benevolently established by the Government.

"For some months we were almost exclusively occupied with surgery, the fame of painless operations having eclipsed the less striking, but even more important, medical relations of the subject ; but these are now becoming more generally known by the public, and medical results have already been obtained of an important and highly encouraging description, and other cases now in hand of the gravest nature, such as palsy, epilepsy, madness, and other painful nervous affections, promise to repay our labours amply. But these cases are so old and inveterate that it requires long treatment to make an impression on them, and protracted observations before we can be sure of our results.

"The surgical cases, for reasons well known to you, are almost all of one description (the removal of the enormous tumours of elephantiasis), but fortunately for the demonstration of the anodyne and narcotic power of mesmerism, the operations have generally been the most severe and dangerous that are required to be performed on the human body. A greater variety of both surgical and medical cases is, however, desirable, and could be easily found in the public hospitals of Calcutta. It is in the practice of large hospitals, with their ever-varying patients and incidents, that the general utility of mesmerism will be best and most speedily illustrated. . . ..

". . . In conclusion, I would beg leave to direct respectfully the attention of the Government to the statistics of the subject, it being a point of much interest to ascertain the ratio of mortality under the old and the new school of surgery. For this purpose I have the honour to append a return of all the mesmeric operations performed by me, now amounting to 133, and I hope the Government will think the subject of sufficient importance to call for the necessary means of comparison from the different hospitals in Calcutta."

Before the end of the year of trial, a petition was sent to the Governor-General, signed by over 300 Native gentlemen of Calcutta, praying for the continuance of the Mesmeric Hospital, on the ground that they had studied the reports, personally witnessed many of the operations and their results, and had satisfied themselves of their value.

Despite the favourable report of the official visitors, and the petition already referred to, the Mesmeric Hospital was closed. A second one, however, entirely supported by voluntary subscriptions, mainly drawn from Native sources, was opened on September 1st, 1848, and Esdaile placed in charge. This was continued for six months, then closed, as the Deputy-Governor appointed Esdaile to the Sarkea's Lane Hospital and Dispensary, for the express purpose of combining mesmerism with the common practice of medicine.

Before Esdaile left India he had performed thousands of painless minor operations and about 300 capital ones. Amongst the latter were nineteen amputations and one lithotomy, but by far the greatest number were for the removal of the enormous scrotal tumours so common in India. Details of some cases will be given in the chapter on "Hypnotism in Surgery"; but his own and more extended account of his work, and the flocking of the Natives to be operated on under the new anæsthetic, form one of the most fascinating pages in the history of medical science. The removal of the larger scrotal tumours was considered so dangerous that few surgeons cared to attempt it. Dr. Goodeve (*Trans. Medical and Physical Society of Calcutta*, vol. vii.) put the mortality at 50 per cent. Although many of Esdaile's cases were particularly formidable ones, upon which other surgeons had refused to operate, his mortality in 161 consecutive cases was only 5 per cent. Further, none of the fatal cases died immediately after operation, all deaths subsequently resulting from fever, cholera, or like causes.

At first Esdaile mesmerised all the patients himself; but, after doing so for six weeks, he became extremely exhausted, and suffered from irritability and sleeplessness. He therefore instructed his Native hospital assistants how to mesmerise, and, except on rare occasions, confined himself to the performance of operations.

Esdaile's mesmeric work was constantly attacked in the Indian medical journals. It was asserted that the coolies of Bengal enjoyed being operated on, and that, knowing Esdaile's hobby, they came from all quarters in order to please him. Esdaile was described as an honest fool, who was deceived by his patients—a set of hardened and determined impostors. In reply, Esdaile drew attention to the following facts :—(1) During the six years previous to 1845, he had only operated on eleven cases of scrotal tumour, but, since using mesmerism, he had had more operations of this kind in a month than took place in all the other Native hospitals in Calcutta in a year. (2) During operation the patients remained perfectly quiet, and showed neither the ordinary nor the physiological signs of pain, *i.e.* the characteristic changes in pulse and pupil did not occur. (3) The same patients showed signs of acute pain when operated on in the waking state. (4) There was no pain after operation, when this had taken place during mesmeric trance, and the patients on awaking generally asked for food. In conclusion, Esdaile pointed out that his patients constantly sent him others, and asked whether it was more likely they had told their friends that they had cheated him into believing they were asleep, or truly assured them that they had had their tumours removed during painless trance.

It was asserted also that if Esdaile's patients were not all impostors, they were certainly all hysterical. Esdaile replied that he did not see how hysteria could have got into his hospitals, where he had never seen it before—coolies and felons not being at all nervous subjects. If that charge were true, fashionable surgeons, who had the disease and antidote ready to their hands, should have no difficulty in performing painless operations. He therefore would soon expect to hear that "Lady Tantrum" had had her arm cut off in a fit of hysterics without knowing it.

Esdaile complained that no account of his painless operations was published in any of the medical journals, and that their editors purposely kept the facts from the profession. Yet in a year's report of the Calcutta Mesmeric Hospital were to be found accounts of 62 capital operations, with 3 deaths, and 640 miscellaneous operations. As all this had been going on regularly for four years, surely it was worthy of mention, if only as an example of epidemic insanity. What reader of English medical journals, he asked, had ever heard of the report of the Mesmeric Committee and Hospital, published by order of the Government, or of the second Mesmeric Hospital in Calcutta, which was still in full operation ?

Chloroform was introduced into India before Esdaile left, and he attempted to show its inferiority to mesmerism. Some of his objections were undoubtedly due to his strong feeling in favour of mesmerism; others arose from the frequency of the disagreeable or dangerous results, which not unnaturally followed the use of a new and little-understood method of inducing anæsthesia. Esdaile found nine cases of death from chloroform reported in the only medical journal he happened to have at hand at the time, and contrasted this with 100 capital operations performed by him in the mesmeric trance. Of the latter only two died within the month—one of cholera and one of tetanus—and there had been neither pain during or after operation, nor disagreeable local or general after-effects.

When the American Congress, of 1853, offered a prize of 10,000 dollars to the discoverer of the anæsthetic powers of ether, described as the earliest anæsthetic, Esdaile sent an indignant protest. He did not claim the reward, but drew attention to the well-known fact that painless mesmeric surgery was daily performed in his hospitals years before ether was heard of.

Although Esdaile's operations formed the most striking part of his work, many of his medical cases are interesting, and some of the more remarkable will be cited in the chapter on "Hypnotism in Medicine." He frequently obtained brilliant results in cases of functional paralysis, but warned both practitioner and patient that time and perseverance were often necessary, especially in long-standing cases. His explanation of the action of mesmerism in diseased conditions will be discussed when dealing with " Theory."

Until he left India in 1851, Esdaile devoted himself entirely to mesmeric work. Not only did this bring him no pecuniary profit, for it involved no increase in his official salary, but he also sacrificed for its sake all private practice and other chances of money-making.

After leaving India, Esdaile settled in Perth, but his interest in mesmerism remained unabated. On September 15th, 1851, he wrote to Elliotson as follows :—

"Before leaving Calcutta, I had the satisfaction of seeing Dr. Webb, Professor of Anatomy, gazetted as my successor at the Mesmeric Hospital."

This was the same Dr. Webb who said, in his introductory lecture at the Medical College of Calcutta :—

"The practicability, which has been daily demonstrated in the Mesmeric Hospital in this city, of performing the most dreadful operations of surgery without pain to the patient, must be regarded as the greatest medical triumph of our day. I cannot recall without astonishment the extirpation of a cancerous eye, while the man looked at me unflinchingly with the other one. In another case, the patient looked dreamily on with half-closed eyes the whole time of the operation, even while I examined the nature of the malignant tumour I had removed, and then, having satisfied myself, concluded the operation."

I was for some time puzzled by the fact that I could discover no mention of Dr. Webb in connection with the Mesmeric Hospital after Esdaile left India, but the following letter from Webb to Elliotson supplied the information :—

"I had risen," wrote Dr. Webb, "so high in the estimation of my friend Esdaile that he made it a last request with the Government that I should succeed to the Mesmeric Hospital. Should you see him, he will learn with surprise that the charge which was promised him and given me, as I understood, was supposed never to have been given, and conferred on some one else who never had a mesmeric case."

In a letter to Elliotson, on September 29th, 1851, Esdaile thus explained why he had left India :—

"My reasons for leaving India were simply that I hated the climate, the country, and all its ways from the moment I set foot in it, and had long determined to quit it at the first practicable moment, which I have accord-

ingly done. Knowing that all the wealth of India could not bribe me to
remain a moment after the expiration of my period of service, I was perfectly indifferent to being called an advertising quack, etc., for addressing
the public through the newspapers—their only source of information—the
medical journals having combined to suppress all evidence on the subject of
mesmerism. I could well afford to laugh at the attempts to injure me and
my practice, the truth being that I did not care a straw about it. If I lived
a few years, I knew that my actions would give the lie to the friendly com-
mentators on my conduct, who gave out that I was agitating for a place in
Calcutta, in order to drive a great trade there like themselves. You may
imagine their astonishment and delight at seeing me give up, almost as soon
as got, what to them is the *summum bonum* of good fortune—a good place
in Calcutta with the prospect of a great practice. . . ."

On December 9th, 1852, Esdaile informed Elliotson that the
inhabitants of the Far North were as susceptible to mesmerism as
those of the Farthest East. Dr. Fraser Thompson, surgeon to the
Perth Infirmary, became a convert, and employed mesmerism in
a variety of diseases. He successfully operated also on some
patients in that institution, but his colleagues promptly called a
meeting of the directors, and stated that they would resign if the
practice of mesmerism were permitted in the hospital.

In March, 1852, Esdaile published a pamphlet on *The
Introduction of Mesmerism as an Anæsthetic and Curative Agent
into the Hospitals of India*, which he dedicated to the members
of the medical profession. In this he complained bitterly of his
treatment by the editors of different medical journals, and of their
determined attempt to suppress all evidence in favour of mesmerism. Professor J. Y. Simpson, of Edinburgh, had written to
Esdaile to the effect that he owed it to himself and his profession
to let his proceedings be known in England. In response to this,
Esdaile sent an account to an English medical journal of 161
scrotal tumours removed during mesmeric trance. The history
of what followed, and Esdaile's opinion of the treatment he
received, I shall give in his own words :—

" My article was not published, and I then sent a more general paper containing a *résumé* of my surgical work. This was rejected for its *unpractical
character !* I have heard that it is given as a reason for not printing my
paper that, though no one now denies my facts, these apply to the Natives of
India only. But, as far as I know, no medical journal has admitted the
reality of *painless mesmeric operations*, even for India, or inserted one of the
numerous European cases reported from London, Paris, Cherbourg, etc. . . .
They will not admit, or permit you even to hear of, such indisputable facts,
through fear of the consequences. But, supposing the Natives of India were

alone concerned, is it of no interest to the surgeon, the physician, the physiologist, and the natural philosopher, to know that the hundred and twenty millions of our Eastern subjects (one would suppose they were monkeys) are so susceptible to mesmeric influence that painless surgical operations, and other medical benefits from mesmerism, are their natural birthright? You have been told all along by your journals that your medical brethren engaged in studying mesmerism are either fools or quacks. But how men like myself, who neither want, nor will accept, private practice, can be reduced to the category of quacks I do not well see. If we are fools, we ought to be encouraged to write ourselves down as such, as the speediest and most effectual way of exposing us. I am convinced that you and I are agreed on one point, namely, in liking to be allowed to judge for ourselves, and that you will not submit to be hoodwinked or led by the nose by persons we pay to keep us well informed of new facts, and the progress made in our profession all over the world. To pretend that there is a *free medical press* in Great Britain is a mockery and a delusion. And the proof of this is that medical men, who pledge their unblemished private and professional reputation for the truth of their statements, are not allowed to be heard by you in your professional organs, if what they advance is contrary to the prejudices and foregone conclusions of the editors. . . ."

After a time Esdaile found the climate of Scotland too cold, a weakness of the lungs having been his reason for going to India in the first instance, and he removed to Sydenham, where he died, on January 10th, 1859, at the age of fifty. He had been married three times, but had no children.

A list of all Esdaile's published works that I have been able to trace will be found in the chapter of References.

JAMES BRAID.

The name of James Braid is familiar to all students of hypnotism, and is rarely mentioned by them without due credit being given to the important part he played in rescuing that science from ignorance and superstition. Regret is usually expressed, however, that he held many erroneous views, which it is claimed the researches of more recent investigators have disproved. The following, as far as I can gather from hypnotic works, and from conversation with those interested in hypnotism, are the opinions almost universally held:—(1) Braid was an English surgeon. (2) He believed in phrenology. (3) He was the discoverer or rediscoverer of the subjective origin of hypnotic phenomena. (4) He knew nothing of suggestion. In all this, one thing alone is correct, namely, that Braid was the rediscoverer of the subjective nature of hypnotic phenomena. This estimate of Braid has arisen from imperfect knowledge of his writings. Few seem to be acquainted with any of his works except *Neurypnology*, or with the fact that this was only one of the first of a long series on the subject of hypnotism, and that later his views completely changed.

James Braid, who was born at Rylaw House in Fifeshire about 1795, was educated at Edinburgh, and qualified there as a surgeon. After practising in Scotland for some years, he removed to Manchester, where he remained up to the time of his death, and gained a high reputation as a skilful physician and surgeon.

On November 13th, 1841, Braid, for the first time, was present at a mesmeric *séance* : the operator was Lafontaine.[1] At that time mesmeric phenomena were generally believed to be due either to mysterious force or fluid, self-deception or trickery. Braid held the latter theory, and on the first occasion saw nothing to cause him to alter his views. At the next *séance*, six days later, he noticed that one subject was unable to open his eyes. Braid regarded this as a real phenomenon, and was anxious to discover its physiological cause ; and the following evening, when the case was again operated on, he believed he had done so. After making a series of experiments, chiefly on personal friends and relatives, he expressed his conviction that the phenomena he had witnessed were purely subjective, and began almost immediately to place these views before the public, his first lecture being delivered on December 27th, 1841.

In 1842, Braid offered a paper on the subject of hypnotism to the Medical Section of the British Association held that year in Manchester. This was refused, whereupon he gave a con-versazione, at which many members of the Association were present, read his paper, and showed cases. His first work on mesmerism was entitled *Satanic Agency and Mesmerism reviewed, in a Letter to the Rev. H. McNeile, A.M., of Liverpool, in Reply to a Sermon preached by him at St. Jude's Church, Liverpool, on Sunday, April 10th, 1842.* McNeile had charged Braid with " refusing to state the laws of nature by the uniform action of which hypnotic phenomena were produced." To this Braid

[1] A description of this *séance* will be found in the Appendix, my attention having been directed to it too late for insertion here.

replied that he had always explained the phenomena on physiological and psychological principles, but that M°Neile had refused
to attend his lectures or to read any account of them. Braid,
who at that time believed in the physical origin of hypnotic
phenomena, referred M°Neile to the theory by which he attempted
to explain certain changes in the central nervous system, more
particularly decreased functional activity, as the result of the
exhaustion of other nerve centres from continued monotonous
stimulation. But, he said, even if his theories did not explain
all the phenomena, surely he might be allowed to employ the
knowledge he had acquired, without being stigmatised from the
pulpit as a necromancer who produced his effects by "Satanic
agency." If a hundred persons started in a steamer, and twenty
became sick, while the remainder escaped, would it be fair to
charge the captain of acting by Satanic agency because the *whole*
were not sick, and because, according to M°Neile, "if it be in
nature, it will operate uniformly and not capriciously ? . . . If
it operate capriciously, then there is some mischievous agent at
work; and we are not ignorant of the devices of the devil."
Would any man but Mr. M°Neile say that, because the captain
gave the signal to heave anchor, to spread the sails, and other
"talismanic tokens" for steering the vessel, and because only
part of the passengers became sick, he was consequently affecting
them through Satanic agency : or that it would alter the matter
one whit because medical men could not assign the true cause
of sea-sickness, or tell why some should be affected by it and
not others ?

In 1843, Braid published *Neurypnology, or The Rationale
of Nervous Sleep*, of which eight hundred copies were sold in
a few months. In this work are to be found his earliest theories.
After having established the subjective origin of the phenomena,
he proposed that they should be called "hypnotic" instead of
"mesmeric," and invented the following terminology :—

Neurypnology, the rationale or doctrine of nervous sleep.
Neuro-hypnotism, or nervous sleep, a peculiar condition of the nervous
system produced by artificial contrivance.

Then, for the sake of brevity, suppressing the prefix " neuro,"
he gave the following terms :—

Hypnotic, the state or condition of nervous sleep.
Hypnotise, to induce nervous sleep.

Hypnotised, put into the condition of nervous sleep.
Hypnotism, nervous sleep.
Dehypnotise, to restore from the state of nervous sleep.
Hypnotist, one who practises neuro-hypnotism.

Braid placed his results and methods before his medical brethren, insisted that they alone ought to use hypnotism, and warned the ignorant against tampering with a powerful agency, which might produce either good or evil according to the manner in which it was managed and applied. Hypnotism, he said, was capable of curing many diseases for which formerly there had been no remedy; but none but a medical man was competent to employ it with advantage to the patient or credit to himself. Braid particularly insisted that hypnotism was not a universal remedy, and stated that whoever talked of such a thing was either a fool or a knave. In reference to his successful therapeutic results, Braid said that he had always tried to dispel mystery, and could teach any intelligent medical man to do what he had done. In skilled hands there was neither pain, discomfort, nor danger associated with hypnotic treatment. Further, he was able to influence a larger percentage of patients by his methods than the mesmerists did by theirs, even with the supposed aid of mysterious agencies.

Braid stated that he had taken every care to avoid deception in his experiments, but, despite this, did not expect his conclusions to be at once accepted. He hoped, however, that his professional brethren would investigate the subject calmly, with an honest desire to arrive at truth, and, having been sceptical himself, he could make allowance for others. A superficial examination of the phenomena was not enough; some theoretical knowledge of the subject was also essential. For example, different patients showed varying susceptibility, and yet many observers expected that all should present uniform hypnotic phenomena. Further, the mental conditions might change slowly or abruptly according to the methods employed, and, from a like cause, widely varying phenomena might be evoked in the same subject at different times. Yet it was not unusual for two observers to be simultaneously demanding opposite test conditions in the same subject.

In many instances, Braid published the written testimony of others in support of his successful treatment of different patients by hypnotism. He explained that the action of certain medical men, who had fraudulently obtained and published false statements in reference to his practice, rendered this necessary.

Braid frequently referred to the almost incredible opposition he had to combat, both at the hands of the orthodox medical practitioner and of the mesmerists. His explanation of this I give in his own words :—

"Throughout the whole of my inquiries my chief desire has been to arrive at what could be rendered most practically useful for the relief and cure of disease ; and I hesitate not to say that, in the hands of a skilful medical man, who thoroughly understands the peculiar modes which I have devised for varying the effects in a manner applicable to different cases, hypnotism, besides being the speediest method for inducing the condition, is, moreover, capable of achieving *all* the *good* to be attained by the *ordinary mesmerising processes*, and *much more*. . . . Of course there is one point which renders hypnotism less an object of approbation with a certain class of society, viz. that I lay no claim for it to produce the marvellous or transcendental phenomena ; nor do I believe that the phenomena manifested have any relation to a magnetic temperament, or some peculiar or occult power, possessed in an extra-ordinary degree by the operator. These are all circumstances which appeal powerfully to the feelings of all lovers of the marvellous, and therefore tell in favour of mesmerism ; and, moreover, seeing that, for conducting the hypnotic processes with any degree of certainty and success, I contend that, in many cases, knowledge of anatomy, physiology, pathology, and therapeutics are all requisite, it is obvious that such requirements must be less calculated to secure the approbation of *non-professional* mesmerists and amateurs, whose magnetic creed taught them to believe that the mere possession by them of the magnetic temperament—of a surcharge by nature, within their own bodies, of a magnetic fluid or odyle—was quite sufficient to enable them to treat any case as efficiently as the most skilful medical man in the universe, simply by walking up to the patient with the *will* and the *good intention* of doing him service, or by adding thereto, occasionally, the efficacy of mesmeric touches, passes, or manipulations. . . . Like the originators of all new views, however, hypnotism has subjected me to much contention ; for the sceptics, from not perceiving the difference between my method and that of the mesmerists, and the limited extent of my own pretensions, were equally hostile to hypnotism as they had been to mesmerism ; and the mesmerists, thinking their craft was in danger—that their mystical idol was threatened to be shorn of some of its glory by the advent of a new rival—buckled on their armour, and soon proved that the *odium mesmericum* was as inveterate as the *odium theologicum*."

Neurypnology was followed by a long series of publications on the subject of hypnotism, and a list of all Braid's writings that I have been able to trace will be given in the chapter of References.

Braid's later theories, it is to be particularly noted, differed widely from his earlier ones; but these will be discussed when dealing with that subject.

In 1852, in the preface to the third edition of *Magic, Witch-craft, etc.*, Braid stated that he now gave his view of all important hypnotic and mesmeric theories, and hoped by this means to make up in some measure for the delay in the publication of another edition of his work on Hypnotism, which had long been out of print and was frequently called for.

"That call," he said, " I hope shortly to be able to respond to, with such fulness of detail as the importance of the subject merits—more particularly with regard to its practical application for the relief and cure of some forms of disease, of which numerous interesting examples will be adduced."

At the conclusion of *The Physiology of Fascination, etc.*, he said :—

" It is my intention shortly to publish a volume entitled *Psycho-Physiology: embracing Hypnotism, Monoideism, and Mesmerism.* This work will comprise, in a connected and condensed form, the results of the whole of my researches in this department of science, and it will, moreover, be illustrated by cases in which hypnotism has been proved particularly efficacious in the relief and cure of disease, with special directions how to regulate the processes so as to adapt them to different cases and circumstances."

Shortly before his death, Braid contemplated publishing a second edition of *Neurypnology* in France: this was never done, nor did the two proposed works above referred to ever see the light.

In the chapter of References I shall give a list of all Braid's works and articles which I have been able to trace. These have long been out of print, and of the former only Nos. 2, 3, 4, 6, and 7 are to be found in the Library of the British Museum. I possess Nos. 1, 2, 5, 6, and 8, as well as most of his articles and two long MS. letters addressed to "M. High-field, Esq., Surgeon," dated respectively 28th October, and 16th November, 1842.[1] These letters, which give an interesting *résumé* of Braid's views on the subjective nature of hypnotic phenomena, contain a description of the hyperæsthesia of the special senses, and of some successful medical cases, together with the denial of

[1] The numbers just quoted correspond with those given in the list of Braid's works and articles in the chapter of References.

the alleged dangers of hypnotism and of the supposed automatism of the subject. Braid published an account of many interesting medical and surgical cases treated by hypnotism. A few of the more important of these will be referred to in the chapters dealing with medical and surgical cases.

In 1859, Dr. Azam of Bordeaux became acquainted with Braid's hypnotic work, and commenced to investigate the subject for himself. An account of his experiments, with much reference to Braid, appeared in the *Archives de Médecine* in 1860. About the same time Broca, who had obtained marvellous results with Braid's methods, read a paper on Hypnotism before the *Académie des Sciences*, which attracted much attention, and Velpeau presented a copy of *Neurypnology* to the same Society. A committee, composed of members of the four sections of the *Institute*, was then formed to report on the subject. On hearing of this, Braid wrote to the *Académie* to say how much pleasure Azam's brilliant results, and the action of the Society, had given him.

From that date, the subject of hypnotism was never lost sight of in France; but it was not until forty years after its original publication that *Neurypnology* was translated by Dr. Jules Simon, who stated that Braid's researches procured for him numerous enemies; but that, despite this, he pursued them with the precision of genius, and was able to add artificial somnambulism to the pathology of the nervous system—a phenomenon which the investigations of the greater number of modern neuro-pathologists have confirmed.

Braid's first translator was W. Preyer, Professor of Physiology at the University of Jena, who, in 1881, published *The Discovery of Hypnotism*. This was a condensation of *Neurypnology*, together with the translation of the pamphlet sent by Braid to Azam in 1860, which had passed into the possession of Dr. Beard of New York, who lent it to Preyer. The same pamphlet is also translated into French, and forms an appendix to Dr. Jules Simon's *Neurypnologie*, which appeared in 1883. In 1882, Preyer published *Hypnotism*, which consisted of a translation of most of Braid's other works.

In 1890, Preyer brought out another work on the subject of hypnotism. This contained a translation of a MS. of Braid's, entitled *On the Distinctive Conditions of Natural and Nervous Sleep*, which now for the first time saw the light. In reference to this, Preyer stated that Braid left his MSS. to his daughter, and that she, on her death, bequeathed them to her brother, Dr. James Braid, jun., who died on November 22nd, 1882. Preyer visited him at Burgess Hill, Sussex, in August 1881, and received the MS. from him.

In addition to the information drawn from Preyer's books, I am personally indebted to him for the gift of various pamphlets by Braid, with some of which I was previously unacquainted.

I published a short account of Braid's work, with a list of his writings, in *Brain*, part lxxiii., Spring 1896. This was followed by other articles with more complete bibliographies in the *Proceedings of the Society for Psychical Research*, part xxx., June, 1896, and in the *Revue de l'Hypnotisme*, vol. xi. pp. 27, 60, 87, and 129. The last article attracted the attention of Professor Bernheim, who wrote a reply to it (*Revue de l'Hypnotisme*, vol. xi. p. 137), in which he attempted to show that Braid was unacquainted with suggestion. This article I answered (*Revue de l'Hypnotisme*, vol. xi. p. 353), giving quotations from Braid's published works, which clearly showed that he not only employed suggestion as intelligently as the members of the Nancy school now do, but also that his conception of its nature was clearer than theirs.

In 1899, an important work on James Braid was published in England. This is entitled *Neurypnology, or The Rationale of Nervous Sleep considered in Relation to Animal Magnetism, and illustrated by numerous Cases of its successful Application in the Relief or Cure of Disease, by James Braid, M.R.C.S., C.M.W.S., etc. A new edition, edited, with an introduction, biographical and bibliographical, embodying the author's later views and further evidence on the subject, by Arthur Edward Waite.* (London, George Redway, 1899.)

The above work comprises (1) a biographical introduction, which gives a short account of Braid's life and a more extended one of his writings ; (2) a reproduction of the original edition of *Neurypnology*, which forms the greater bulk of the volume ; (3) an appendix of editorial notes, chiefly drawn from Braid's later works ; and (4) a bibliography of Braid's writings.

Although *Neurypnology* is historically interesting, it must not be forgotten that it was written almost immediately after Braid commenced his hypnotic work, and that later his views

underwent a complete change. The French translation of
Neurypnology is more valuable than Mr. Waite's, as in an
appendix of 36 pages it reproduces Braid's last MS., which
gives a summary of his more matured theories.

The bibliography, to which Mr. Waite attaches great
importance, only imperfectly reproduces those just referred to,
which I myself published at earlier dates. Apparently, too,
Mr. Waite himself believes in animal magnetism, metallo-
therapeutics, phrenology, and clairvoyance, but when he attributes
to Braid a belief in these things, he shows that he has absolutely
failed to grasp the spirit and significance of his teaching.

Braid died suddenly on March 25th, 1860, according to
some accounts from apoplexy, according to others from heart
disease; he left a widow, son, and daughter. He maintained his
active interest in hypnotism up to the end; and three days
before his death sent his last MS. to Dr. Azam, with the following inscription: "Presented to M. Azam, as a mark of esteem
and regard, by James Braid, Surgeon, Manchester, March 22nd,
1860." Sympathetic notices of Braid's death appeared in the
local papers and different medical journals, all of which bore
warm testimony to his professional skill and high personal
character. The *Lancet* drew attention to the fact that, though
he was best known in the medical world by his theory and
practice of hypnotism, he had also obtained wonderfully successful results in operations in cases of club foot and other deform-
ities, which brought him patients from every part of the
kingdom. Up to 1841, he had operated on 262 cases of
talipes, 700 cases of strabismus, and 23 cases of spinal
curvature.

(B) LATER HISTORY OF HYPNOTISM.

Although the justness of Braid's views as to the subjective
origin of mesmeric phenomena was generally admitted, and
despite the attention drawn to his theories and practical work
by such well-known men of science as Professors Carpenter and
John Hughes Bennett, the practice of hypnotism apparently -

ceased in England after Braid's death. At the present day, however, hypnotism has found a place in the medical practice of every country in Europe, the pioneer to whom this result is mainly due being Liébeault, of Nancy.

DR. A. A. LIÉBEAULT.

Liébeault was born in 1823, and commenced to study medicine in 1844. He read a book on animal magnetism, in 1848, which impressed him greatly, and a few days later he successfully mesmerised several persons. He received his M.D. in 1850, and shortly afterwards started country practice.

He worked hard, and was often in the saddle making his rounds at 2 A.M. In 1860, he began to study mesmerism seriously, just at the time that Velpeau communicated Azam's experiments to the *Académie de Médecine*. In order to find subjects Liébeault took advantage of the parsimonious character of the French peasant. His patients had absolute confidence in him, but they had been accustomed to be treated in the ordinary manner. He therefore said to them : " If you wish me to treat you with drugs, I will do so, but you will have to pay me as formerly. On the other hand, if you will allow me to hypnotise you, I will do it for nothing." He soon had so many patients that he was unable to find time for necessary repose or study. In 1864, he settled at Nancy, lived quietly on the interest of his capital, and practised hypnotism gratuitously among the poor.

For two years he worked hard at his book, *Du sommeil et des états analogues, considérés surtout au point de vue de l'action de la morale sur le physique*, but of this one copy alone was sold. His colleagues regarded him as a madman; the poor as their Providence, calling him "the good father Liébeault." His clinique was crowded with patients; he cured many who had vainly sought help elsewhere, and few left him without having received benefit. In 1882, he cured an obstinate case of sciatica, of six years' duration, which Bernheim had treated in vain for six months. In consequence of this, Bernheim came to see him and his work. This was a great event in the life of the humble doctor. At first Bernheim was sceptical and incredulous, but soon this changed into admiration. He multiplied his visits, and became a zealous pupil and true friend of Liébeault. In 1884, Bernheim published the first part of his book, *De la Suggestion*, which he completed, in June 1886, by a second part, entitled *La Thérapeutique Suggestive*. From that date Liébeault's name became known throughout all the world. The first edition of his book was quickly bought up, and doctors flocked from all countries to study the new therapeutic method.

In the summer of 1889, I spent a fortnight at Nancy in order to see Liébeault's hypnotic work. His clinique, invariably thronged, was held in two rooms situated in a corner of his garden. The interior of these presented nothing likely to attract attention; and, indeed, any one coming with preconceived ideas of the wonders of hypnotism would be greatly disappointed. For, putting aside the methods of treatment and some slight differences probably due to race-characteristics, one could easily have imagined oneself in the out-patient department of a general hospital. The patients perhaps chatted more freely amongst themselves, and questioned the doctor in a more familiar way than one is accustomed to see in England. They were taken in turn, and the clinical case-book referred to. Hypnosis was then rapidly induced in the manner which will be described under " Methods," suggestions given and notes taken, the doctor maintaining the while a running commentary for my benefit.

Nearly all the patients I saw were easily and rapidly hypnotised, but Liébeault informed me that the nervous and hysterical were his most refractory subjects.

As I was a stranger, an exception was made in my favour, and I was shown a few hypnotic experiments; but cure alone seemed the sole object of his work. The quiet, ordinary, everyday tone of the whole performance formed a marked contrast to the picture drawn by Binet and Féré of the morbid excitement shown at the Salpêtrière. The patients told to go to sleep apparently fell at once into a quiet slumber, then received their dose of curative suggestions, and when told to awake, either walked quietly away or sat for a little to chat with their friends : the whole process rarely lasting longer than ten minutes. The negation of all morbid symptoms was suggested ; also the maintenance of the conditions upon which general health depends, *i.e.* sleep, digestion, etc. I noticed that in some instances curative suggestions appeared to be perfectly

successful, even when the state produced was only that of
somnolence. The cases varied widely, but most of them were
either cured or relieved. No drugs were given; and Liébeault
took especial pains to explain to his patients that he neither
exercised nor possessed any mysterious power, and that all he
did was simple and capable of scientific explanation.

Two little incidents, illustrating the absence of all fear in
connection with Liébeault and hypnotism, interested me greatly.

A little girl, about five years old, dressed shabbily, but
evidently in her best, with a crown of paper laurel-leaves on her
head, and carrying a little book in her hand, toddled into the
sanctum, fearlessly interrupted the doctor in the midst of his work
by pulling his coat, and said: "You promised me a penny if I got
a prize." This, accompanied by kindly words, was smilingly given,
incitement to work having been evoked in a pleasing, if not scientific
way. Two little girls, about six or seven years of age, no doubt
brought in the first instance by friends, walked in and sat down
on a sofa behind the doctor. He, stopping for a moment in his work
made a pass in the direction of one of them, and said : "Sleep,
my little kitten," repeated the same for the other, and in an
instant they were both asleep. He rapidly gave them their
dose of suggestion and then evidently forgot all about them. In
about twenty minutes one awoke and, wishing to go, essayed by
shaking and pulling, to awaken her companion—her amused
expression of face, when she failed to do so, being very comic.
In about five minutes more the second one awoke, and, hand in
hand, they trotted laughingly away.

Braid anticipated many of the most important observations
of the school of Nancy; but we ought not, on that account, to
undervalue the services of that school, and more especially those
of its founder—Liébeault. Braid's researches were undoubtedly
the exciting cause of the hypnotic revival in France; but, as we
have seen, little or nothing was known of any of his works
except *Neurypnology*, and his last MS., which contained some of
his later views, was not published in that country until
1883. Liébeault independently arrived at the conclusion that
the phenomena of hypnotism were purely subjective in their
origin, and to him we owe the development of modern
hypnotism.

Another point in reference to their careers is worthy of note.

Braid's views at once brought him fame. His books sold rapidly, the demand for them exceeding his power of supply. The medical journals were open to him, to an extent which may well excite envy in those interested in the subject at the present day. Liébeault's book, on the contrary, remained unsold; his statements only found sceptics, his methods of treatment were rejected without examination, and he was laughed at and despised by all. From the day he settled in Nancy, in 1864, until Bernheim—some twenty years later—was the means of bringing him into notice, Liébeault devoted himself entirely to the poor, and refused to accept a fee, lest he should be regarded as attempting to make money by unrecognised methods. Even in his later days fortune never came to him, nor did he seek it. And his services—services which he himself, with true modesty, described as the contribution of a single brick to the edifice many were trying to build—only began to be appreciated when old age compelled him to retire from active work. Though his researches have been recognised, it is certain that they have not been estimated at their true value, and that members of a younger generation have reaped the reward which his devotion of a lifetime failed to obtain.

The term " School of Nancy " has been applied to Liébeault and his colleagues; but, as Professor Beaunis points out, they do not claim to have originated a school, and, though they agree on certain points, differ widely on others.

Other Continental Workers.—In 1878, while Liébeault's work was practically ignored, Charles Richet asserted that the phenomena of hypnotism were genuine. In the same year, Charcot drew public attention to the subject, and he and his followers formed what has been called the Salpêtrière School. Charcot's researches attracted attention in this country, but his observations were not confirmed; and the interest in hypnotism for which he was responsible practically died away, or, if his experiments were quoted, it was only in order to discredit hypnotism.

In Germany, about 1880, Heidenhain and others interested themselves in hypnotism, but the influence of their work was not lasting.

In 1882, Bernheim, who, as we have seen, had become a convert of Liébeault, commenced to hypnotise all the hospital patients who came under his care. His work was carefully

watched—from the physiological side—by Professor Beaunis—
from the legal one—by Professor Liégeois. In the first four years
about 5000 cases were recorded, hypnosis being obtained in 75
per cent. A few years later the number had increased to 10,000,
and the percentage of successes to 85. Of the medical men, who
now came to Nancy from all countries, most, if not all, were
convinced of the genuine nature of hypnotism, and many commenced to study and practise it on their own account. The
history of the growth and development of this movement is so
fully given in the last English edition of Moll's *Hypnotism*, that
it is unnecessary to describe it in detail. In most European
countries hypnotism now plays an important part, while many
of those who practise it are well known by their contributions to
other departments of medicine. Hypnotism has also found its
way into university class-rooms, and has occupied a prominent
place at numerous medical congresses, more particularly the
International Congresses of Experimental Psychology.

It possesses also a rich literature. Max Dessoir, in his
Bibliography of Modern Hypnotism, published in 1888, and
augmented by an Appendix in 1890, cites 1182 works by 774
authors, and since then the number has largely increased. Several
journals, notably the *Revue de l'Hypnotisme* and the *Zeitschrift
für Hypnotismus*, occupy themselves almost exclusively with the
subject, while others, such as the *Annales de Psychiatrie*, contain
from time to time important contributions to its psychological side.

England.—To the Society for Psychical Research we owe the
first attempt, since Braid's time, to subject hypnotism to rigorous and
far-reaching scientific investigation. This Society was established
in 1882, for the purpose of investigating those obscure phenomena
which alone, amongst all other natural phenomena, had remained
uninvestigated by modern science. It is expressly stated that
membership of the Society does not imply the acceptance of any
particular explanation of the phenomena investigated, nor any
belief as to the operation in the physical world of forces other
than those recognised by physical science.

The President of the Society is Sir Oliver Lodge, F.R.S., while
his predecessors were Sir William Crookes, F.R.S., Henry Sidgwick, Balfour Stewart, F.R.S., William James, and the Right
Hon. A. J. Balfour, F.R.S. Amongst past and present Vice-
Presidents and members of the Council were to be found : Henry

Sidgwick, Oliver J. Lodge, F.R.S., A. Macalister, M.D., F.R.S., William James, F. W. H. Myers, J. J. Thomson, F.R.S., W. F. Barrett, F.R.S.E., the Right Hon. A. J. Balfour, F.R.S., the Right Hon. G. W. Balfour, Lord Rayleigh, F.R.S., Walter Leaf, Litt.D., and J. Venn, D.Sc., F.R.S.

In the list of members appear Professors Ramsey, Beaunis, Bernheim, Bowditch, Stanley Hall, Th. Ribot, Liégeois, Lombroso, Charles Richet, Drs. Max Dessoir, Féré, Liébeault, Schrenck-Notzing, Pierre Janet, Wetterstrand, and many other well-known names.

At an early date in the existence of the Society, a Committee was appointed for the purpose of investigating hypnotism; the subjects for experiment being almost invariably healthy men. The Reports of the Committee were published from time to time in the *Proceedings* of the Society, besides valuable articles by the late Edmund Gurney and Frederic Myers. The views of the former were markedly in advance of those held at that time, while Myers' attempts to explain the phenomena of hypnotism by the intelligent and voluntary action of a secondary or subliminal consciousness, still remains the most important of recent contributions to the theoretical side of the subject.

The commencement of the present revival of hypnotism in England, from its medical side, was apparently due to Dr. Lloyd Tuckey who happened to be in the neighbourhood of Nancy in August, 1888, and visited Liébeault out of curiosity. He then went to Amsterdam and Paris to see the cliniques there, and on his return commenced to employ hypnotism amongst his own patients. His most important work is *Psycho-Therapeutics*, now in its third edition.

Dr. Kingsbury, of Blackpool, was one of Dr. Tuckey's earliest followers, and, in 1891, published *The Practice of Hypnotic Suggestion.*

Scotland.—In 1890, Dr. Felkin published *Hypnotism, or Psycho-Therapeutics*, while Dr. George Robertson, Superintendent, Murthly Asylum, Perth, has written several articles on the subject, the most important being "*The Use of Hypnotism among the Insane,*" *Journal of Mental Science*, 1892.

Ireland.—In 1891, Sir Francis Cruise published a pamphlet entitled *Hypnotism*, in which he drew the attention of the profession to the value of the work being done at Nancy. Since then he has successfully used hypnotism in the treatment of dipsomania, kleptomania, etc., as well as in various functional nervous disorders. Nothing else has apparently been published in Ireland on the subject; but Sir Francis claims to have made several converts, who employ hypnotism in their practice.

The list just given by no means exhausts the names of those who practise hypnotism, but simply refers to some of the earlier workers who drew attention to the subject by their writings.

In 1891, the British Medical Association appointed Sir William Broadbent, Sir William Gairdner, Drs. Clouston, Drummond, Kingsbury, Needham, Conolly Norman, Suckling, Hack Tuke, Outterson Wood, and Yellowlees to act as a Committee " to investigate the nature of the phenomena of hypnotism, its value as a therapeutic agent, and the propriety of using it." At the Annual Meeting, in 1892, the Committee presented the following report, which, it is to be noted, was unanimous:—

"The Committee, having completed such investigation of hypnotism as time permitted, have to report that they have satisfied themselves of the genuineness of the hypnotic state. No phenomena which have come under their observation, however, lend support to the theory of 'animal magnetism.'

"Test experiments which have been carried out by members of the Committee have shown that this condition is attended by mental and physical phenomena, and that these differ widely in different cases.

"Among the mental phenomena are altered consciousness, temporary limitation of will-power, increased receptivity of suggestion from without, sometimes to the extent of producing passing delusions, illusions, and hallucinations, an exalted condition of the attention, and post-hypnotic suggestions.

"Among the physical phenomena are vascular changes (such as flushing of the face and altered pulse rate), deepening of the respirations, increased frequency of deglutition, slight muscular tremors, inability to control suggested movements, altered muscular sense, anæsthesia, modified power of muscular contraction, catalepsy, and rigidity, often intense. It must, however, be understood that all these mental and physical phenomena are rarely present in any one case. The Committee take this opportunity of pointing out that the term hypnotism is somewhat misleading, inasmuch as sleep, as ordinarily understood, is not necessarily present.

"The Committee are of opinion that as a therapeutic agent hypnotism is frequently effective in relieving pain, procuring sleep, and alleviating many functional ailments. As to its permanent efficacy in the treatment of drunkenness, the evidence before the Committee is encouraging, but not conclusive.

"Dangers in the use of hypnotism may arise from want of knowledge, carelessness, or intentional abuse, or from the too continuous repetition of suggestions in unsuitable cases.

"The Committee are of opinion that when used for therapeutic purposes its employment should be confined to qualified medical men, and that under no circumstances should female patients be hypnotised, except in the presence of a relative or a person of their own sex.

"In conclusion, the Committee desire to express their strong disapprobation of public exhibitions of hypnotic phenomena, and hope that some legal restriction will be placed upon them.

F. NEEDHAM, *Chairman.*
T. OUTTERSON WOOD, *Hon. Sec."*

This report was referred back for further consideration. In 1893, it was again presented, with the addition of an important appendix, consisting " of some documentary evidence upon which the report was based." This comprised—

"1. Details of a series of valuable investigations carried out by Mr. J. N. Langley, M.A., F.R.S. (Lecturer on Physiology in Cambridge University), in conjunction with Mr. Wingfield, B.A. On the death of Dr. Ross of Manchester, Mr. Langley joined the Committee, and placed these details at its disposal.

"2. A report by Dr. G. M. Robertson, who, acting as Dr. Clouston's representative, visited Paris and Nancy for the *special purpose* of investigating and reporting upon the methods employed at these two schools.

"3. A report by Dr. Yellowlees, approved by Professor Gairdner.

"4. Reports by Drs. Robertson, Fleming, Kingsbury, Draper, and Hack Tuke.

"4a. A *résumé* of cases treated by Dr. T. Outterson Wood.

"Dr. Hack Tuke, in presenting the report, said he hoped the adoption of the report would, among other things, give a stimulus to the movement for putting a stop to public exhibitions of hypnotism."

A Dr. Brown moved that the report should lie on the table. The amendment was seconded.

It was suggested that the amendment should be altered so as to read that the report be received only, and the Committee thanked for their services.

The resolution to receive the report was carried.

HISTORY OF MY OWN PRACTICE.

My first introduction to the subject was indirectly due to James Esdaile. As we have seen, after leaving India he lived for some time in my native town, Perth, and many of his experiments were seen and afterwards reproduced by my father,

the late Dr. J. P. Bramwell.   These experiments, which as a boy
I witnessed from time to time, deeply impressed me; and I eagerly
devoured such books on the subject as my father possessed,
notably Dr. Gregory's *Animal Magnetism* and a translation of
Reichenbach's work.

When a student at Edinburgh, my attention was again drawn
to hypnotism by Professor John Hughes Bennett.   A *résumé* of
Braid's work and theories formed a regular part of his course of
physiology, and he confidently asserted that one day hypnotism
would revolutionise the theory and practice of medicine.

Soon after leaving Edinburgh I became busily engaged in
general practice, and hypnotism was almost forgotten until I
learned that it had been revived in the wards of the Salpêtrière.
Of the methods and theories in vogue there I knew nothing, but
determined, if opportunity occurred, to go to Paris to study them.
Before this chance arrived, however, a case occurred in my own
practice in which hypnotic treatment was apparently indicated.[1]
Although I told my patient how little I knew of the subject, I
had no difficulty in hypnotising him.   My success encouraged
me to persevere—at first cautiously amongst personal friends,
and then more and more boldly amongst my patients in general.

On March 28th, 1890, I gave a demonstration of hypnotic
anæsthesia to a large gathering of medical men at Leeds.   This
was reported in the *British Medical Journal* and the *Lancet*,[2] and,
in consequence, so many patients were sent to me from different
parts of the country that I decided to abandon general practice,
and to devote myself to hypnotic work.

As I was well aware of the fate that had awaited earlier
pioneers in the same movement, I naturally expected to meet
with opposition and misrepresentation.   These have been encountered, it is true; but the friendly help and encouragement
received have been immeasurably greater.   I have also had many
opportunities of placing my views before my professional brethren,
both by writing and speaking, opportunities all the more valued
because almost always unsolicited.   My interest in hypnotism has
brought me in contact with many medical men in other countries,
and I owe a debt of gratitude for the kindness and courtesy
invariably shown me by those whose cliniques I have visited
in France, Germany, Belgium, Sweden, Holland, and Switzerland.

[1] Case No. 80, pp. 238-9.   [2] Pp. 164-7.

Braid from Pereira's *Materia Medica*. The operator was Dr. O'Shaughnessy, of Calcutta, and the alleged induction of hypnosis was an accidental one. The following is the account referred to :—" At 2 P.M. a grain of the resin of hemp was given to a rheumatic patient. At 4 P.M. he was very talkative, sang, called loudly for an extra supply of food and declared himself in perfect health. At 6 P.M. he was asleep. At 8 P.M. he was found insensible, but breathing with perfect regularity, the pulse and skin natural, and the pupils freely contractile on the approach of light. Happening by chance to lift up his arm—the professional reader will judge of my astonishment," observed Dr. O., " when I found that it remained in the posture in which I had placed it. The patient had become cataleptic. We raised him to a sitting posture, and placed his arms and legs in every imaginable attitude. A waxen figure could not have been more pliant. He continued in this state till 1 A.M., when consciousness and voluntary motion quickly returned." A similar experiment was made with another patient, with like results.

According to Dr. von Schrenck-Notzing, of Munich, Cannabis Indica markedly facilitates the induction of hypnosis; if the toxic condition is not too pronounced, suggestions given as in hypnosis are carried out; the resulting hallucinations being more distinct and brilliant than the spontaneous ones. The following is an illustrative case :—

. The subject, aged 22, was healthy, and had never been previously hypnotised. At 6 P.M. he was given about a grain and a half of the extract of Cannabis Indica. At 7 P.M. he was excited, felt intoxicated and his face was flushed. Pulse 104. At 8 P.M. he felt overpowered with fatigue, was compelled to lie down and could not keep his eyes open. Schrenck-Notzing then placed his hand upon the patient's forehead, and successfully suggested cataleptic rigidity of the arm, analgesia of one arm and hyperæsthesia of the other, hallucinations of sight, hearing and taste, change of personality; and also a post-narcotic suggestion which was carried out the following day.

Chloroform.—Amongst those who have successfully used chloroform in the induction of hypnosis, Rifat and Herrero deserve especial mention. The latter, who is Professor of Clinical Medicine at Valladolid, gave an extremely interesting account of his experiments at the First International Congress of

Hypnotism (Paris, 1889). He selected six subjects, whom he had failed to hypnotise by ordinary methods, and, in their case, was able to confirm the statement of Dr. Rifat, of Salonica, that the narcotism of chloroform, at the end of the period of nervous excitement, and in the moments which precede the stage of delirium, is a condition quite as suggestible as that of hypnotic somnambulism. With four of these subjects, either from individual peculiarities or from too rapid administration of the chloroform, the period of susceptibility was so short that it hardly afforded time for making suggestions.

The experiment was repeated the following day with two subjects, a couple of days later with the others; and precautions were taken with the object of prolonging the period of suggestibility. After four or five inhalations of chloroform one patient passed into a suggestible condition resembling somnambulism, and, at the suggestion of Herrero, remained in this state for two hours after the inhaler had been removed. The three others required half the time, and less than half the chloroform, to arrive at the same condition they had reached in the former experiments. One of them was told, while in this condition of pseudo-chloroformic somnambulism, that in the future half a minute's looking at Herrero's eyes would be sufficient to produce this state; the suggestion was successful. Under similar circumstances, the others were told to oppose less and less resistance to the action of the narcotic. Five days later, the one who had responded most slowly to this suggestion went to sleep almost immediately, when the inhaler, either dry or moistened with a little alcohol, was applied to his nostrils. Four subjects, who had resisted hypnosis, were thus easily converted into excellent somnambules by suggestions made during chloroform narcosis; and, at the same time, the necessity for giving chloroform was removed by suggestion.

According to Herrero, this proved that chloroform could overcome unconscious resistance to hypnosis, but did not show that it could remove the conscious resistance opposed by the will. Shortly after making these experiments, however, he had amongst his patients a lady suffering from mania. Her doctor in Madrid had previously tried to hypnotise her every day for a month without success, and she now looked upon hypnotism as a satanic art and firmly refused to have anything to do with it.

Herrero considered this a good test case and, without mentioning a word about hypnotism, succeeded in persuading her to take chloroform. In less than five minutes, fifteen grammes produced the suggestible period of anæsthetic sleep; therapeutic suggestions were then given, and also others for the purpose of changing the chloroform narcosis into hypnosis. The next day three grammes were sufficient to produce the suggestible period; the following day it appeared when only the dry inhaler was used. On the fourth day she went to sleep by looking at Herrero's fingers and, during the two months she remained under treatment, hypnosis was always induced in this way, and generally instantaneously. Herrero says that since then he has often changed chloroform narcosis into hypnosis, and has only failed on one occasion, when he was compelled to abandon the attempt owing to the opposition of the patient's relatives. In conclusion, he expresses his conviction that, by means of chloroform and suggestion during the proper period of narcosis, one can always succeed in inducing hypnotic somnambulism, despite any resistance opposed consciously or unconsciously by the patient.

Alcohol.—Schrenck-Notzing sometimes employs alcohol for the induction of hypnosis, and, in addition, claims to have changed intoxication into hypnosis. AUG 31 1918

Chloral, Morphia.—Bernheim finds repeated doses of chloral or injections of morphia useful, when the ordinary methods of inducing hypnosis have failed.

Sometimes, when only slight hypnosis can be obtained by the usual means, narcotic drugs have proved useful in deepening the condition. Schrenck-Notzing relates a case in which he induced slight hypnosis with difficulty, but failed to obtain any response to curative suggestions; similar suggestions given during deep sleep resulting from chloral were successful.

Natural Sleep.—Many authorities claim to have changed natural into hypnotic sleep. According to Wetterstrand, it is often very easy to put oneself *en rapport* with sleeping persons, especially with children. The following is his method:—One hand is laid carefully and lightly on the sleeper's forehead, the body is gently stroked with the other, and, in a subdued voice, the patient is told to go on sleeping. When questioned he replies, and *rapport* is established. If his arm is raised it is often found to be cataleptic, or may be made so by suggestion.

Wetterstrand thinks this method of inducing hypnosis of much practical value and claims to have often used it successfully.

Moll was once able to change the afternoon nap of a gentleman, whom he had often hypnotised, into hypnosis without awaking him. He mentions that Baillif, Gscheidlen, Berger, Bernheim, and Forel have succeeded in changing natural sleep into hypnosis, even in persons who had not previously been hypnotised, or who had been refractory in the waking state.

According to Beaunis, it is easy by similar methods, to change natural somnambulism into hypnosis.

Schrenck-Notzing says he has frequently succeeded in inducing hypnosis from natural sleep, and also from hysterical attacks of sleep. One or two instances are also recorded by Esdaile and Schrenck-Notzing, in which post-epileptic and other forms of coma have been changed into hypnosis.

(C) MY OWN METHODS.

These have varied widely. At first I attempted to induce hypnosis mainly by mechanical means : at that time I was ignorant of what had been written on the subject by Liébeault and other members of the Nancy school, and had not observed the methods of other operators.

After seating the patient in a comfortable chair, I arranged a small moveable mirror above his eyes, and placed a lamp in such a way as to throw a bright light upon it. The patients were told to look fixedly at the mirror as long as they could keep their eyes open. In some instances the eyes closed rapidly and hypnosis quickly appeared ; in others, even after half an hour's gazing, there was no apparent result. When this was the case, I requested them to shut their eyes, and made passes without contact over the face and upper part of the body, at the same time adding a few suggestions. Hypnosis was induced in every instance, but sometimes much perseverance was necessary, and in one case success was only obtained at the sixty-eighth attempt. At that time the patients were all drawn from my own practice, and the induction of hypnosis, which at first had often been tedious and difficult, soon became easier with increased experience. Mechanical aids were gradually discarded : the patients simply looked at my eyes for a few seconds, while I made energetic suggestions. I now held a clinique three times a week, and sometimes hypnotised from thirty to sixty patients in an evening. I passed rapidly from one to the other, saying to each in turn: "Look at my eyes! Your eyelids are getting heavy, you cannot keep them open, they are closing now, they are fast!" As the eyelids closed, which they almost invariably did at once, I made an energetic pass in the direction of the. patient's face and said: "Sleep!" With two exceptions, success was obtained in every case, and in nine out of ten in the time necessary to utter the words just quoted. The patients were still nearly all drawn from my own practice, but, unlike my earlier cases, few suffered from severe illness and many were hypnotised for operative purposes only.

Shortly after the hypnotic demonstration at Leeds, on March 28th, 1890,[1] I commenced to receive a different class of patients, all of whom were strangers to me. Most of them suffered from neurasthenia, hysteria, or ' other forms of functional nervous trouble; but in addition there were many cases of dipsomania and some of genuine insanity. In all, the illness was of long duration and other methods of treatment had been employed without benefit. To my surprise and disappointment, a small percentage alone were hypnotised by the method so successfully employed amongst my own patients. At first the fresh cases were treated along with others already hypnotised; .but this, instead of aiding me as formerly, seemed to increase my difficulties, as the new patients found others sleeping around them a disturbing element. Each patient was then taken singly, and fixed gazing at a mirror in a darkened room again resorted to. In addition, I frequently made them look at my eyes while I made verbal suggestions. I also procured one of Luys' revolving mirrors, but found it worse than useless. The instrument was driven by clockwork, but could not be stopped until it ran down, and there was no method of regulating its speed. It made a loud and disagreeable noise, which from time to time became more marked and irregular, and irresistibly suggested an infernal machine on the point of exploding! I had another constructed without the faults which characterised that of Luys. This too was driven by clockwork, but could be arrested at any time and its speed regulated, while the

[1] Pp. 164-7.

E

sound was uniform and soothing. With this mirror I succeeded
in easy cases, such as could have been hypnotised by any other
method, but it was no help in difficult ones. By one or another
of these methods I hypnotised about 75 per cent of my patients,
but in many instances only after repeated trials. After a time
mechanical means were again almost entirely abandoned ; and I
relied more and more on verbal suggestion and careful study of
the patient's mental condition.

The following is now my usual method :—I rarely attempt
to induce hypnosis the first time I see a patient, but confine myself to making his acquaintance, hearing his own account of his
case, and ascertaining his mental attitude with regard to hypnotism.
I usually find, from the failure of other methods of treatment,
that the patient is more or less sceptical as to the chance of his
being benefited. In most cases also he has either read misleading
sensational articles on hypnotism, or his friends have painted its
dangers in striking colours. I endeavour to remove erroneous
ideas, and refuse to attempt to induce hypnosis until the patient
is satisfied of the safety and desirability of the experiment. I
never tell a patient that I am certain of being able to hypnotise
him, but always explain how much depends upon his own mental
condition and power of carrying out my directions. I then say :
"Presently I shall ask you to look at my eyes for a few seconds,
when probably your eyelids will become heavy and you will feel
impelled to close them. Should this not happen, I shall ask you
to shut them, and to keep them closed until I tell you to open
them. I shall then make certain passes and suggestions, but I
do not wish you to pay much attention to what I am saying or
doing, and above all you are not to attempt to analyse your
sensations. Your best plan will be to create some monotonous
drowsy mental picture and to fix your attention upon that. You
must not expect to go to sleep. A certain number of hypnotised
persons pass into a condition more or less closely resembling
sleep ; few do so at the first sitting, however, and you must only
expect to feel drowsy and heavy." After these explanations, and
having darkened the room and instructed any spectators to remain
quiet, I place my patient in a comfortable chair and request him
to look at my eyes, at the same time bringing my face slightly
above and about ten inches from his. The patient's eyes sometimes close almost immediately. Should they not do so, I continue

to look steadily at him and make suggestions. These are twofold; the patient's attention is directed to the sensations he probably is experiencing, and others, which I wish him to feel, are suggested. Thus: "Your eyes are heavy, the lids are beginning to quiver, the eyes are filling with water. You begin to feel drowsy, your limbs are becoming heavy, you are finding it more and more difficult to keep your eyes open, etc." Sometimes this produces the desired result; the eyes close and the first stage of hypnosis is induced. If this does not take place, I direct the patient to close his eyes, and make passes over the head and face, either with or without contact, repeating meanwhile appropriate verbal suggestions. This is continued for half an hour. No stereotyped method is employed, however, the process being varied with different patients, or with the same patient at different times, to suit the particular needs of special cases. To ensure success, it is necessary to understand the mental condition of the patient, to gain his intelligent co-operation, and to create a clear picture of hypnosis together with the expectation of its appearance.

In a few instances I have attempted to change natural sleep into hypnosis, but so far without success. I have occasionally employed galvanism, and have also given chloroform, chloral, bromide and various other drugs, but generally with negative results.

I have hypnotised several patients who were completely deaf: some of these were unacquainted with the deaf and dumb alphabet, and writing was the only means of communication. The necessary explanations and instructions were given beforehand in this way, as also the suggestions which were to be fulfilled during and after hypnosis.

For the first few years of my hypnotic practice, I never made curative suggestions until hypnosis had been induced. I changed my methods, however, after having observed in Continental cliniques that suggestions were frequently responded to in cases of slight, or even doubtful, hypnosis. Now, in addition to attempting to induce hypnosis in the manner just described, I combine this with curative suggestions. Thus, from the very first treatment the patient is subjected to two distinct processes, the object of the one being to induce hypnosis, that of the other to cure or relieve disease; and frequently the latter is successful before the patient can be described as genuinely hypnotised.

(D) SELF-HYPNOSIS AND SELF-SUGGESTION.

Putting aside the question of self-hypnosis amongst fakirs and other religious fanatics, I am not acquainted with many instances in which the primary hypnosis has been induced by the subject himself. Braid, however, stated that he hypnotised himself on more than one occasion, and successfully suggested the disappearance of rheumatic pain. Professor Forel, of Zurich, and Dr. Coste de Lagrave have also succeeded in hypnotising themselves, and the latter can influence himself in many ways by suggestion; thus, he states he is able to get rid of pain, fatigue, mental depression, etc.

Shortly after commencing hypnotic work, I found that patients, who had been deeply hypnotised, could be instructed to reinduce the condition at will. Here, suggestions during hypnosis were not necessary for the production of its phenomena; they were equally efficacious when made beforehand in the waking state. The subject was able to suggest to himself when hypnosis should appear and terminate, and also the phenomena which he wished to obtain during and after it. This training was at first a limited one; the patients, for example, were instructed how to get sleep at night or relief from pain. They did not, however, always confine themselves to my suggestions, but originated others and widely varying ones, regarding their health, comfort, or work. In several instances they made use of self-hypnosis for operative purposes, and astonished their dentists by remaining insensible to the pain of having their teeth extracted. In some instances this power has been retained for over twelve years.

I have also observed the phenomena of self-hypnosis in healthy persons who had been hypnotised for experimental purposes. Here, the subjects, when awake, could suggest to themselves that muscular rigidity, local and general analgesia, hallucinations, etc., should appear during hypnosis; and then hypnotise themselves at will, when the phenomena duly appeared. During self-hypnosis the subjects were either *en rapport* with every one or only with certain individuals, according to the suggestions they had made to themselves beforehand.

Even in slight hypnosis self-suggestion is not without influence, although its results are neither so striking nor so far-reaching as in the case of somnambules.

CLASSIFICATION OF METHODS OF INDUCING HYPNOSIS.

The methods by which hypnosis is induced have been classed as follows :—(1) Physical Methods; (2) Psychical Methods; (3) those of the Magnetisers.

The modern hypnotiser, however, whatever his theories may be, borrows his actual technique from Mesmer and Liébeault with equal impartiality, and thus renders classification well nigh impossible. Thus, the members of the Nancy school, while asserting that everything is due to suggestion, do not hesitate to use physical means. The passes with contact employed by Mesmer are almost exactly reproduced by Wetterstrand. Fixed gazing generally precedes or accompanies suggestion, and, when these fail, Bernheim does not scruple to have recourse to narcotics.

As to physical methods, it is more than doubtful whether these have ever succeeded when mental influences have been carefully excluded, and the subjects have been absolutely ignorant of the nature of the experiment. No one was ever hypnotised by looking at a lark-mirror, until Luys borrowed that lure from the bird-catchers and invested it with hypnotic powers. On the other hand, any physical method will succeed with a susceptible subject who knows what is expected of him.

METHODS OF TERMINATING HYPNOSIS.

The hypnotic state tends to terminate spontaneously. In slight hypnosis this usually happens as soon as the operator leaves the patient; in more profound stages it may not occur until after the lapse of several hours. The methods of artificially terminating the condition may be divided as follows :—(1) Physical, by means of various sensorial stimuli ; (2) Psychical, by direct or indirect suggestion.

(1) **Physical.**—Esdaile's method of terminating the mesmeric state consisted in blowing sharply on the patient's eyes, rubbing the eyelids and eyebrows, or sprinking cold water on the face.

Sometimes these methods failed, and then the patient was allowed to sleep quietly until the condition terminated naturally.

On one or two occasions patients undergoing surgical operations came out of the trance before the operation was completed ; Esdaile's investigations led him to believe this was due to the action of cold.   In hot weather the patients were operated on almost naked, and it was observed that those who were completely anæsthetic when tested in the mesmerising room, where they were covered up in bed, became more or less conscious when placed in the operating room, and the blankets removed. Patients in the mesmeric trance, who were insensible to the loudest noises, the cutting of inflamed parts, the application of nitric acid to raw surfaces, and other painful surgical operations, became fully conscious when their naked bodies were exposed for a few minutes to the cold air.   Subsequently this mistake was avoided, and no further cases occurred in which the trance terminated before the close of the operation.

At the commencement of his hypnotic practice, Braid used to awaken his patients by directing a current of cold air upon their faces, but he afterwards abandoned this in favour of suggestion.

According to Pitres, pressure upon certain parts of the body, called by him *zones hypno-frénatrices*, will terminate the hypnotic condition.   The forcible opening of the eyes has also been used as a method of awakening.

(2) **Psychical.**—The members of the Nancy school *suggest* during hypnosis that the subject shall awake[1] at a given signal, as, for example, when the operator utters the word "Awake," or counts "One, two, three." The nature of the signal itself is of little or no importance, the essential point being that the subject shall understand its import.

The method just described is the one I usually adopt, and I have rarely experienced the slightest difficulty in awaking my patients.   In a few instances, where deep hypnosis had been obtained at the first attempt, the patients did not awake instantaneously in response to suggestion, and afterwards remained somewhat drowsy and heavy.   When this occurred, I at once re-hypnotised the patient and repeated the suggestion that he should

---

[1] The word "Awake" is simply used for convenience and must not be taken as implying that the hypnotic condition is one of sleep. The supposed connection between hypnosis and sleep will be discussed later.

immediately respond to my signal, and that on awaking no trace of drowsiness should remain. A very little training of this kind produced the desired result.

Theoretical Explanations of the Effects produced by different Methods of terminating Hypnosis.—According to Moll, the awaking from hypnosis, like that from natural sleep, occurs in two ways : (1) from mental causes and (2) from sense-stimulation. In the opinion of Forel, however, and certain other members of the Nancy school, the stimulation of the special senses only awakens the patients when it acts as an indirect suggestion, the physical stimulus being simply the signal for awaking.

Dr. Crocq, of Brussels, on the other hand, draws attention to the fact that Bernheim and Beaunis say that the subject can generally be awakened by verbal suggestion, but, if this is not sufficient, that it can then be effected by blowing two or three times upon the eyes. The blowing, he says, according to these authors, then becomes a stronger suggestion than a verbal command. It appears to Dr. Crocq a contradiction to attribute the immediate awaking of the subject by blowing upon the eyes to suggestion, when one has just failed to arouse him by repeated verbal commands. One cannot in justice raise the objection that blowing upon the eyes is an unconscious suggestion, seeing that this has succeeded where direct suggestion has just failed. Again, when a subject, who knows nothing of hypnotism nor of what you wish him to do, is put to sleep for the first time, blowing upon his eyes will awake him without anything to this effect having been suggested to him. Blowing, therefore, appears to possess a particular property which provokes awakening.

While Braid believed that the mental effect, resulting from the indirect physical action of mechanical means, could be checked or reversed by stronger and more direct verbal suggestion, he still held, and I think justly so, that physical impressions were capable of producing both physical and mental results. Forel, on the contrary, denies the physical influence of mechanical processes, on the ground that suggestion is capable of altering their supposed action. He says : " Blowing on the face no longer awakens my subjects, because I have suggested that this would remove pain instead of arousing them." From this he concludes that the act of blowing produces no result, and considers this a powerful argument against the Somatic school.   Would it not be equally logical to contend that the prick of a pin produced no physical effect, because the subject, rendered insensible to pain by suggestion, had been taught to regard the pin-prick as a signal to evoke some other condition ?   Forel ignores too completely the artificial character of the hypnotic state.   Doubtless hypnotic subjects can be trained to inhibit certain sensations, and to regard others as the signals for the manifestation of various phenomena; but we are not justified in concluding from this that all the ordinary physical impressions spontaneously cease to be appreciated in hypnosis.   Further, in slight hypnosis and in untrained subjects, the action of physical impressions can be readily observed, and a loud noise, or the prick of a pin, will speedily terminate the condition.   Finally, Esdaile's patients referred to above had clearly not been taught that cold was to arouse them in the midst of an operation.

CHAPTER IV.

(1) **Average Susceptibility.**—In April, 1892, Schrenck-Notzing published the result of his First International Statistics of Susceptibility to hypnosis. Fifteen observers in different countries furnished returns which showed, without reference to sex, age or health, that they had tried to hypnotise 8705 persons, with 519 failures : *i.e.* only 6 per cent were uninfluenced.

Van Eeden and van Renterghem, from May 5th, 1887, to June 30th, 1893, attempted to hypnotise 1089 persons, and only failed with 58, or 5·33 per cent.

Liébeault informed me that he had no complete record of the thousands of cases he had treated during his hypnotic practice of over thirty years, but that, from 1887 to 1890, he had tried to hypnotise 1756 cases, his failures only amounting to a fraction over 3 per cent.

From 1882 to 1886, Bernheim attempted to hypnotise 5000 of his hospital patients, and succeeded with 75 per cent. A few years later the number had risen to 10,000, and the successes to over 80 per cent.

Bérillon, out of 250 cases in children, hypnotised 80 per cent at the first or second attempt.

Up to March, 1890, Wetterstrand's cases amounted to 3209, and of these only 105, or 3·7 per cent, were uninfluenced. Amongst the failures 75 had only been tried once or at most twice. By the end of January, 1893, the number of his hypnotic patients had reached 6500, while the percentage of failures had decreased.

In the first year of his hypnotic practice, Forel endeavoured to hypnotise 205 patients, many of whom were insane. He

57

succeeded in 171 cases and failed in 34; but in the last 105 the failures fell to 11 per cent. In 1898, he informed me that he had tried to hypnotise about 1000 persons and had succeeded with over 95 per cent.

Amongst my earlier patients the average susceptibility varied from 100 per cent in one group to 78 per cent in another. These groups illustrate the fact that susceptibility to hypnosis is influenced by many widely differing causes, and that, unless these are carefully noted, general statistics on the subject are apt to be misleading. The first group comprised patients drawn from my own general practice at Goole; the second, strangers who had come to me from a distance.

Group I. — Many of the patients in this group were hypnotised in the hurried rounds of a large general practice : unless the case was of special interest no notes were taken, and I have no complete record of the numbers treated, which roughly speaking amounted to about 500. The following table, however, gives the first 100 consecutive cases which were treated at my own house, the results in every instance being recorded at the time :—

Table A.

Total Number, 100 ; Male, 27 ; Female, 73.
Greatest Age, 76 years ; Lowest Age, 4 years ; Average Age, 23·42 years.

Results.

Refractory, 0 ; Slight Hypnosis, 12 ; Deep Hypnosis, 40 ; Somnambulism, 48.
Hypnotised at First Attempt, 92 ; After Repeated Trials, 8.
Average Number of Trials in these Eight Cases, 4.
Average Number of Sittings in the 100 Cases, including Attempts at Hypnosis, 10.

This table, I think, fairly represents the results obtained in the 500 cases referred to. It is to be noted, however, that although no failures are recorded in the 100 examples just cited, I was unable to hypnotise 2 out of the total 500 treated.

Group II. — The following table gives the first 100 consecutive cases in which the patients were not drawn from my own practice. In every instance the results were recorded at the time :—

Table B.

Total Number, 100 ; Male, 42 : Female, 58.
Greatest Age, 70 years ; Lowest Age, 9 years : Average Age, 34 years.

Results.

Refractory, 22 ; Slight Hypnosis, 36 ; Deep Hypnosis, 13 ; Somnambulism, 29.

Hypnotised at First Attempt, 51 ; After Repeated Trials, 26.

Average Number of Trials in these 26 cases, 15.

Average Number of Sittings in the 100 cases, including Attempts at Hypnosis, 35·9.

Remarks.—These two tables form a marked contrast. Table A contains no refractory subjects, while in Table B these amount to 23. In A also a larger proportion passed into the deeper stages, and this difference is further accentuated by the fact that the average number of sittings in B greatly exceeded that in A. Further, it is probable that the number of somnambules in A could easily have been increased. In many instances no direct attempt was made to produce somnambulism : *i.e.* amnesia on awaking was not suggested. At a later date, I found that several members of this group could be rendered somnambulic at a single sitting, although they had not previously passed into that stage and had not been hypnotised for many months. It is to be noted that while in A 92 were hypnotised at the first attempt, in B the number only amounted to 51. Again, the number of trials required to induce hypnosis, when this did not appear at the first attempt, only averaged 8 in A, whereas it reached 15 in B. Amongst the refractory patients in B the number of unsuccessful attempts varied from 3 to 156, the average being 38·20.

The means employed for inducing hypnosis is described in the chapter upon " Methods." It is important to note that in B these were usually numerous, varied and prolonged, while in A, on the contrary, they were generally short and simple.

These tables will be again referred to in discussing the different causes which influence susceptibility.

(2) **Susceptibility in reference to the Depth of Hypnosis.**
—No uniform classification of hypnotic stages exists, and thus it is difficult to compare the various statistics on the subject. I will, however, quote some of them here, at the same time referring the reader to the chapter on " Stages " [1] for fuller information as regards classification.

[1] Pp. 150-155.

The following results were obtained in the 8705 International cases recorded by Schrenck-Notzing :—

Refractory . 519, or 6 per cent.   Hypotaxis   . 4316, or 49 per cent.
Somnolence . 2557, or 29 „   Somnambulism, 1313, or 15 „

In 1089 cases treated by van Eeden and van Renterghem of whom 529, or 48·57 per cent, were men, and 560, or 51·42 per cent, women, we find the following results :—

Refractory . 58, or 5·33 per cent.   Deep Sleep . 445, or 40·87 per cent.
Slight Sleep . 466, or 40·87 „   Somnambulism 120, or 11·61 „

Liébeault gives the result of 755 cases, thus :—

	Men.	Women.	Total.	Proportion per cent.	
				Men.	Women.
Somnambulism . .	54	91	145	18·8	19·4
Very profound Sleep	21	34	55	7·3	7·2
Profound Sleep . . .	108	163	271	37·6	34·8
Light Sleep . . .	52	99	151	18·1	21·1
Somnolence . . .	21	50	71	7·3	10·6
Uninfluenced . .	31	31	62	10·8	6·6
Total . .	287	· 468	755		

The above table is restated by Beaunis in order to show the influence of age upon the different stages :—

Age. Years.	Somnam- bulism.	Very Deep Sleep.	Deep Sleep.	Slight Sleep.	Somnol- ence.	Not in- fluenced.
Up to 7 . .	26·5	4·3	13·0	52·1	4·3	0
7–14 . .	55·3	7·6	23·0	13·8	0	0
14–21 . .	23·2	5·7	44·8	5·7	8·0	10·3
21–28 . .	13·2	5·1	36·7	18·3	17·3	9·1
28–35 . .	22·6	5·9	34·5	17·8	13·0	5·8
35–42 . .	10·5	11·7	35·2	28·2	5·8	8·2
42–49 . .	21·6	·4·7	29·2	22·6	9·4	12·2
49–56 . .	7·3	14·7	35·2	27·9	10·2	4·4
56–63 . .	7·2	8·6	37·6	18·8	13·0	14·4
63 and over .	11·8	8·4	39·9	20·3	6·7	13·5

Beaunis draws attention to the fact that this table shows clearly that somnambulism is reached more frequently in children than in adults.

The statistics of Dr. Ringier, of Zurich, give similar results; between the ages of 7 and 14 his somnambules amounted to 52·94 per cent, and from 14 to 21 years to 42·31 per cent.

These figures are in marked contrast to those of the general statistics which disregard age. Thus, of the 8705 cases recorded by Schrenck-Notzing, and of the 1089 given by van Eeden and van Renterghem, nearly the same proportion, *i.e.* 15 and 11·61 per cent, became somnambules. The percentage of somnambules in Liébeault's 755 cases was 18·8 in men and 19·4 in women, while Braid found that only 10 per cent of his patients became somnambules.

In my groups, as we have seen, the number of somnambules was remarkably high, reaching 48 per cent in Table A and 29 per cent in Table B. Further, in A deep hypnosis was obtained in 48 per cent, slight hypnosis in 12 per cent, while none were refractory.

(3) **Nationality.**—Race, apparently, has no influence upon susceptibility. Liébeault's extraordinary success led to the assumption that the French were peculiarly susceptible, but the statistics of Wetterstrand, of Stockholm, compare favourably with the results obtained at Nancy, while Dr. Grossmann, of Berlin, asserts that he hypnotises 93 per cent of his patients, and lays stress on the fact that most of them are hard-headed North Germans. Dr. Morier told me that he found Colonial patients in South Australia as susceptible as those of European origin. Esdaile asserted that there was no difference in susceptibility between the Scotch and the Natives of India, and hypnotic anæsthesia was induced as readily in Perth Infirmary as in the Government hospitals in Calcutta. Most of my patients were English, and their susceptibility, as far as Table A is concerned at all events, has not been exceeded elsewhere.

(4) **Sex.**—Sex has little or no influence on susceptibility. Wetterstrand finds both sexes equally easy to influence, while in Liébeault's statistics the difference in favour of women amounts to only 1 per cent. Dr. Hugh Wingfield, when Demonstrator of Physiology at Cambridge, hypnotised 152 undergraduates, and only failed in about 20 per cent of the total number tried.

As there was never more than one attempt made with the same
subject, this undoubtedly underrates the susceptibility. Esdaile's
patients, with very few exceptions, were males, and Liébeault and
others have remarked upon the ease with which soldiers and
sailors can be hypnotised.

My own observations agree with these. In Table A all the
males were hypnotised, the only refractory cases in the entire
group of about 500 being two females, both hysterical.

(5) **Age.**—According to most authorities, children are more
easily hypnotised than adults. Wetterstrand found that all
children from 3 or 4 to 15 years of age could be influenced
without exception: his youngest successful patient being $2\frac{1}{2}$
years old. Bérillon, out of 250 cases in children, hypnotised
80 per cent at the first attempt. Liébeault also found them
peculiarly susceptible, and one of his statistical tables records
100 per cent of successes up to the age of 14. In adult life,
age, apparently, makes little difference; in the same table we find
that from the ages of 14 to 21 the failures were about 10 per
cent, and from 63 years and upwards about 13 per cent. The
following figures illustrate the influence of age upon susceptibility
in 744 of Liébeault's patients :—

Up to 7 years of age . .	Total 23.	No failures.	
From 7 to 14 years of age .	„ 65.	„	
„ 14 to 21 „ .	„ 87.	Failures 9, or 10·3 per cent.	
„ 21 to 28 „ .	„ 98.	„ 9, or 9·1 „	
„ 28 to 35 „ .	„ 84.	„ 5, or 5·9 „	
„ 35 to 42 „ .	„ 85.	„ 7, or 8·2 „	
„ 42 to 49 „ .	„ 106.	„ 13, or 12·2 „	
„ 49 to 56 „ .	„ 68.	„ 3, or 4·4 „	
„ 56 to 63 „ .	„ 69.	„ 10, or 14·4 „	
„ 63 and upwards . .	„ 59.	„ 8, or 13·5 „	

Generally speaking, I have found children more susceptible
than adults, my youngest successful case being 3 years of age.
On the other hand, I have met with failures within the ages that
Liébeault and Wetterstrand found invariably susceptible.

(6) **Social Position.** — Drs. Döllken (Marburg) and Carl
Gerster (Munich) state that a marked difference exists between
the lower and higher classes, the latter being more easily hypnotised. Bernheim claims to have succeeded with many patients
belonging to the upper classes, while Wingfield, as we have seen,
hypnotised 152 undergraduates at the first attempt. Forel, on

the other hand, draws attention to the fact that the bulk of
Liébeault's patients belonged to the working classes, and states
that unprejudiced, uneducated people are as a rule easily
hypnotised.

As far as my observations go, the induction of hynosis is not
influenced by the social position of the patient. It is true that
susceptibility was less marked in Table B than in Table A,
while at the same time the majority of cases in the former were
of a higher rank than in the latter. On the other hand, causes
which undoubtedly influence susceptibility adversely were more
marked in B, and, when these were absent, social position had
apparently no effect.

(7) **Physical Condition.**—According to Moll, Liébeault, and
others, good general health favours the induction of hypnosis.
Many of my most successful cases were strong healthy males,
who were easily hypnotised for operative and experimental
purposes. As already seen, undergraduates, soldiers and sailors
generally proved good subjects.

(8) **Sense-Stimulation.**—Fixed gazing, the sudden flashing of
a bright light, revolving mirrors, monotonous sounds, the application
of hot plates to the head, galvanism, and monotonous stimulation of
the cutaneous nerves by means of passes, have all been employed
in the induction of hypnosis. What part these methods play in
increasing susceptibility; how much is due to direct physical,
how much to indirect mental, influence, it is difficult to determine.
In Table A, where with few exceptions hypnosis was easily
induced, they were hardly employed at all, while in Table B,
especially in the refractory cases, they were used to a much
greater extent.

(9) **Mental Condition.** — (a) *General Intelligence.*—Gerster
states that fools are the least susceptible to hypnosis, whereas the
intelligent man with the well-balanced brain is more or less easily
influenced. Moll, also, finds the dull and stupid difficult. Dr.
von Krafft-Ebing, of Vienna, and Bernheim hold similar views:
the former states that intelligent subjects can be readily hypnotised, and the latter claims to have succeeded with many
highly educated persons; while Forel asserts that every mentally
healthy man is naturally hypnotisable. With these opinions I agree;
for I have found the stupid and unimaginative more difficult to
influence than those possessing fair intelligence.

(b) *Volition and Attention.*—It is sometimes stated that
feebleness of will facilitates the induction of hypnosis, but this
Moll declares to be erroneous. The subjects must be able to
arrest their thoughts and direct them into a particular channel—
an indication of strength, not weakness of will. This opinion is
shared by Krafft-Ebing; while Forel considers that subjects who
cannot remain mentally passive, and who analyse their own
sensations, are difficult to influence. Braid considered that there
was a direct relation between the power of concentrating the
attention and susceptibility. Fixed gazing alone would not excite
hypnosis; the attention must be concentrated on some non-
exciting object or idea—this was the primary and imperative
condition. Amongst my own patients, I have usually observed
that strength of will, and power of concentrating the attention,
favoured the induction of hypnosis, while their absence had an
opposite effect.

(c) *Faith.*—Faith alone has apparently little effect on susceptibility. I have failed with subjects who firmly believed I
could hypnotise them, and that they were specially susceptible.
On the other hand, I have succeeded with many who were convinced that they could not be influenced. Liégeois says it is not
necessary for the subject to have faith, as the magnetisers used
to assert, but he must loyally observe the prescribed conditions.
Forel states that people who laugh and say that they cannot be
hypnotised are often easily influenced: those who a moment or
two before had regarded hypnotised persons as impostors, and the
operator as a dupe, were often quickly hypnotised before they
realised what was taking place.

(d) *Self-Suggestion.*—A determination to resist the operator
renders the induction of hypnosis impossible. Here the failure
is due to conscious self-suggestion. Some of my unsuccessful cases
of dipsomania, who only agreed to be treated under the pressure
of their relatives, afterwards confessed that they had resisted
every attempt to induce hypnosis. The involuntary self-
suggestion of the patient is a still more common obstacle; but to
this I will refer when dealing with morbid states.

(e) *Imitation.*—Many operators attach much importance to
the influence of imitation upon susceptibility, and for this
reason attempt to hypnotise fresh patients in the presence of
others who are put to sleep before them. Liébeault invariably

hypnotised his poorer patients in the presence of each other, and refractory subjects amongst his private ones were always brought to his clinique in the hope that they might be influenced through imitation. Van Eeden and van Renterghem usually hypnotise more than one patient at a time in the same room. Bernheim hypnotises his hospital patients in the wards, and thus the others see what he is doing. Forel says it is advantageous to hypnotise another person in the presence of the patient, and attributes much of Wetterstrand's success to the fact that he generally treats a number of patients simultaneously.

With these opinions I do not entirely agree. In Table A susceptibility was probably increased by imitation, but the patients in Table B found that the presence of others embarrassed them and distracted their attention. I now almost invariably treat each patient separately. Before beginning, however, I occasionally hypnotise an old patient in the new one's presence ; and possibly this sometimes facilitates matters by removing fear, and creating a vivid picture of the desired condition.

(*f*) *Behaviour of Spectators.* — As Moll has stated, it is extremely important that spectators should maintain silence and especially refrain from expressing doubt or mistrust in any way, as the least word or gesture may thwart the attempt to induce hypnosis. For example, I was once asked to hypnotise a patient suffering from grave and long-standing nervous disease. His medical man, in introducing me, assured him that I had the power of compelling him to do whatever I liked, even to making him sign a cheque for £20,000 in my favour. Needless to say, I failed to induce hypnosis. The third attempt was more promising ; but at its conclusion the same medical man remarked to the patient that he was evidently one of those persons whom it was impossible to hypnotise !

(10) **Morbid Mental and Physical Conditions.**—(*a*) *Mental Excitement and Fear.*—Fear, with its attendant mental excitement, usually prevents the induction of hypnosis. In England at the present day nearly every one has read, and been more or less influenced by, various unfounded newspaper stories regarding the dangers of hypnotism. The public generally has accepted the misleading statement that hypnosis is characterised by unconsciousness and suspended volition ; and while patients are under the influence of these ideas it is difficult or impossible

F

to hypnotise them. In such cases no attempt to induce hypnosis
should be made at the first interview. The true nature of the
hypnotic state should be explained, and the patient's fears
removed. Above everything he should be made to understand
that his volition will not be interfered with. Forel, too, holds
that mental excitement is unfavourable to the production of
hypnosis, and fear renders it impossible. Thus, he says, the first
attempt to induce hypnosis frequently fails because the patients
imagine that extraordinary things are going to happen to them.

(b) *Insanity, Hysteria, etc.*—According to Bernheim, it is a
mistake to think that the nervous, weak-brained, or hysterical
are easy to influence; on the contrary it is often difficult or
impossible to hypnotise those suffering from mental disorders.
Moll states that the hysterical are particularly difficult to
hypnotise. This is largely due to the spirit of contradiction
which exists in such patients, and the opposing self-suggestions
that result from it. If we take, he says, a pathological condition
of the organism as necessary for hypnosis, we shall be obliged to
conclude that nearly every one is not quite right in the head.
On the contrary, it is now generally agreed that the mentally
unsound, particularly idiots, even if not wholly insusceptible, are
still very much more difficult to hypnotise than the healthy.
Wetterstrand states that one of the best somnambules he ever
saw was remarkable for good health and freedom from nervousness. Further, he invariably found that the most difficult to
influence were the hysterical, restless, and egotistical, who were
unable to concentrate their thoughts and attention.

Gerster says the daily press echoes the statement that it is
only the "credulous" and feeble-minded who can be hypnotised;
the opposite, however, is correct. According to Forel, all
experienced operators agree that the insane are undoubtedly the
most difficult to hypnotise. With patience and perseverance
some of the milder forms of mental disorder may be influenced;
but it is extremely difficult to hypnotise those who are suffering
from grave insanity. Here, owing to the continuous cerebral
irritation, and the fact that the attention is fixed exclusively
upon diseased ideas, it is almost impossible for suggestion to find
an entrance into the brain. As we have seen, Esdaile's patients
were regarded as hysterical, but he pointed out that hysteria
was unknown in his hospitals. Braid found patients with very

mobile brains difficult to influence, and entirely failed with idiots, despite much perseverance.

My personal observations accord with these views. Nearly all my difficult and refractory cases suffered from some form of nervous disease; and I have, as a general rule, found that the difficulty in inducing hypnosis bore a direct proportion to the gravity and duration of the mental disturbance. The tables already referred to illustrate this. In A, 2 cases were experimental and 22 were hypnotised for minor operations: both the former and most of the latter were in good health, while the majority of the remainder neither suffered from grave disease, nor had been ill long.

In Table B, there were 12 experimental and 2 operative cases, all in good health. The remainder suffered from grave and long-standing disease, such as insanity, dipsomania, hysteria, neurasthenia, and the like.

As the existence of nervous diseases apparently lessens the susceptibility to hypnosis, I now propose to consider the different conditions associated with these affections which apparently form obstacles to success.

(a) *Attention.*—I have hitherto failed to hypnotise idiots, apparently because they possess little spontaneous and no voluntary attention. The condition of the attention in hysteria, neurasthenia, and certain types of insanity forms a serious, but not insuperable, obstacle to the production of hypnosis. It is necessary, first, that the patient should attend to and understand the operator's description of the phenomena of restfulness, drowsiness, lethargy, etc., which it is desired to evoke, and, secondly, that he should be able to fix his attention on some inanimate object or monotonous train of thought. In the cases just referred to this result is particularly difficult to obtain. The patient's attention is concentrated upon his own diseased condition, and he is constantly watching, analysing, and exaggerating his symptoms. Sometimes, as in hysterical melancholia and certain forms of obsession, the patient is a prey to a continued flow of unhappy thought, which he is incapable of arresting. At others, the physical condition renders hypnosis difficult, since the various forms of hysterical tremor and spasm absorb the attention, and make mental quietude impossible. Pain is also an obstacle.

(b) *Duration of Illness.*—Prolonged illness is undoubtedly unfavourable to the production of hypnosis. Here the morbid symptoms have become ingrained, as it were, while the failure of all previous treatment has rendered the patients hopeless.

(c) *Self-Suggestion.*—The conditions just referred to give rise to various forms of self-suggestion antagonistic to the operator. Thus, the failure of other forms of treatment excites the self-suggestion that hypnotism will also prove unsuccessful. The patients, who are constantly analysing their own sensations, are also self-suggestionists who are only interested in themselves. One of my patients, for example, who had suffered from hysterical neurasthenia for twelve years, finally regarded all her symptoms as the result of medical treatment. Thus, pain in the head was due to galvanism, in another part of the body to massage—in fact a number of localised painful regions were labelled with the names of the medical men who had attended her. Hypnotism was not more fortunate. Not only did fixed gazing speedily produce headache and nausea, but passes made behind the patient's back at a distance of 20 feet—though with her knowledge—frequently excited actual vomiting.

(11) **Natural Somnambulism and Hysterical Sleep.**—I have had no opportunity of attempting to induce primary hypnosis during either of the above-mentioned states. Beaunis and other authorities, however, consider that susceptibility to hypnosis is increased during natural somnambulism. Gerster found that children who, without being actual somnambules, talked and answered questions in their sleep, could be easily hypnotised. Schrenck-Notzing states that hysterical attacks of sleep favour the induction of hypnosis, and that the one condition can be changed into the other.

(12) **Natural Sleep.**—Beaunis, Moll, Wetterstrand, Schrenck-Notzing, Gscheidlen, Baillif, Berger, Bernheim, Forel, Gerster, and other observers, assert that natural sleep increases the susceptibility to hypnosis, and cite many instances in which the one has been changed into the other. A like opinion was expressed at an earlier date by Bertrand. I have, however, been unable to confirm these observations. In several instances I have attempted to change natural sleep into hypnosis by the method described by Wetterstrand, but always without success. The cases, however, were all difficult ones in which many unsuccessful attempts had previously been made.

(13) **Narcotics.**—Various narcotic drugs have been employed from very early times as a means of increasing susceptibility to hypnosis. Esdaile and Braid cited opium, hemp, aconite, hyoscyamus, laurel leaves, wine, ether and chloroform amongst the substances which were supposed to have this effect. Bernheim finds that susceptibility is increased by repeated doses of chloral and injections of morphia. Claude Perronnet states that chloroform, belladonna, ether, stramonium and hyoscyamus favour the production of hypnosis. According to Schrenck-Notzing, the general influence exercised upon the nervous system by narcotics markedly increases susceptibility. He, like Braid, considers Cannabis Indica the best drug for this purpose, but he has also found chloroform, morphia, sulphonal, bromide of potassium, paraldehyd and alcohol useful. Rifat states that susceptibility is so enormously increased by the action of narcotic remedies that, by their means, hypnosis ought to be obtained in almost every instance. Some authorities, particularly Herrero, attach much importance to the influence of chloroform. Wetterstrand does not always succeed in inducing hypnosis by the aid of chloroform; but in several instances, when other methods had failed, it enabled him to obtain profound somnambulism. Forel has only tried on two occasions to change chloroform narcosis into hypnosis; both attempts failed, but the cases were extremely difficult ones.

I have employed chloroform in three instances without success. In the first case, a lady about 40 years of age, suffering from hysterical neurasthenia, chloroform was administered on several occasions; suggestions being given until deep narcosis was obtained, and also while this was passing off. In the second case, a girl aged 12, suffering from moral insanity, chloroform was also administered. In the third case, a patient in the National Hospital for Nervous Diseases, several attempts were made to induce hypnosis under the influence of chloroform; but these invariably failed : later, when the patient came to my own house, I succeeded in hypnotising her by ordinary methods. I have occasionally given chloral, bromide and Cannabis Indica, but without any definite increase of susceptibility. These negative results, however, all occurred in extremely difficult cases.

(14) **Operator.**—While the subjective nature of hypnotic phenomena is accepted, most authorities still attach importance

to the personal influence of the operator. Bernheim asserts that
every hospital physician ought to be able to hypnotise 80 per cent
of his patients; and that, if he cannot do this, his failure results
from lack of experience or of other qualities necessary for success.
Forel agrees with this opinion, with the limitation, however,
that the insane be excluded from the statistics.

According to Moll, it is absolutely indispensable that the
operator should possess practical experience of the methods of
inducing hypnosis, and at the same time be acquainted with the
varying mental conditions of mankind. It is only, he says, by
experience and power of observation that one is enabled to choose
the method the most likely to succeed. Easy subjects can be
hypnotised by any one, but the difficult by the experienced
operator alone. The influence of one person over another is
dependent on the individuality of both. Thus A, for example,
can be hypnotised by B, while he remains refractory to the
efforts of C. On the other hand, D can be hypnotised by C, but
not by B. Moll compares this influence to that which exists
between teacher and pupil, and to other natural relationships.
The successful operator, he says, must be calm, tactful, and patient.
It is thus much easier to write prescriptions than to spend hours
daily in the attempted induction of hypnosis.

In Krafft-Ebing's opinion, the application of suggestion is a
complicated psychological process and not mere talking. Schrenck-
Notzing considers that while the technique can be learnt by
study and practice, the physician who is a good psychologist will
always be the most successful in influencing his patients. The
individuality of the operator is of greater importance than
mechanical and artificial methods.

Forel says the operator must be enthusiastic, patient, confident, and fertile of resource in varying his methods. The
greatest obstacle to success is lack of interest and of personal
initiative; and those who try to hypnotise mechanically by a
given plan frequently fail. The operator must be free from
distrust and nervousness, and not easily depressed or fatigued:
it is essential that he should understand, and know how to manage,
the mental condition of his patients. He must be able to obtain
their consent to the attempted induction of hypnosis; tactfully
remove their fears by explaining that nothing unnatural or
mystical is going to take place; keep them from becoming

mentally excited or nervous; and remove the idea that sleep is necessary for the success of the experiment.

Verbal suggestion is the method now mainly relied on for the induction of hypnosis; and both the character of the suggestions, and the manner in which they are conveyed undoubtedly influence susceptibility. The skilful operator arouses in the patient's mind the image or picture of the hypnotic state, and at the same time evokes the expectation of its appearance. He directs the patient's mind to the sensations he is actually experiencing, and utilises these as the starting-point from which he suggests others which he wishes him to feel.

In Forel's opinion, something more is wanted in the operator than patience and perseverance. He must be able to inspire his patients with the same qualities; and it is by no means an easy matter to persuade a patient to undergo a hundred or more unsuccessful attempts to induce hypnosis. Forel also draws attention to the fact that at Nancy, where a number of patients are hypnotised in one room, the operator makes his suggestions in a loud voice and thus they are heard by every one. Wetterstrand, on the contrary, whispers his suggestions softly to each patient in turn, and this, Forel thinks, increases susceptibility.

(15) **Number of Attempts.**—Lloyd Tuckey says: " My practice is to make three or four attempts to hypnotise and, if no effect is produced, I feel that the subject is not susceptible. I have occasionally, in special cases, made five or six attempts, but so far I have almost invariably found that if no effect is produced at the third sitting it is useless to make further efforts, at least for some time to come." Very different views are held by other observers. According to Forel, much time and perseverance is often necessary in obstinate cases, and with these the attempts should be repeated frequently and with short intervals between them.

Moll holds that the repetition of the process is an important factor in the induction of hypnosis; the chance increasing enormously with the frequency of the sittings. He has, he says, sometimes made forty or more attempts without result and then, by further repetitions, finally succeeded in many of the cases. Wetterstrand rarely induces hypnosis at the first attempt, and, although he usually does so at the third or fourth, has sometimes found as many as seventy sittings necessary. In one case Dr.

Oskar Vogt, of Berlin, only succeeded in obtaining somnambulism after 500, and in another after 700 sittings. In many of my cases which yielded the best therapeutic results, hypnosis was only obtained after repeated failures. In extreme instances the number of these amounted to over 100.

Conclusion.—As a general rule I have found the nervous, ill-balanced and hysterical the most difficult to influence; and healthy people, who possessed the power of concentrating their attention, the easiest. Exceptions have occurred, however, and I have sometimes, though rarely, succeeded at the first attempt in inducing deep hypnosis, and even somnambulism, in patients suffering from hysteria; and this despite the presence of pain, muscular tremor or spasm.

Beyond this, however, and the effect of the other causes just referred to, the varying susceptibility to hypnosis is still difficult to explain. For example, I have seen nothing elsewhere which equalled the susceptibility of my own patients at Goole. Further, although my therapeutic results of late years have not fallen below those obtained in the second group of patients treated at Goole—those not drawn from my own practice—the apparent susceptibility to hypnosis has been much less.

It is difficult to estimate correctly the conditions responsible for these varying results, and I cannot believe that there was any inherent peculiarity in the inhabitants of Goole, which rendered them specially susceptible to hypnosis. The following facts, however, are worthy of note :—

(1) Before beginning hypnotic work, I had already been sixteen years in general practice at Goole, and had gained my patients' confidence.

(2) At that time hypnotism had not been discussed in newspaper and magazine articles, and no dread as to its results had been excited.

(3) As already stated, most of my earlier patients were hypnotised either for operative purposes, or for the relief of illness, which was neither grave nor of long standing.

The difference in susceptibility, between the first and second groups referred to above, may be explained by the fact that the conditions which characterised the former were absent from the latter. Thus, those of the second group were all strangers to me, and nearly all suffered from grave and long-standing disease.

The patients I have treated of late years, however, are of exactly the same type as those of the second group. Notwithstanding this, my percentage of cases of profound hypnosis has fallen to the average given by Schrenck-Notzing's statistics. I can only account for this by the alteration in method already referred to. Formerly, curative suggestions were not given until hypnosis was induced; now they are employed from the very beginning, and I frequently find that recovery takes place before the patients show any symptom of undoubted hypnosis. My first aim is no longer the hypnotic state, but direct hypnotic cure.

Whether all the patients, who recover under this form of treatment, have been really hypnotised is a question which will be discussed later. If hypnosis, as Bernheim says, is nothing but suggestion, then, in that sense, they have been hypnotised. On the other hand, if we accept Braid's conception of hypnosis, we must answer the question in the negative.

CHAPTER V.

HYPNOTIC phenomena were formerly supposed to owe their origin to purely physical stimuli. As we have seen, metals and magnets, when applied to the subject's skin, or even held at some distance from his body, were alleged to produce extraordinary and varying results. These statements, now generally regarded as entirely fallacious, will be again referred to in discussing hypnotic theories.

On the other hand, phenomena such as those about to be described are now held to be due to *suggestion*. The importance, however, of the part played by suggestion is varyingly estimated by different authorities; some assert that it explains the phenomena, others hold that it is simply the artifice used to excite them. This point, an important one in reference to hypnotic theory, will also be discussed later.

It must not be supposed that the phenomena about to be described arise in the order in which they are placed; the arrangement is a purely artificial one adopted for convenience' sake. Later, attempts at classification will be discussed in the chapter on "The Different Stages of Hypnosis." Meanwhile, it should be understood that all the phenomena cited cannot be elicited in every subject. In slight hypnosis the phenomena are neither so varied nor so striking as those occurring in deeper stages; but most, if not all, tend to show a control of the organism in excess of that exerted by volition acting in the normal state.

(I.) THE PHYSIOLOGICAL PHENOMENA OF HYPNOSIS.

(A) Changes in the Voluntary Muscular System.

The first muscular change observed in hypnosis is usually a sudden or gradual closing of the eyes. The appearance of the lids varies; sometimes they are closed more tightly than natural by muscular spasm, at others they are not quite shut, and a portion of the eyeball remains visible. When closed, the eyelids either remain motionless, or quiver as long as the hypnosis lasts. In some instances, just before or immediately after the closure of the lids, the eyeballs roll upwards—usually, however, quickly returning to the normal position. Occasionally the eyeballs turn inwards as well as upwards; in one case I observed both were turned to the left. In many cases of deep hypnosis, however, the eyes remain open, not only in the state itself, but also while it is being induced; and it is to be noted that most, if not all, of these changes really depend upon the methods employed by the operator.

In a certain proportion of hypnotic subjects the limbs can be bent at the joints like soft wax, and maintain any position in which they are placed; this condition is termed *flexibilitas cerea.*

According to Bernheim, *catalepsy* can be induced in all subjects who have passed the first stage. The amount of muscular contraction varies widely, sometimes being barely sufficient to maintain an upraised limb in position, at others passing into a tonic contracture of nearly all the voluntary muscles. Moll asserts that a cataleptic posture was maintained for seventeen hours in one instance, and also cites a case of Berger's, where a young girl, although continually watched, was said to remain in this condition seven hours without perceptible change. At the same time, Moll admits that dynamometric investigations do not give very definite results; he thinks they show a slight decrease of muscular power in hypnosis. Binet and Féré state that a cataleptic subject cannot remain in a constrained position for more than ten or fifteen minutes, and that a similar feat might be performed by a strong man. Notwithstanding this, they think the following important differences exist between suggested and voluntary muscular contraction. An arm made rigid by suggestion drops slowly and gently, and records a perfectly straight tracing on Marey's apparatus; the respiratory tracing being also normal. In similar experiments in the waking state, the hand and arm soon tremble, and the breathing becomes hurried and irregular.

Carpenter stated that a marked *increase of muscular power* was frequently induced by suggestion. One of Braid's subjects, who was so muscularly feeble that for years he had been unable to lift a weight of twenty pounds, took a quarter of a hundred-weight upon his little finger and swung it round his head with the utmost ease.   On another occasion, he raised half a hundred-weight as high as his knee on the last joint of his forefinger.

Continued movements, sometimes of a complicated nature, may be induced in hypnosis and maintained for a longer or shorter period.

Various *changes of personality* can be suggested during hypnosis, when the control of the muscular movements, necessary for representing the different parts, is frequently apparently greater than that possessed by the subjects in their normal state.

Echolalia.—According to Berger, hypnotised subjects are capable of repeating everything like phonographs.   The most interesting instance of this phenomenon is cited by Braid.   One of his subjects, a young work-girl, who did not know the grammar of her own language and was entirely ignorant of music, correctly accompanied Jenny Lind in several songs in different languages, and also in a long and difficult chromatic exercise which was specially improvised in order to test her.

Many observers have noticed an *absence of muscular tedium.* Thus, when uncomfortable positions are suggested or assumed during hypnosis, the fatigue and pain which usually follow excessive muscular exertion are apparently absent.

Paralysis.—The different voluntary muscles may be paralysed singly or in groups.   In some cases the paralysis is apparently due to the fact that the muscles necessary for the performance of any given movement do not contract; in other instances the necessary muscles act, but are overpowered by the violent con-traction of the antagonistic ones.

According to Drs. Paul Richer and Gilles de la Tourette, of Paris, hypnotic paralyses are characterised by the following features which distinguish them from those of an organic nature, viz. complete laxity of the limbs, exaggeration of tendon reflexes, spinal trepidation, loss of muscular sense, exaggeration and modification of the muscular contractions provoked by the galvanic current, and vasomotor troubles.   These observations have not been confirmed by the Nancy school.   Moll, for example, after repeated experi-ments, found no difference between the electric excitability of the nerves and muscles in the hypnotic and the normal states.

Most of the muscular phenomena just referred to are supposed to have been excited by direct verbal suggestion, while, as regards the remainder, the exclusion of suggestion is not proved. According to the Salpêtrière school, however, certain abnormalities appear in the voluntary muscles during the respective stages of hypnosis, which are not of psychical origin, and arise independently of suggestion in response to physical stimuli. These are :—

(1) **Lethargy.**—The limbs are relaxed and fall by their own weight ; the tendon reflex is increased. There is neuro-muscular hyperexcitability, *i.e.* the muscles tend to contract under the influence of mechanical stimuli, whether applied to tendon, or nerves of supply, or the muscles themselves. Excitation of the antagonistic muscles causes the contracted ones to relax.

(2) **Catalepsy.**—Every position given to the limbs is maintained for some time ; there is neither tendon reflex nor increase of muscular irritability.

(3) **Somnambulism.**—Gentle stimulation of the skin causes rigid contraction of the underlying muscles, which does not cease when the antagonistic ones are excited, but disappears when the original stimulation is repeated. Further, the muscles do not contract if subjected to the same stimuli which excite them when the subject is in the lethargic condition.

The phenomena just described are now generally regarded as artificial in their origin, but this point will be discussed under " Theory."

Remarks. — All the new *reflexes* described by Charcot, Heidenhain, and others are apparently due to suggestion and training ; and, as Moll has pointed out, the supposed alteration in the ordinary tendon reflexes is open to doubt. Thus, there is an increase in the patellar reflex when the muscles are completely relaxed by suggestion, and a decrease when they are rigid.

According to Moll, the continued and other forms of muscular contractions observed in hypnosis take place either without or against the will of the subject. In the former case they are executed easily and steadily ; in the latter, they are characterised by strong muscular contractions and trembling, indicating ineffectual resistance to the will of the operator, and thereby showing an increased depth of hypnosis. The phenomena Moll describes do not, I think, warrant his conclusions as to the state of the subject's volition. This will be discussed more fully later : meanwhile, I may point out that the operator may have unconsciously suggested an unsuccessful resistance to the execution of the movement.

In order to induce the muscular movements, the subject, says Moll, must thoroughly understand what the operator wishes. While Moll admits that the common and most natural way of effecting this is by telling the subject what he should do, *i.e.* the method of "verbal suggestion," he, at the same time, states that verbal suggestion is made more effectual by means of the operator's gestures. Further, he asserts that certain muscular phenomena, such as catalepsy, cannot always be excited by mere verbal suggestion, and then mesmeric passes are necessary in order to produce them. These views cannot be accepted unquestioned. Braid long ago pointed out that the passes and gestures of the operator, together with the placing of the hypnotised subject in different attitudes, constituted only a clumsy and indirect method of arousing in his mind the idea of certain muscular movements; whereas the very same idea and consequent movements were more easily excited by direct verbal suggestion.

It is true that the hypnotised subject's powers of perception are frequently increased, thus enabling him to interpret indirect suggestions which might be meaningless to him when awake. Further, his power of hearing, comprehending, and responding to direct verbal suggestion is also greater than in the normal state. All these gestures, passes and other indirect suggestions, appear to me very much in the light of "baby language" or comic pantomime. If we wish to induce a normal individual to escape from danger, as, for example, the presence of a lion, we tell him that one is near, and that he ought to get out of the way as quickly as possible. We should not dream of attempting to influence him by going down on all fours and roaring; and I see no reason for conveying suggestions to hypnotised subjects in similar ridiculous ways. Moll himself admits that mesmeric passes are only responded to when the individual knows what they are intended to effect. He also states that while centrifugal passes excite contractions and centripetal ones dissipate them, such action is apparently due to unintentional suggestion, as he has often found their effects reversed. Surely the recognition of this fact should have prevented Moll from attributing a greater power to passes than to verbal suggestion.

Although Moll asserts that the voluntary muscles are entirely under the influence of external suggestion during hypnosis, he also describes conditions in which suggestion is stated to have little or no effect. He divides hypnotised subjects into two groups according to their condition : (1) Active ; this state on superficial observation might be mistaken for the waking one. (2) Passive ; characterised by muscular relaxation. In both there is, he says, resistance to suggestion. Thus, in No. 1, when a continued movement has been suggested, Moll finds it impossible, in some instances, to at once counteract the first suggestion by a second—the movement being continued despite the operator's command. In No. 2, in spite of all suggestions, the subjects let their arms drop after they have been raised, and do not respond to questions. Moll asserts—the italics are his own—that : " *One of these two functional abnormalities of the muscles exists in all hypnotic states,*" *i.e.* a movement which has been excited by suggestion cannot always be terminated in the same way, or a suggested movement may remain unfulfilled. None of Moll's three contradictory propositions can be accepted without examination. Thus, (*a*) the voluntary muscles are not entirely under the influence of suggestion during hypnosis. A subject, who will execute movements which are indifferent or agreeable to him, will invariably refuse to perform those which are repugnant to his moral sense. (*b*) I have always found that suggested contractures and continued movements ceased at command, unless the order was given in such a way as to be misinterpreted by the subject, or he had been previously trained by the methods of the stage performer. (*c*) Again, I have only found instances of extreme muscular relaxation, and refusal to respond to suggestions, amongst those who had been trained by passes, gestures and other similar methods. The effects of this training, however, could always easily be removed by suggestion, whereupon the subjects would now promptly answer questions and execute movements. Braid demonstrated how the slightest change in the operator's voice might vary or reverse the result of his commands. Thus the suggestion, that a subject should try to stop a continued movement, might be made in such a way that the varying emphasis on the word *try* might convey three different ideas to his mind, viz. : (1) that he was to continue the movement ; (2) that he was to continue, but apparently attempt to stop it ; (3) that the movement should cease. In reference to

continued movements and muscular contractures which cannot at
once be dissipated by suggestion, Moll states decidedly that these
phenomena must be distinguished from " suggestion."   Suggestion
produces a particular muscular action, but does not explain its
long duration.   It cannot be supposed, he says, that an idea
which I implant in the subject should have more effect than the
idea he himself originates, and, thus, if there are phenomena
which are characteristic of hypnosis, their existence proves that
the external and the self-suggested idea affects the functions
differently ; or else that the muscles in hypnosis are influenced
by something besides suggestion, *i.e.* the tendency to contracture.

Thus, according to Moll : (1) Hypnosis is characterised by
a tendency to muscular contracture.   (2) Suggestion does not
explain the duration of the contractures.   (3) It is unreasonable
to suppose that differences exist between the operator's suggestion
and the self-suggestions of the subject.   All these statements are
open to question : (1) Neither muscular contraction nor relaxation
characterises hypnosis ; each in turn may be excited, but neither
arises spontaneously.   (2) Suggestion, strictly speaking, is only
the method used to excite hypnotic phenomena, and does not
explain any of them ; but, in the sense in which Moll uses it, it
does explain the long-continued contraction.   The contraction
continues because the subject has accepted the idea that it should
do so : it ceases when his muscles become exhausted, or when his
brain receives the fresh idea that it should stop.   The power of
maintaining the contracture beyond the limits of normal strength
is, of course, another matter, and one which suggestion does not
explain.   (3) The waking self-suggestions of the subject often
differ widely in their results from those of the operator given in
hypnosis.   This does not show a difference in the suggestions
themselves, but in the conditions under which they are made.

Voluntary Muscles.   Summary.—As far as my personal
observations go, there are few, if any, changes in the voluntary
muscles which are absolutely characteristic of hypnosis ; and none
which arise independently of direct or indirect suggestion.   The
most noticeable phenomenon is the long maintenance of an uncomfortable posture, associated with extreme muscular rigidity, and
the subsequent absence of fatigue.   As most, if not all, of the
muscular feats of hypnosis could be reproduced by trained
unhypnotised persons, the phenomena are only worthy of note

when it can be clearly proved that they are beyond the hypnotic subject's waking powers.

(B) Changes in the Involuntary Muscular and Vasomotor Systems.

Pulse.—The induction of hypnosis is sometimes accompanied by an acceleration of the pulse. This, although regarded as a characteristic phenomenon by some authorities, appears to be due to emotional causes alone; for, although it frequently appears the first time hypnosis is induced, it rarely occurs afterwards. During deep hypnosis, when the subject is allowed to rest undisturbed by suggestions of any kind, the pulse sometimes falls spontaneously.

I have seen many instances in which the frequency of the pulse was altered by suggestion. In some cases it was only necessary to state quietly that the pulse should beat faster or slower; in others the suggestion was not successful unless it was associated with an emotional one. Thus, to quicken the pulse, the subject was told that he was hurrying to catch a train; to produce slowing, something depressing was described.

The following case is an example of the former class, *i.e.* that in which the alterations were produced by simple suggestion. I hypnotised the subject, Mrs. A., aged 40, and the results of the suggestions were recorded by Dr. Alcock, of Goole, who reported as follows: "Dudgeon's sphygmograph was employed, but all possible precautions were taken to prevent the errors which are sometimes associated with its use. Thus, the position of the instrument, and the adjustment of the tension apparatus, were not altered in any way from the beginning to the close of the experiments, and all the tracings were taken at one sitting, rapidly one after the other. Without suggestion in the waking state, the pulse was 80 and the tracing normal; the aortic and dicrotic notches were well marked, and both occurred during and on the down-stroke. The subject was then hypnotised and increased rapidity suggested, when the pulse rose to 100. The tracings showed a decrease in the aortic notch, almost to the verge of extinction; while the dicrotic notch became more prominent, and appeared rather as a separate wave on its own account, than as a part of the down-stroke. In other words, the down-stroke more

G

nearly reached the base-line before the dicrotic wave commenced. These tracings apparently showed that decreased tension was associated with increased speed. Slowing of the pulse was then suggested, when it fell to 60, and tracings the reverse of those just referred to were now recorded. The aortic notch occurred almost immediately after the up-stroke was finished, and the following wave appeared as a rounded hump, approaching the initial up-stroke in height. The dicrotic notch began early in the down-stroke and the dicrotic wave was well marked. These tracings apparently showed that decreased speed was associated with increased tension. The subject was then told that her pulse should beat at its normal rate, when it again rose to 80. There was now no difference between the tracing, and that taken before hypnosis had been induced or suggestions given. The respiration remained unchanged throughout the experiments." In another case, where Professor Waller was the recorder, I easily obtained an alteration of 20 per cent in the pulse rate by suggestion.

Moll, Beaunis, and many others record similar alterations in the rapidity and tension of the pulse. Beaunis believes that these changes are brought about by suggestion acting directly upon the inhibitory centres of the heart. Moll, on the other hand, thinks we should hesitate before accepting this conclusion. The action of the heart is influenced both by respiration and by ideas which affect the emotions, and thus the phenomena are probably an indirect result of suggestion. As we have seen, in some cases the phenomena in question could not be induced unless respiratory changes and emotional states had previously been excited, and to these doubtless Moll's objections apply. Where neither respiratory changes nor emotional states were evoked, Beaunis' explanation appears more probable.

Respiration.—With the exception that respiration sometimes remains unchanged in hypnosis during violent muscular exertion, there is little of note to record. It is true that the respiration can be accelerated, slowed or temporarily arrested, by suggestion, but similar phenomena can be induced voluntarily in the waking state.

Bleeding.—Bourru, Burot, Mabille, Jules Voisin, Artigalas, Remond, Hulst and others report cases in which bleeding from the skin has been induced by suggestion. In some instances the subjects were carefully watched during the whole of the experiments, and precautions were taken to prevent fraud. In others this was evidently not the case; and, in addition, the operators rubbed the skin with a blunt instrument.

Dr. Hulst (America) asserts that he caused a subject's nose to bleed by suggestion; but, as she suffered from frequent epistaxes, the possibility of coincidence is not excluded.

Local Redness of the Skin.—Forel records several cases in which he produced local redness of the skin by suggestion. In one instance this appeared at the end of five minutes; the subject being carefully watched all the time by Forel and other medical men.

Beaunis reports similar cases, and asserts that all precautions were taken to eliminate mal-observation or fraud.

Schrenck-Notzing cites an interesting experiment which he, and Dr. Rybalkin, of St. Petersburg, made upon Camille, Liébeault's celebrated somnambule. They suggested to her in the waking state that the skin below her ear was red and inflamed, and that she had evidently been bitten by an insect. In about three minutes there appeared a patch of erythema with a distinct rim.

Blistering, etc.—At Nancy, in 1885,—in the presence of Liébeault, Bernheim, Liégeois, Dumont and Beaunis—Focachon hypnotised a subject, strapped a piece of gummed paper upon the back of her left shoulder and suggested that this should produce a blister. On the following day several blisters appeared, which suppurated freely.

Forel records similar experiments with one of his nurses. The blister suppurated for eight days, and seven weeks later the place was still discoloured.

On February 21st, 1890, Rybalkin hypnotised a boy, aged 16, suggested that he should touch an unlighted stove with his arm, and that a blister should form at the seat of contact. The arm was then bandaged, and the subject put to bed and watched. Three hours later there was considerable swelling, accompanied by redness; next morning two large and many small blisters had formed.

Krafft-Ebing has published a case, that of Ilma S., in which he and Dr. Jendrássik, of Buda-Pesth, assert that they produced blisters and marks like burns by suggestion. When an object was pressed upon the subject's skin and suggestions of heat made, a blister or eschar like that of a burn appeared, the exact size and

form of the object used. If, however, the object was pressed
upon the left side of the body, the mark appeared in a reversed
position on a corresponding part of the right side, and there only.
The subject was hysterical and suffered from right hemianæsthesia.

Hulst states that with one of his subjects, a girl aged 22, he
succeeded on three occasions in producing local inflammation of
the skin, with the formation of superficial sores.

I have never been able to produce a blister by suggestion.
In several instances, however, I have seen local redness of the
skin appear, under circumstances which apparently excluded fraud
or mal-observation.

Cases are also recorded in which suggestion is stated to have
prevented blistering under circumstances where this would otherwise have occurred. Thus, similar blisters were placed on each
forearm of Focachon's subject, and it was suggested that the one
on the left should produce no effect. Next day the right arm
alone was blistered.

Delbœuf made the following experiment with his subject J.
After obtaining her consent in the waking state, he hypnotised
her, extended her arms on a table, and suggested that the right
should be insensible to pain. Each arm was then burnt with a
red-hot bar of iron, 8 millimetres in diameter, the extent and
duration of its application being identical in both. There was
pain in the left arm alone. The burns were bandaged and J.
sent to bed. During the night the pain in the left arm continued,
and next morning there was a wound on it 3 centimetres in
diameter, with an outer circle of inflamed blisters; on the right
there was only a defined eschar, the exact size of the iron and
without inflammation or redness. The day following the left
arm was still more painful and inflamed. Analgesia was then
successfully suggested, when the wound soon dried and the inflammation disappeared.

Changes of Temperature.—In the case of Ilma S., Krafft-
Ebing and Jendrássik claim not only to have changed her
temperature, but even to have produced the exact degree
suggested.

Dr. Dumontpallier, of Paris, recorded a case in which he
obtained a local increase of temperature of 3° centigrade. Dr.
Lehmann, of Copenhagen, also claims to have obtained an increase
of temperature by suggestion, while Drs. Marès and Hellich, of

Prague, state that they have reduced the temperature from 37° C. to 34·5°. In the latter two cases the respective suggestions of heat and cold were made.

Dr. Levillain, of Paris, records a case where Charcot is said to have produced the *œdème bleu des hystériques* by suggestion. The subject was told that her hand would swell, become blue and turn cold. The hand increased to nearly double its former volume and presented all the appearance of "blue œdema"; its temperature fell 3° C. lower than the rest of the body. Suggestion quickly caused the symptoms to disappear.

I have never succeeded in changing the temperature in hypnosis. On one occasion I suggested to an extremely good somnambule that the skin of his arm should become burning hot. The subject at once complained of pain and heat, but, although the suggestions were energetically continued for about half an hour, there was no increase of temperature; suggestions of cold were equally unsuccessful in lowering it. The observations were made by Professor Waller, and the instrument employed was infinitely more sensitive than the ordinary clinical thermometer.

Remarks.—The evidence as to the production of blistering and changes of temperature by suggestion is by no means conclusive. In none of the cases which have come under my notice have sufficient precautions been taken to eliminate the possibility of fraud or mal-observation. Thus, in Focachon's cases, the subject was alone and unwatched the whole night. Krafft-Ebing appears to have taken the temperature in the axilla with an ordinary clinical thermometer. This method is obviously untrustworthy, as hysterical subjects have frequently succeeded in raising the temperature by rubbing the thermometer. On March 25th, 1895, I received the following reply from Dr. Hulst, in reference to the precautions that had been taken in his case: " The experiments I made were not well controlled and fraud cannot be positively excluded. I want to confess, however, that I have had some doubts with regard to the blistering experiments with my subject—not so much because I doubt her honesty, but because the burning sensation which she experienced may have induced her to rub or scratch unconsciously ; yet I never saw her do so."

In the *Zeitschrift für Hypnotismus*, vol. iv., 1896, Schrenck-Notzing gives the following account of experiments made with Eva S. The subject was apparently hysterical, and showed

increased vasomotor excitability in the waking state; slight
pressure on the skin almost immediately produced redness.
During hypnosis, Drs. Flach and Offner produced erythema of
the skin by gently rubbing it with a cold key, which they told
the subject was red-hot.   Parish, the author of *Illusions and
Hallucinations*, then joined the experimenters and apparently
induced blistering by simple verbal suggestion.   The experiment
repeated under more stringent conditions, was again successful.
At the suggestion of Schrenck-Notzing, the subject was brought
to Munich, and, in the presence of Parish, Rudinger, Clausner,
Moritz, Löwenfeld, Mueller, Hoffmeyr, Schrenck-Notzing, Kopp,
Minde, Billinger, Hirschberger, and Albrecht, a fresh attempt was
made to produce blistering.   At 6.45 P.M. the subject was undressed
and put to bed, and the left hand and arm bandaged.   A portion
of skin on the back of the right forearm, between the wrist and
the elbow, was selected for the experiment.   The right arm was
then enclosed in a wooden box, with an opening in the top
through which the portion of skin selected could be seen.   With
this exception, the entire arm, hand and box were enveloped in
a complicated series of bandages, with which sheets of paper had
been incorporated.   The subject was then hypnotised and the
blister suggested.   She was continually watched until 6.15 P.M.
of the following day.   At times the subject appeared to fall into
a natural sleep; at others she was awake and restless, and complained of itching and burning.   At the termination of the
experiment, the bandages on both arms were found to be so far
loosened that the subject could move her fingers.   Perforations,
resembling pin-pricks, were observed both in the layers of paper
and the bandages, but none of these were found at the place
selected for blistering, which was protected by the wooden box.
Schrenck-Notzing found a hairpin near the bed, and the subject
had been seen to lay her right arm over her head upon the
pillow, and also to move both arms a good deal.   The experiment
was repeated under still more stringent conditions; the arm was enveloped in a plaster of Paris bandage and the subject closely watched
for twenty-four hours.   The results were entirely negative.·

Schrenck-Notzing justly calls attention to the amount of
freedom allowed to subjects in these and other similar experiments which are now regarded as classical.   Thus, Focachon's
subject, who was alone all night, might have mechanically

irritated her skin in the first experiment, and in the second held the blister away from it and so prevented its action.

Menstruation.—Forel states that he has succeeded in exciting or arresting menstruation by suggestion. He has also caused it to appear at a given moment by post-hypnotic suggestion, and regulated its duration and intensity. Most of these experiments were made upon his female asylum attendants, who were subjected to careful examination.

I have rarely attempted to alter the normal menstrual function by suggestion, but have frequently done so when irregularities existed. Examples of these from my own practice, and those of others, are to be found under "Menstrual Disorders."

Action of the Bowels.—Many instances are recorded in which action of the bowels has been excited or arrested by suggestion. Braid claims to have made the first observation of this kind. A girl, aged 14, suffering from constipation, was told by Braid during hypnosis that her bowels would act in five minutes. He awoke her and the suggestion was carried out at the time indicated. She was again hypnotised, and the experiment successfully repeated. At a later date, Braid stated that he had made many similar suggestions in other instances, and with unvarying success.

According to Moll, the peristaltic action of the bowels can generally be easily excited by suggestion; and in some instances the effect of aperients can be checked in the same way. These statements are confirmed by the observations of Beaunis, Forel, Krafft-Ebing and many others.

Urine.—Wetterstrand asserts that with one of his patients, suggestion not only removed difficulty in micturition, but also largely augmented the amount of urine secreted. Generally speaking, however, the cases cited as showing suggestive alterations in the secretion of urine are neither numerous nor conclusive. All that is proved in most instances is that the patient emptied the bladder in response to suggestion.

Lachrymal Secretion.—Most observers record cases in which the lachrymal secretion has been excited in hypnosis. This is usually done either by suggesting emotional states, or a sensory delusion such as a pungent smell. Beaunis asserts that he has excited the lachrymal secretion of one eye by suggestion, while the other remained normal.

Perspiration.—The only instances I know of in which perspiration has been altered by suggestion will be cited under " Medical Cases."

Secretion of Milk.—Several cases are recorded in which the secretion of milk has been increased or arrested by suggestion. One of the earliest is cited by Esdaile. His sister-in-law, when weaning a child, suffered from the accumulation of milk in her breasts, which rendered them painful and swollen. Esdaile hypnotised her and in half an hour she was free from pain. Next morning the breasts were soft and comfortable, and there was no further secretion of milk.

An experiment, the reverse of this, is related by Braid. He hypnotised a patient who was nursing, and suggested an increased secretion of milk in one breast. On awaking she had no recollection of what had been done, but complained of a feeling of tightness and tension in the breast. Her husband then told her that Braid had been trying to increase the secretion of milk. She was sceptical as to the result, as her child was fourteen months old and the milk had almost disappeared. Her breast, however, almost immediately became distended with milk, and a few days later she complained that her figure was deformed in consequence. Braid again hypnotised her and successfully repeated the experiment with the other breast. The patient suckled her child for six months longer, the supply of milk being more abundant than it had been at any time since her confinement.

The following case is reported by Grossmann :—B., aged 20, primipara, suckled her child for a fortnight and then ceased to do so, as she had to leave home. Three weeks later she returned and wished to again nurse the child, but the secretion of milk had ceased absolutely in the right breast and almost entirely in the left. The patient was hypnotised, and the sensations associated with the flow of milk suggested. In three minutes, the veins of the left breast became enormously congested and milk began to flow from it. At first, repeated pressure failed to produce a single drop from the right breast, but when the suggestions were repeated milk was secreted freely. Some hours later the breasts were still full, though the patient had not attempted to suckle the child.

Grossmann, evidently unaware of Esdaile and Braid's cases, cites this as the first instance in which alteration in milk-secretion had been caused by suggestion.

Dr. Hassenstein, of East Prussia, reports a case in which the secretion of milk entirely ceased owing to emotional causes, and was rapidly restored by suggestion.

(C) Changes in the Special Senses, Muscular Sense, Common Sensations and Appetites.

(1) INCREASED ACTION.

Sight.—I have seen the range of vision, both distant and near, increased by suggestion in subjects whose sight was normal. Sometimes, however, the improvement was due to the disappearance of a spasm of the accommodation, and an interesting example of this class is cited under " Medical Cases." [1]

One of the most remarkable instances of increased vision is described by Dr. Bergson (France). The subject read letters reflected in the operator's eye, the image of which was only $\frac{1}{250}$ of an inch high.

Hearing.—In deep hypnosis, I have invariably found that the hearing could be rendered more acute by suggestion ; the range, as tested with the stop-watch, being frequently double that of the normal state. Similar observations are recorded by others ; and Beaunis, in addition, succeeded in accelerating the time of reaction to auditory sensations.

In the *Zeitschrift für Hypnotismus*, for 1896, Dr. Inhelder, formerly assistant physician to Professor Forel, published ten years' experiments with male and female warders in the night watching of suicidal and homicidal lunatics. The warders were hypnotised, trained to sleep by the bedside of dangerous patients, and to awake the instant the latter attempted to get out of bed. Sounds which had no reference to the warder's duties were inhibited by suggestion, while those which it was important they should hear were rendered more acute.

In addition to their ordinary routine of hard work, these warders sometimes performed night duty for six months at a stretch, without being unduly fatigued. The results, as far as the patients were concerned, were also uniformly successful and no accident of any kind occurred. When I visited Forel, in 1892, he successfully repeated this experiment for my benefit.

---

[1] Pp. 191-4.

Smell.—The experiments of Braid and other observers show that hyperæsthesia of the sense of smell can frequently be induced by suggestion. One of Braid's subjects, when blindfolded in a room full of people, could identify any person known to him by the sense of smell alone. If allowed to smell a glove, he could afterwards recognise its owner, but his power of performing these feats disappeared when his nostrils were plugged.

Muscular Sense.—The following experiments were made with Mrs. A., and recorded by Dr. Alcock. Four pill-boxes, new and identical in appearance, were selected, and a 2-drachm weight placed in each. To three, however, other weights were added, giving an ascending series of 20 grains at a time. The boxes, lettered underneath S, I, N, G, respectively, were nearly the same weight, viz. S, 38 grains; I, 36 grains; N, 35 grains; G, 37 grains. The weights in the first experiment were, therefore: S, 2 drachms 38 grains; I, 2 drachms 56 grains; N, 3 drachms 15 grains; G, 3 drachms 37 grains. At first the subject was tested in the waking state, when it was found that she was unable to discriminate between S and G, a difference of 1 drachm 2 grains. She was then hypnotised, hyperæsthesia of the muscular sense suggested, and the following precautions taken. On each occasion the boxes were first mixed; then one was selected at random and the distinguishing letter only noted after the experiment. The subject was blindfolded; her arms were extended and the palms of the hands turned upwards. A box was placed on each hand, and she was asked to say " Right " or " Left," accordingly as she considered which hand supported the heavier box. She was never told whether she had made a correct estimate or not, and never saw, either before, during or after the experiments, the contents or lettering of the boxes. Until the conclusion of the experiments, I knew nothing of the boxes selected or their contents.

EXPERIMENT No. I.

S and N ; differing in weight grains 37.			Result—Correct.
I " G ;	"	"	41.	"	"
S " I ;	"	"	18.	"	"
N " G ;	"	"	22.	"	Wrong.
S " I ;	"	"	18.	"	Correct.
S " I ;	"	"	18.	"	"
N " G ;	"	"	22.	"	"
S " G ;	"	"	59.	"	"
I " N ;	"	"	19.	"	"

EXPERIMENT No. II.

This was identical with the first, with the exception that the added weights gave an ascending series of 10 grains at a time. The weights of the boxes, therefore, were as follows: S, 2 drachms 38 grains; I, 2 drachms 46 grains; N, 2 drachms 55 grains; G, 3 drachms 7 grains. Increased sensibility was then suggested, with the following result:—

S and G;	differing in weight grains 29.			Result—Correct.
S „ N;	„	„	17.	„ „
S „ I;	„	„	8.	„ „
I „ N;	„	„	9.	„ Wrong.
I „ N;	„	„	9.	„ Correct.
S „ I;	„	„	8.	„ Wrong.
S „ I;	„	„	8.	„ Correct.
S „ I;	„	„	8.	„ „
N „ G;	„	„	12.	„ „
N „ G;	„	„	12.	„ „

In a third experiment, the weights ascended by 5 grains at a time, and next-door neighbours in the series were tried. In that instance, exactly the same numbers of failures and successes were recorded.

Miss M., one of my subjects, who could only play a few dance tunes upon the piano with her music before her and in the absence of strangers, when hypnotised, blindfolded and deprived of her music, played the same tunes much more brilliantly before a room full of people.

Braid recorded cases of hypnotised subjects who were able to write neatly, crossing the t's and dotting the i's, even when most effectual precautions were taken to prevent their seeing what they were doing. They could go back a line, strike out a false letter and write the correct one in its proper place. One subject could accurately correct the mistakes in a whole page, but, if the relative positions of the paper and table were changed, all the alterations would be wrong, as they were placed according to the original position of the paper.

Braid believed that the phenomenon of *echolalia*, to which reference has already been made, was due in great measure to improvement in the muscular sense.

Common Cutaneous Sensibility.—The following experiments

were made with Mrs. A., and the results again recorded by Dr. Alcock. The ordinary method, with a pair of blunt-pointed compasses, was employed, and the parts selected were the hands placed behind the subject's back, and the region over the eyebrow. Precautions were taken to prevent the subject seeing what was done, or being influenced by unconscious suggestion on the part of the operator. Thus she was never asked: "Do you feel one or two points?" but was told beforehand to say "One" or "Two," as she imagined herself to be touched by one or two points. I hypnotised the subject and made suggestions of increased cutaneous sensibility; but, as I sat with my back towards her, I saw nothing of the experiments, and only learnt the results afterwards. The following were the distances required in order that the points could be appreciated as distinct :—

Right palmar hypothenar eminence. Before suggestion. Half an inch.
   ,,   ,,   ,,   After   ,,   Quarter of an inch.
Back of left hand along length of first finger. Before suggestion. Seventeen
                      lines.
   ,,   ,,   ,,   ,,   After suggestion. Nine lines.
Just over left eyebrow and parallel to it. Before suggestion. One inch.
   ,,   ,,   ,,   After   ,,   Half an inch.

Berger also records similar experiments, which were repeated and confirmed by Moll.

Thermo-sensibility.—The following experiments were made with Mrs. A., and the results again recorded by Dr. Alcock. Two test-tubes were nearly filled with tepid water, and a few drops of cold added to one of them. Mrs. A. then took a tube in each hand and was told to guess which was the warmer. The experiment was repeated and varied in several ways, when it was found that she could discriminate between minute differences of temperature, which we ourselves could not detect, and which she could not appreciate in the normal state.

Braid and later observers also cite cases of increased sensitiveness to changes in pressure and temperature. According to the former, some subjects recognised objects placed half an inch from their skin; others walked about in absolute darkness without striking against anything, because they recognised the position of objects by alterations in the resistance of the air and in the temperature.

Appetites, Hunger and Thirst.—I have observed many

instances in which suggestion induced hunger in patients suffering from a morbid loss of appetite. I have also seen healthy subjects, who had just partaken of a hearty meal, again make an equally good one when hunger was suggested to them.

(2) Decreased, Arrested and Distorted Action.

The activity of the special senses may be decreased by suggestion, or their action may be entirely arrested, and the subject rendered insensible to visual, auditory and other sense-impressions.

Sensory delusions, hallucinations as well as illusions, can also be evoked in the same way.

Liégeois classifies hallucinations as follows :—

(1) **Positive.**—The subject sees hallucinatory objects, and these act in the same way as if they were real in preventing the view of other objects.

(2) **Negative.**—An object disappears in response to suggestion and then apparently ceases to hide other objects.

(3) **Retroactive.**—Here it is suggested to the subject that he has heard or seen imaginary things ; on awaking he remembers them and believes in their reality.

(4) **Deferred.** — The appearance of the hallucination is delayed by suggestion and appears at the date fixed. This form will be dealt with more particularly under post-hypnotic suggestions.

(5) **Hallucinations of Memory.**—These will be discussed when dealing with the general question of memory in hypnosis.

(6) **Changes of Personality.**—Here the subjects assume the rôle suggested, and speak and act in accordance with their conception of the part. This Liégeois considers to be a veritable hallucination.

Motor Hallucinations.—While the subject is at rest, if he is told that he is making certain movements, the physical phenomena usually associated with them appear. According to Beaunis, this is a true hallucination ; an act which is not performed is believed by the subject to be executed, because the idea of it is aroused in the ideomotor centres.

Moll asserts that visual hallucinations are more easily evoked when the subject's eyes are closed, as the act of opening them is apt to terminate the hypnosis. Illusions, in his opinion, are more readily suggested than hallucinations.

My experience does not accord with Moll's. I have never found any difficulty in inducing sensorial hallucinations in deeply hypnotised subjects, no matter whether their eyes were open or shut.

There is an important point in reference to certain negative hallucinations, viz., that the object must first be seen in order *not* to be recognised. One can, for example, place a minute mark on one of twelve otherwise exactly similar pieces of paper, and suggest to the subject that he shall not see the marked one. Here, before the negative hallucination can take place, the subject must first select the particular paper by recognising the mark.

When a negative hallucination is suggested, the subject frequently adds a positive one on his own account. Thus, if an object is obliterated by suggestion, and a second one moved behind the first, he apparently still sees the second. The memory of the latter has been transformed into a visual hallucination.

Binet and Féré believe that a suggested visual hallucination produces the same optical phenomena as a real image. A prism, they say, doubles it, and complementary colours give their natural resultant. Bernheim points out, and my experiments agree with his, that this only occurs in trained subjects who know what they are expected to see.

Anæsthesia and Analgesia.—According to Moll, complete analgesia is extremely rare in hypnosis, although authors, copying from one another, assert that it is common. There is an immense difference, he says, between pricking the subject with a needle and using the faradic brush. The pain caused by the use of the latter is so great, especially when considerable electric force is used, that very few hypnotised persons can bear it.

I have generally been able to induce profound anæsthesia or analgesia when the stage of somnambulism has been reached, and, unlike Moll, have found such subjects completely insensible to powerful applications of the faradic brush. To one, acutely sensitive to pain in the normal state, analgesia alone was suggested, when she watched and discussed the application of the brush, and described the tactile sensations associated with it. Pain was entirely inhibited. In such cases, the corneal and conjunctival reflex is either absent or can be abolished by suggestion. The nose and throat also can be rendered insensible, and subjected to careful examination without pain or discomfort to the subject. Some interesting experiments of this kind were made for me by Dr. Greville Macdonald. Given deep hypnosis, analgesia and anæsthesia are equally easy to induce, and can be evoked simultaneously and separately in the same subject. One arm, for example, may be made anæsthetic and the other analgesic, and the latter condition even associated with a hyperæsthesia of tactile sensations. Further examples of anæsthesia and analgesia are given under "Surgical Cases."

Hunger and Thirst.—Debove, Fillassier, and others record experimental cases in which the desire for food and drink was removed by suggestion; the subjects abstaining from both for a considerable period, without the inconvenience which they would have otherwise experienced.

(II.) THE PSYCHOLOGICAL PHENOMENA OF HYPNOSIS.

(A) Post-Hypnotic Suggestions.

Under ordinary circumstances, the instant hypnosis is terminated all the phenomena which have characterised it immediately disappear. In response to suggestion, however, one or more of these phenomena may manifest themselves in the subject's waking life. This is brought about in two ways. (1) Where the operator suggests that one or more of the phenomena shall persist after waking. For example, the analgesia successfully suggested in all my operative cases was continued by this means after hypnosis was terminated. The same thing can be done in experimental cases, and muscular contractures, alterations in the special senses, or hallucinations thus continued from the hypnotic to the waking state.

(2) The most interesting class of post-hypnotic suggestions, however, are those in which the appearance of the phenomena has been delayed until some more or less remote time after the termination of hypnosis. The production of sleep at night, the prevention of the return of periodic pain, the excitation of the

action of the bowels, or of the menstrual flow, are examples of
this from the therapeutic side; while post-hypnotic appreciation
of time, automatic writing, delayed hallucinations, etc., are
examples from the experimental side. The mental condition of
the subject during the fulfilment of post-hypnotic suggestions
will be referred to in discussing memory, and again dealt with
under "Theory."

(B) Rapport in Hypnosis.

In deep hypnosis, particularly in the somnambulistic state,
the phenomenon called *rapport* generally appears. The subject
responds to the operator alone; and, while the latter's slightest
gesture or softest whisper is instantly obeyed, he remains inert
though others may stimulate him by speaking loudly or acting
roughly. The following case illustrates this :—

I hypnotised C., a soldier in good health, in the presence of
Mr. Ernest Hart, Drs. Hack Tuke, Outterson Wood, Wingfield
and others. Mr. Hart said that he could wake C. and asserted
that this was the easiest thing in the world to do. He shook C.
and told him to wake up, but with no result. He then asked me
to leave the room, alleging that my presence prevented his success.
I did so and closed the door after me, but remained close to it. I
heard Mr. Hart say : "Wake up. Dr. Bramwell has gone home ;
we are all going away and the room will be locked up for the
night." Mr. Hart and the others then left the room, walking
very loudly, and joined me in the passage. Mr. Hart then
suddenly slipped back into the room and shut us out. Five
minutes after, he admitted that he could not waken C. We
returned to the room and I whispered to C. : "Wake up." He
at once did so.

Next day, during hypnosis, I asked C. what Mr. Hart had
done to him while they were alone in the room. He said Mr.
Hart had forcibly lifted his eyelids and rubbed his eyeballs with
his fingers. A week later the experiment was repeated, when
Mr. Hart and others employed every means they could think of
to arouse C. These attempts failed, but he again awoke the
instant I requested him to do so.

I could easily cite many other instances of a similar nature which have been observed by myself and others. It is not necessary to do so, however, as I propose to show, in discussing this question in the chapter on "Theory," that the phenomenon is a purely artificial one, the result of training by the operator, or of self-suggestion on the part of the subject.

(C) Consciousness in Hypnosis.

Only 10 per cent of Braid's subjects passed into a condition resembling sleep, followed by amnesia on waking. The lost memory could generally be restored by suggestion in subsequent hypnoses; but, in a few instances, Braid was unable to thus recall the events of hypnotic life, and thought that when this happened the subjects had passed into a deeper and more unconscious stage, which he termed hypnotic coma.

According to the Salpêtrière school, the stage of lethargy is characterised by loss of consciousness.

Bernheim's observations and statements as to hypnotic consciousness are somewhat contradictory. Thus, he asserts that the profoundest somnambules show consciousness when stimulated by questions, and afterwards can recall what has passed. From this he concludes that consciousness always persists during every phase of hypnosis. He describes, however, other somnambules who are supposed to have lost consciousness. These, he says, fall into a profound and heavy sleep, and are incapable of remembering anything on awaking — even if tormented by questions during hypnosis, they remain inert.

Remarks.—Generally speaking, the hypnotic condition—whether slight or deep—is a conscious one. This is obviously true as regards the lighter stages, where the subject not only realises all that is taking place around him, but can also recall it when the hypnotic state is terminated. In profound somnambulism also the subjects can usually recall in subsequent hypnoses all that has passed in previous ones; sometimes, however, they may undergo operations and perform acts of which they are unconscious. Thus, (a) in surgical cases, where anæsthesia has been successfully suggested, the patients are unable to recall anything about the operations, either when awake or in subsequent hypnoses. If analgesia alone is suggested, they can revive tactile, but not

H

painful sensations. The fact that this unconsciousness of pain is real and not a negative hallucination, is proved by the absence of shock, the persistence of analgesia after awaking, and the unusual rapidity of the healing process.

(*b*) Under certain circumstances the events of profound hypnosis cannot be recalled by suggestion. If the subject is told to sleep deeply, and to be unconscious of everything until awakened by the operator, two widely differing conditions may be observed : (1) Despite the commands of the operator, the subject at once manifests consciousness if any experiment, of which he disapproves, is attempted. (2) If, however, he is neither questioned nor touched, he generally takes no notice of anything said or done around him. On awaking, he frequently has no recollection of what has passed, and suggestion in hypnosis sometimes fails to revive the lost memory.

(*c*) The hypnotic subject can be trained to perform automatic acts. If some simple movement is suggested, of which volition does not disapprove, it may after a time become *automatic, i.e.* after having been frequently voluntarily and consciously performed, it may be executed unconsciously as a genuine automatic act in response to the habitual stimulus which has excited it. The memory of this act—one which has apparently not aroused consciousness—cannot be evoked in subsequent hypnoses.

(D) Spontaneity in Hypnosis.

Moll believes that he has observed spontaneous mental and physical action even in the deepest forms of hypnosis. At the same time, he admits that he is unable to prove that these apparently spontaneous acts did not result from some external stimuli, which might have been so slight as to escape observation. He states that he has been struck by the absence of independent currents of thought in deeply hypnotised subjects.

The first difficulty met with in attempting to discuss "spontaneous" action is the ambiguity attached to the word itself. According to Moll, in order that an act or thought should be spontaneous it must arise independently of external stimuli. From that point of view, an effect may occur without a cause or a phenomenon without a generator. It is more logical, however, to admit that previous sensations have been registered and that volition is a resultant of past, as well as of present, sensations.

For practical purposes, in discussing spontaneity we may divide the mental and physical phenomena into two groups: (1) Where the phenomena are not due to the suggestions of the operator, or to impressions received from the outer world during hypnosis. (2) Where the phenomena have been excited by stimuli received during hypnosis, but where their character has not been definitely determined by these stimuli, *i.e.* where the response to the given sensations has been, as it were, chosen by the subject.

Group 1.—Of this class a typical example will be given in discussing automatism, *i.e.* the dressmaking problem solved by D. When I hypnotised her I knew nothing about her difficulties. The solution of the problem came into her mind while she was resting quietly in a condition of profound hypnosis with her eyes shut—at a time when no suggestions of any kind, either direct or indirect, were being made to her.[1]

Other somnambules also stated, when questioned in subsequent hypnoses, that they occasionally, although rarely, thought of the events of their waking life when hypnotised, and arranged plans for the future. More extended investigations, carried out on the same lines, would probably show that somnambules possess more independent mental activity than they are generally credited with. It must be remembered, moreover, that the suggestions of the operator tend to curtail the mental activity of the subject. Thus, in the " deep " stage, they are usually told to sleep and to think of nothing, while in the " alert " stage they are generally occupied in carrying out more or less complicated suggestions.

All the phenomena of self-hypnosis already referred to—and further discussed under " Theory "—fall under *Group* 1. For, although we can identify the stimuli which excited them, these arose before hypnosis took place and originated with the subject himself.

Group 2.—Examples of this group are very numerous. Thus, I suggested to E. during hypnosis that he should open his eyes and act as if he were awake. He was to go into another room, where he would find Dr. F. and entertain him until I joined them. When I entered the room, F. told me that E. had given him an interesting account of the hypnotic operations at Leeds, and of a lecture and demonstration I had given at York. E. had been

[1] P. 320.

present on both occasions and was one of the patients operated on. When I told F. that E. was in the hypnotic state he would not believe it. I awoke E.; he had no recollection of what he had said or how he had got into the room. He was rehypnotised and questioned, when he recalled my instructions and how he had carried them out. I asked him why he had chosen hypnotism as the topic of conversation. He replied that he was sure Dr. F. had come to find out about it, and so he chose that subject as he thought it would interest him.

Miss D.'s description—which will be given in the chapter on "Theory"—of being doctored by her mother is another example of this kind.[1]

Under this group also fall all the cases in which subjects have resisted disagreeable suggestions. Here the response to the external stimuli was opposite or different to that desired by the operator, and in this sense was spontaneous on the part of the subject. This form of "negative spontaneity" shows itself both in action and thought; the subjects not only oppose physical resistance to the suggestions, but, if questioned, give their reasons for doing so.

(E) Memory in Hypnosis.

Memory in relation to hypnotic states varies widely and is influenced by the depth of the hypnosis, the personality of the subject and the suggestions of the operator.

Memory in hypnosis may be :—

(I.) *Unchanged.*—In this group, the subjects when hypnotised can recall the events of normal life, and on awaking remember all that has passed during hypnosis.

In some instances, however, where the memory is apparently unchanged, closer examination shows that it has either been increased or diminished. Of this the two following cases are examples :—

(a) I had frequently hypnotised Miss G., and could influence not only her voluntary muscles but also her special senses. On awaking she could always recall what had passed, despite suggestions to the contrary. At a later date, I found I could induce analgesia. Touching the cornea, passing needles into the flesh, and probing the nose and vocal chords were unaccompanied

[1] P. 321.

by pain or disagreeable sensations. On awaking, *despite suggested amnesia*, the subject could recall all the tactile sensations associated with these operations, but was unable, even in response to suggestion, to revive any memory of pain.

(*b*) Certain changes in the voluntary muscles and the special senses could be induced in Mrs. H., all of which she remembered on awaking. Analgesia, however, could not be induced. Though her memory was apparently unchanged, experiment revealed the existence of a sub-conscious one, superior to the normal. I suggested, during hypnosis, that she should fall asleep the first time Mr. K. *called* and shook hands with her. On awaking, she remembered what had been said. A week or two passed without her seeing him, then one day Mr. K. *met her at my house* and shook hands with her. She did not fall asleep. Both the subject and I had forgotten the exact terms of the suggestion, and believed it had been a failure. Some time afterwards, however, Mr. K. called at the subject's own house, when she fell asleep the moment he shook hands with her. She was not thinking of the suggestion at the time.

(II.) *The subjects can recall during hypnosis the events of waking life and those of previous hypnoses—with a clearness corresponding to their powers of memory in the normal state—but, on awaking, the incidents of hypnosis are more or less forgotten.*

In this group the subjects usually assert that they are able to remember all that has passed during hypnosis. Questioning, however, reveals the fact that their memory is not nearly so perfect as they believe it to be. Further, what they do recall soon fades, thus resembling ordinary dreams, which, although vivid on awaking, are often quickly forgotten.

(III.) *The subjects can recall during hypnosis the events of previous hypnoses, as well as those of normal life, and on awaking remember little or nothing of what has occurred.*

The hypnotic memory just referred to surpasses the normal one : the improvement shows itself (*a*) in an increased power of recalling impressions received during hypnosis, and (*b*) in reviving the lost impressions of normal life.

The following are examples of group (*a*):—

(1) During hypnosis, I read some verses twice to Miss S. which were new to her, and suggested that she should recall them on awaking. The experiment was successful, despite the fact

that her normal memory was so bad that it was almost impossible for her to learn anything by rote.

(2) Miss D., as we shall see, was able to recall in subsequent hypnoses complicated series of figures, which had been read to her once or at most twice in hypnosis—a feat quite beyond the powers of her normal memory.[1]

The following are examples of group (b):—

(1) As already stated, Miss M., an imperfectly educated girl, could play a few tunes upon the piano, but only with her music before her. When hypnotised and blindfolded she played them much more brilliantly. As she would never play before strangers when awake, and did so when hypnotised, this showed not only an improvement in memory, but the absence of various inhibitions due to nervousness and shyness.

The improvement of memory as to remote events is still more interesting; and this I have frequently demonstrated in the following manner:—(2) Certain subjects were first questioned in the normal state as to the earliest events they could remember, when it was generally found they could recall nothing which had happened before the age of five or six. They were then hypnotised and, starting from the first event in their lives they could recall, it was suggested that they should revive the memory of earlier and earlier incidents. Some of the subjects related what they stated had happened at the age of two, and one described a children's party given on the first anniversary of her birthday.

(3) Sometimes I suggested a modified change of personality *i.e.* that the subject had become a child again and was learning to write. By this means samples of handwriting were obtained, beginning with the first pothooks and altering in character as increased age was suggested : these the subject was unable to produce in the normal state. On awaking, the subjects remembered nothing they had told me. When I, in my turn, related the incidents, some recognised them and wondered how I knew what they themselves had long forgotten ; others recalled nothing.

As far as the facts themselves are concerned, older relatives confirmed the statements made by the subjects. This, however, does not exclude possible error. The subject, who thought she recalled the first anniversary of her birthday, may only have remembered an account she had heard at a later date, but, as no

[1] Pp. 119-139.

recollection of this was to be found in the normal consciousness, its revival would indicate an improvement, although not so far-reaching a one, in memory.

In Dr. Morton Prince's case, referred to under "Theory," [1] the subject was able to recall during hypnosis events of which the normal consciousness possessed no knowledge—notably those that had occurred during the delirium of fever.

The increase in hypnotic memory is closely related to the depth of the hypnosis, and reaches its fullest development in somnambulism, which is characterised by post-hypnotic amnesia. Moll, Krafft-Ebing and many others also cite cases of improvement in hypnotic memory, which more or less closely resemble the examples just given.

The recollection during hypnosis of the events of waking life, and of those of previous hypnoses, rarely occurs spontaneously in the untrained subject. The questions of the operator, however, readily evoke these memories, and his indirect suggestions produce the same result. Thus, when a disagreeable suggestion is given, the subject is able to recall, despite the wishes of the operator, the feelings, sentiments or prejudices of his waking life, and, acting in accordance with these, rejects the suggestion. The subject, on the other hand, who has been frequently hypnotised and taught to revive lost memories by suggestion, soon comes to do so spontaneously. When hypnosis is induced, especially its "alert" stage, the subject takes up his hypnotic life at the point at which he left it when last hypnotised; and the memories of past hypnoses and of waking life are at once restored, or at all events reappear, just as ordinary memories would, with every association of ideas that is brought about by his surroundings. Subjects in the "deep" stage, who are apparently unconscious of whatever is passing around them which does not directly concern them, frequently pass into the "alert" stage when anything is said or done which does interest them. Their memory then revives; and, as in the case of Miss D. already referred to, they spontaneously join in the conversation.

Cases are said to have occurred in which the forgotten dreams of normal sleep have been spontaneously recalled in hypnosis, but this I have been unable to confirm.

It has been attempted during hypnosis to revive the me

[1] Pp. 394-6.

of what has occurred during the administration of an anæsthetic, such as ether or nitrous oxide gas, but the experiments of this kind with which I am personally acquainted were failures. Further, I have never succeeded during hypnosis in recalling the events of normal sleep. With one subject, whose hypnotic memory of the events of waking life was exceptionally good, I carried out the following experiment :—He was in the habit of falling asleep every Sunday afternoon in his arm-chair; and on these occasions he was read to aloud, the sentences being repeated again and again. I afterwards hypnotised him and suggested that he should recall what had been read. The experiment, though frequently repeated, was invariably unsuccessful.

As far as my experience goes, the loss of memory associated with non - hypnotic double personality cannot be restored by suggestion. I have, however, only experimented with one case. The subject, like Félida X.,[1] passed spontaneously into a second state of consciousness, and could recall nothing in the normal state of what she had said or done during the attacks. During hypnosis there was a marked improvement in memory as regards the events of waking life, but suggestion failed to revive anything which had happened in the attacks.

Post-Hypnotic Amnesia.—All hypnotic stages, except the slightest, are characterised by a decrease of memory on awaking, which usually corresponds to the depth of the hypnosis. Sometimes the subject recalls and retains a certain proportion of the incidents of his hypnotic life; at others he remembers everything on waking, but forgets it all a few minutes after; finally, he may have absolutely no recollection of anything he has said or done during hypnosis. This stage, characterised by complete amnesia on waking, is termed "somnambulism," and in it *the phenomena of deepest hypnosis can be excited by suggestion, i.e.* one can obtain alterations in the special senses as well as in the muscular system. This amnesia after hypnosis, however, is sometimes reached in slight stages, when alterations in the voluntary muscles can alone be induced; in other instances it is absent in the deeper ones, characterised by alterations in the special senses. One subject, for example, may be unable on awaking to recall that the muscles of his arm had been rendered rigid, while another may distinctly remember a sensory hallucination.

[1] Pp. 385-6.

According to Bernheim, subjects who cannot remember the events of hypnosis on awaking are sometimes also unable to recall what immediately preceded hypnosis. Although this phenomenon can be produced by suggestion, I have never seen it arise spontaneously.

The two most important points as to post-hypnotic amnesia are (1) the circumstances under which the condition arises, and (2) those associated with the restoration of the lost memories.

(1) It is difficult to determine whether post-hypnotic amnesia ever appears without either direct or indirect suggestion. The majority of those, who have passed into the stage in which their special senses can be influenced by suggestion, remember on awaking nothing of what has taken place. Here, although the operator may have made no direct suggestion of amnesia, indirect suggestion is not excluded. With nearly every one, the idea of hypnosis represents a kind of sleep with subsequent forgetfulness; and this is so ingrained that the majority of those in whom hypnosis short of somnambulism has been induced, assert that they have not been hypnotised, because they have not been asleep. This point of view often remains unshaken, despite the explanations of the operator. Further, in those who have been deeply hypnotised without subsequent amnesia, this phenomenon can generally be excited by a single direct suggestion of the operator.

(2) In cases of complete post-hypnotic amnesia, I have never seen the lost memories spontaneously revived in the waking state, nor restored by association of ideas—even when this has been of the most direct kind and the subject has been informed of the events of hypnosis. My observations have led me to accept Beaunis' conclusion that the lost memories of hypnosis possess this distinctive and essential characteristic: that they cannot be revived by chance association of ideas, and therefore are fundamentally different from those of the waking state.

Bernheim, Moll, Heidenhain and others hold different views. According to these authorities, the lost memories of hypnosis can be restored in the following ways:—(A) By direct association of ideas; *e.g.* the subject is told something of what has happened and recalls the rest. (B) By chance association of ideas acting just as they would do in normal life. (C) By the operator's touch. Bernheim says: "I lay my hand on the subject's forehead to concentrate his attention; he thinks deeply for an instant, with-

out falling asleep, and all the latent memories arise with great
precision." (D) By the operator simply asserting to the subject
in the waking state that he is to remember. (E) By means of
the dreams of normal sleep.

The restoration of the lost memories of hypnosis during
normal sleep is a phenomenon I have never observed; and, as
far as I am aware, the only instances on record are two cited by
Bernheim.   Before accepting the spontaneous revival of lost
hypnotic memories, one must be sure of two things: (a) that in
the cases cited the post-hypnotic amnesia was complete, and (b)
that no new hypnosis was induced.

(a) In cases short of somnambulism, where the subject
remembered some of the events of hypnosis on awaking, and then
more or less quickly forgot them, it is possible that the lost
memories may have been restored by the association of ideas, and
also that similar memories might be revived in normal dreams.
Such instances are widely different, however, from those in which
the subject has forgotten all the events of hypnosis on awaking:
these, I believe, are quite unaffected by association of ideas or
dreams.

(b) Fifty years ago, Braid drew attention to the fact that lost
memories were revived when the operator placed his hand on the
subject's body, and thus helped him to concentrate his attention.
Braid recognised, however, that the condition induced was a fresh
hypnosis; but this, the all-important point, Bernheim apparently
fails to grasp.   All trained somnambules can recall the events of
hypnosis in response to the simple statement of the operator,
"Now you remember."   The phrase "Now you remember" equals
in value the word "Sleep," or any other signal for inducing
hypnosis.   In response to it, the subject passes into the hypnotic
state and relates the events of past hypnoses.   When his story
is finished, and his attention directed into some other channel,
the normal state reappears and he forgets all he has just said.

(IV.)—*The subject may be unable, even in response to suggestion,
to recall during hypnosis certain events of past hypnoses.*

Attention has already been drawn to the fact that the subject
can revive the past impressions of hypnosis, better than his
ordinary self can recall similar ones of waking life.   This statement, however, only applies to the hypnotic events of which the
subject has been conscious.   Impressions may be received which

do not reach hypnotic consciousness; these cannot be recalled in subsequent hypnoses. They are of two kinds :—

(1) Those received during profound hypnotic conditions. As already stated, when a somnambule is told to sleep deeply and to hear nothing except the operator's voice, and that only when addressed to him, he may or may not be able to recall in subsequent hypnoses what has taken place. If anything is said which concerns him, he may apparently remain unconscious, or, like Miss D., pass into the "alert" stage and join in the conversation. In both cases he is able to recall what has taken place. Further, he will successfully resist any experiments which are disagreeable to him; and he knows in subsequent hypnoses what they were and why he opposed them. On the other hand, if nothing is said or done which in any way interests the subject, he usually remains unconscious, and can generally recall nothing in subsequent hypnoses.

(2) Further, the subject may be unable to recall, during subsequent hypnoses, specially selected sensations inhibited during "alert" as well as "deep" stages. The familiar example is the inhibition of pain for operative purposes. Anæsthesia may be suggested, when the patient can revive neither painful nor tactile sensations; or analgesia alone may be induced, when the patient can recall the steps of the operation, but has no memory of pain. That this inhibition of pain is a real, not an apparent one, is proved by the following facts :—(1) Not only do the patients remain passive during operation, but the physiological signs of pain are absent, *i.e.* there is neither dilatation of pupil, nor increase of pulse. (2) There is no corneal reflex. (3) Powerful applications of the faradic brush elicit no signs of pain. (4) Shock is absent. (5) Pain on awaking can be prevented by post-hypnotic suggestion. (6) The healing process is abnormally rapid.

Again, certain sounds may be inhibited, which subsequently cannot be recalled. For example, Forel's warders, as we have already seen,[1] who slept by the bedside of homicidal lunatics, heard nothing unless the patients attempted to get out of bed. All other sounds failed to disturb them and could not be recalled, while the absence of fatigue in this form of night-watching also demonstrated the genuine nature of the inhibition.

Braid recognised three main conditions of post-hypnotic memory :—(1) The subjects afterwards remembered the events of

[1] P. 89.

hypnosis. (2) They forgot on awaking the events of hypnosis, but recalled them in subsequent hypnoses. (3) After the deeper stage, which he called "hypnotic coma," memory was lost and not revived in subsequent hypnoses.

According to Bernheim, the hypnotic condition in all its stages is a conscious one; and, when amnesia follows on awaking, the lost memories can be revived in various ways, including that of simple affirmation by the operator. The subject can then recall everything that has been said and done by himself and others; nothing is forgotten. Bernheim states that the hypnotic coma of Braid does not exist. Subjects, he says, who remain inert during hypnosis, and are without apparent memory on awaking, are really conscious all the time. In support of this, he asserts two things:—(1) The operator, by stimulating the subject by questions, etc., can always elicit signs of consciousness during hypnosis; he can always make the subject come out of his torpor. (2) On awaking, the subject can be made to recount all that has passed. These statements are only partially correct. It is true, no matter how profound the hypnosis, that the operator can at once arouse the subject's attention and keep it alert. If he does so, the deep stage which I have described does not appear. On the other hand, such a stage can be induced and may be maintained under the conditions I have described, *i.e.* in the absence of sensations interesting or disagreeable to the subject. In such cases, as the subjects can recall nothing when questioned in subsequent hypnoses, the conclusion that this particular stage was not a conscious one appears reasonable. This view is further strengthened by the fact that particular sensations, notably pain, can be entirely inhibited and never exist for consciousness at all.

While Bernheim asserts that consciousness is never lost and that memory can always be revived, he formerly described (*Suggestive Therapeutics*, p. 8) a condition which I have never observed, and of which he now denies the existence (*Revue de l'Hypnotisme*, vol. xii. p. 143). Speaking of somnambules, he says: "Others, on the contrary, fall into a deep, heavy sleep and remember absolutely nothing on waking. While they are asleep they can be questioned in vain—tormented with questions : yet they remain inert."

Under certain circumstances, subjects are said to be unable to recall during hypnosis events which happened at an earlier period in the same hypnosis.

Of this class two groups of cases are cited :—(a) Changes of personality. According to Moll, and some other authorities, when changes of personality are suggested during hypnosis these are associated with loss of memory, *i.e.* a subject as Napoleon does not remember what he did as Frederick the Great. This partial amnesia is an artificial one accidentally created by suggestion, and in subsequent hypnoses the subject can recall what he said and did when playing both rôles.

(b) Alternating memories without change of personality. Gurney described two stages of hypnosis, distinguished from each other by entirely different memories. In stage A the subject knew nothing of stage B, and in B nothing of A.[1] I have never seen these stages arise spontaneously ; but have artificially created them by suggestion, and found that the subjects could recall in subsequent hypnoses all that had been said and done in both stages.

(V.) *Owing to suggestion, the subject may have forgotten in hypnosis the events of waking life.*

As already stated, there is a tendency to recall in hypnosis the events of waking life. This develops with time and training, until at length the subject possesses even a richer store of the memories of waking life than he does in the normal state. Suggestion may partly or entirely suspend or destroy this memory, and so create an artificial amnesia. Hence, the subject may in hypnosis recall nothing of waking life, or only certain selected incidents which have not been excluded by suggestion. The lost memories can be restored by suggestion ; and thus the condition differs from the so-called amnesia we have just discussed in the last section. There, the subject could not recall what he had never experienced ; here, in response to suggestion, he forgets what he formerly knew, and later again recalls it by the same means.

(VI.) *Owing to suggestion, the subject may be unable to recall in hypnosis the events of previous hypnoses.*

Here the changes in memory correspond to those just described under section V. The memories of previous hypnoses, which would have arisen either spontaneously or in response to suggestion, are prevented from doing so, either in whole or in part, by the suggestions of the operator. This amnesia can be at once abolished by further suggestion.

[1] Pp. 396-7.

According as arranged by the operator, the two forms of amnesia just described may either occur separately, or may be combined in the same subject. In the latter case the subject will be unable to recall in hypnosis the events of waking life, and those of previous hypnoses.

(VII.) *Owing to suggestion, the subject may have forgotten on awaking some or all the events of waking life.*

This amnesia may occur in various ways :—

(*a*) It may apparently be complete. The subject is then unable to recall anything connected with his waking life, and may even have lost the sense of his own identity. All memory of previous hypnoses is also forgotten.

(*b*) The amnesia may be limited by suggestion. Here the subject cannot remember selected events and ideas of his past life. For example, he may be unable to recall certain words or letters ; or may remember them, and yet be unable to utter them or write them down. This power of suggesting post-hypnotic amnesia is sometimes of therapeutic as well as of experimental value. For instance, one of my patients, a nervous girl, was much frightened by seeing a friend in an epileptic fit and was unable to dismiss the scene from her mind. This was blotted out by suggestion and although several years have passed since then, its memory has never arisen either in the normal state or in hypnosis.

(*c*) The amnesia just described may be modified by the post-hypnotic suggestion that the memories of hypnosis alone be continued into the waking state. The subject then forgets in waking life the events of his past normal life, and remembers those of his past hypnotic life which he would otherwise have forgotten.

(VIII.) *Owing to suggestion, the subject in the normal state may be unable to recall certain selected events in waking life, which took place after hypnosis terminated.*

Of this class Forel's warders again afford an example. He found that some of them were greatly distressed by the purposeless noises of the insane, and suggested, during hypnosis, that they should only hear those sounds in the waking state which were necessary for the performance of their duties. All others were inhibited and never existed for the waking consciousness; and thus suggestion in subsequent hypnosis failed to revive them.

(IX.) *Owing to suggestion, the subjects may recall in hypnosis, or in the waking state, the sensory hallucinations of earlier hypnosis.*

For example, the subject may remember in hypnosis a hallucinatory dog which he believes he has seen in a former hypnosis and, as the result of suggestion, this memory may be prolonged into waking life.

(X.) *The subject may recall during hypnosis the events of previous hypnoses and those of waking life, the latter to a greater extent than he could do in the normal condition; and by suggestion this memory may be retained on awaking.*

Here amnesia has been prevented by suggestion, and there is now no break in the memory of the hypnotised subject. It is true he cannot recall inhibited sensations which have never existed for consciousness, such as those described under No. IV. Apart from this, the only alteration is one of improvement. In the waking state the subject now remembers past events which he was unable voluntarily to recollect, but the memory of which has been revived in hypnosis. He also recalls the impressions he received during hypnosis—impressions which he would not have been able to revive so vividly had they been made in the waking state. He remembers, for instance, the piece of poetry which has been read to him twice during hypnosis, and which he would have required to have heard read many times in the normal state, in order to retain an equally clear recollection of it.

(XI.) *Memory in Relation to Post-Hypnotic Suggestions.*

According to most authorities, post-hypnotic suggestions, even when executed some time after awaking, are not carried out in the normal condition; there is, in effect, a new hypnosis or a state closely resembling it. In support of this, they rely mainly on the alterations which take place in memory; as a rule post-hypnotic acts are forgotten immediately after fulfilment.

According to Moll, the conditions under which post-hypnotic acts are carried out vary widely. He summarises them as follows :—(1) A state in which a new hypnosis, characterised by suggestibility, appears during the execution of the act, with loss of memory afterwards and no spontaneous awaking. (2) A state in which no symptoms of a fresh hypnosis are discoverable, although the act is carried out. (3) A state with or without

fresh susceptibility to suggestion, with complete forgetfulness of
the act and spontaneous awaking. (4) A state of susceptibility
to suggestion with subsequent loss of memory.

At first I believed that all post-hypnotic acts were forgotten
immediately after fulfilment. Later, I noticed many exceptions to
this rule, but these—with the exception of those occurring in so-
called " waking somnambulism "—have been confined to one class,
viz. that where the removal of morbid symptoms has been successfully suggested. Thus, if I successfully suggest to a patient, who is
suffering from insomnia, to sleep eight hours the following night,
he remembers that he has done so. The same thing happens
when constipation or amenorrhœa is cured by suggestion; and
yet the same patients may be unable to recall experimental post-
hypnotic suggestions, such as rigidity of the muscles. Why
they should remember the former and forget the latter is a
question by no means easy to answer. The explanation may
possibly be found in the fact that the suggested sleep, for
example, is not so much the direct outcome of the suggestion
as of the removal of the morbid conditions on which the insomnia
depended.

The different phenomena described by Moll as associated with
post-hypnotic states are largely the result of training. The
following experiment illustrates this. I suggested to O. that ten
minutes after awaking she should commence to rotate her hands.
I awoke O., who then carried on a conversation with me and
another person who was present. At the end of ten minutes she
carried out the suggestion. I asked her why she moved her
hands. She replied: " I fancy you told me to when I was asleep."
" Do you remember my having done so ? " " No." " Can you
recall anything which happened when you were hypnotised ? "
" No." A fresh experimental suggestion of a simple and un-
objectionable nature was made, but was not carried out. I then
said to O: " Stop moving your hands." She did so. I talked
about something else for a moment or two and then asked her
why she had moved her hands. She denied having done so and
was unable to recall anything about it. She remembered, however,
everything else that had taken place while the experiment was
being carried out. I rehypnotised O. and gave her the same
post-hypnotic suggestion and then aroused her. While she
executed it, I succeeded, by varying my suggestions and making

them more forcible, in getting her to accept fresh suggestions and
to recall the memories of the previous hypnosis.

(XII.) *Memory in " Waking Somnambulism."*

The term "waking somnambulism" is applied by Beaunis
to a condition in which a subject, who has been previously
deeply hypnotised, will accept suggestions similar to hypnotic ones,
without having on that occasion been subjected to any hypnotic
process, or having passed through any state resembling sleep or
trance. The following is a typical example:—I say to N.,
who has not been recently hypnotised, but who is a somnambule:
"I am going to prick your arm with a needle and you will feel
no pain." I pass the needle deeply into his flesh, while he looks
on smilingly. I ask: "Doesn't this hurt you?" "No." "Do
you know what I am doing?" "Yes." Except for the
suggested analgesia N.'s condition apparently in no way differs
from the normal. His eyes are open and his movements natural
He not only talks to me, but to others around him, and answers
questions and reasons just as he would do when awake. I now
abandon the experiment and turn his attention in another
direction. A moment or two afterwards I ask him: "Are you
sure it did not hurt you when I pricked your arm?" He
replies: "What do you mean? You never pricked my arm."
He has entirely forgotten the incident. Beaunis considers this
condition a hypnotic one for two reasons: (1) the subject will
receive other suggestions of a hypnotic nature; (2) the suggestions are forgotten immediately after fulfilment. With the first
proposition I entirely agree, for I have observed that all
subjects, in whom deep hypnosis has previously been induced,
will subsequently exhibit the same range of phenomena in
response to suggestion in the apparently waking state. The
condition termed "waking somnambulism" is undoubtedly a
hypnotic one, but there are some slight points of difference
between it and the usual form of hypnosis induced in the same
subjects by ordinary methods. In ordinary somnambulism all
the events of hypnosis are forgotten on awaking, and can only
be recalled in fresh hypnoses. In the cases of waking somnambulism which I have observed, sometimes the suggestions were

I

forgotten almost immediately, at others they were remembered for a longer period, and in some cases were recalled after the lapse of weeks. The subject of one of these experiments was questioned in hypnosis as to her memory of suggestions carried out in a state of waking somnambulism. She replied : " Sometimes I forgot them quickly, sometimes remembered them for an hour or two, never longer." When I reminded her that she had recalled one at the end of a month, she replied : " Oh yes ! You made the suggestion just before I left your room, and I talked it over with my mother on my way home." Here the recollection of the event was complicated by the subject's verbal description of it, and possibly by her mother's comments.

With another subject, I noticed a difference between the mental attitude as to hallucinations suggested in hypnosis and those created in waking somnambulism. On several occasions she saw a cat in response to suggestion. She was always delighted with the imaginary animal, believed it to be a real one, and showed great pleasure in playing with it. At a later date, in the apparently waking state, I successfully suggested a similar hallucination. She said : " I see that cat, but it is not real. I know it is only an imaginary one you have made me see."

The occasional persistence of the memory of post-hypnotic acts, and the recognition of the artificial nature of a hallucination, are the only differences I have discovered between waking somnambulism and the " alert " stage of ordinary somnambulism. Both conditions are hypnotic ones ; and the slight apparent differences between them are probably due to unconscious training by the operator, or to the self-suggestions of the subject.

(F) Hypnotic and Post-Hypnotic Appreciation of Time.

As already stated, I commenced to employ hypnotism as a therapeutic agent in 1889, and in less than two years treated over 500 patients ; of these 48 per cent became somnambules, *i.e.* were unable, when hypnosis was terminated, to recall the events of hypnotic life. Having observed that the curative effect of suggestion was increased by prolonged hypnosis, I frequently suggested to my patients that they were to remain in that state until a given hour—usually that of their next meal—and then left them. Although rarely present at the conclusion of the experiment, I obtained ample and trustworthy evidence that hypnosis invariably terminated at, or within a few minutes of, the hour indicated, and thus accidentally discovered that deep hypnosis was associated with an increased appreciation of time. These observations—the by-product of therapeutic work—led to careful experiment with somnambules, the majority of whom were males and all in good health. The following were the usual suggestions given: (1) A simple act was suggested during hypnosis, which was to be carried out at a given time before that state terminated. (2) The subject was told during hypnosis that this state was to cease at a specified future hour. (3) The performance of some simple act at a given hour after the termination of hypnosis was suggested. (4) Awaking from natural sleep at a given hour was suggested during hypnosis. (5) The subject was told in the waking state that he was to pass into the hypnotic condition at a given hour, remain hypnotised for a specified time, and perform certain simple acts at stated intervals; then pass again into the normal state and remain in it for a specified time, and again pass into the hypnotic condition. These experiments, continued from 1889 to 1902, have been frequently repeated before competent observers. The majority of the suggestions were executed at the moment indicated, while in the remainder the error in time appreciation rarely exceeded five minutes. In many instances, except those referred to in group No. 4, the subjects were carefully watched from the beginning to the end of the experiment.

Similar phenomena have been observed by nearly all who have done practical hypnotic work; and I have seen experiments, resembling those just cited, reproduced in various foreign cliniques. Two, formerly regarded as the most remarkable of their kind, were made by Beaunis and Liégeois. In one of these a visual hallucination appeared after a suggested interval of 172 days, and in the other after 365. The late Professor Delbœuf, however, pointed out, in reference to all such experiments, that even in the longest a fixed date had been impressed upon the subject's mind. Thus, Beaunis' subject was told that the 172nd day was New Year's Day, and Liégeois' was impressed by the fact that the suggestion was to be executed in a year from the time it was given. The experiments, therefore, did not involve the carrying out of a suggestion after the lapse of so many days, which the subjects were supposed to count as they passed, but simply on the arrival of a fixed and easily recognised date. This objection applies with great force to my earlier cases. In every instance a specified hour was suggested; and, in order that the subjects might be conveniently watched, the time involved rarely exceeded a few hours. This point will be again referred to in treating of the theoretical explanation of the appreciation of time. Meanwhile, I wish to draw attention to the experiments made by Delbœuf, with the object of eliminating an easily recognised fixed date from the suggestions.

Delbœuf's Experiments.—These occupied a week, from Saturday, October 2, to Saturday, October 9, 1886. His subjects were his two maid-servants, J. and M., sisters, aged respectively 20 and 23. All the experiments were of a similar character; from time to time during hypnosis the subjects were told that they were to do something at the expiration of a certain number of minutes, an interval of waking life always intervening between the suggestion and its fulfilment :—

Exp.[1] 1.—Sat., Oct. 2, 1886; subject J.; time 6 A.M. *Sug.*: At the expiration of 350 m. J. was to ask Delbœuf if she should harness the donkey. Delbœuf's wife was ill and went out in an invalid carriage drawn by a donkey, but J. had nothing to do with it; thus her question would be unusual. *Res.*: The impulse to ask the question came into J.'s mind at the time it was due, but she successfully resisted it.

Exp. 2.—Subject M.; time 8 A.M. *Sug.*: At the expiration of 350 m. M. was to ask Madame Delbœuf if she would like to go out. Under the circumstances the question would be an unusual one. *Res.*: At 1.50, the hour indicated, M. was impelled to ask the question, but as she happened to be in the village on an errand, was unable to do so. She returned at 2.30 and carried out the suggestion.

Exp. 3.—Mon. ; subject J.; time 9.15 A.M. *Sug.*: In 900 m., i.e. at 12.15 A.M., J. was to go into the bedroom of one of Delbœuf's children and pull his ear. *Res.*: Suggestion was carried out 95 m. too soon.

Exp. 4.—Subject M.; time 9.25 A.M. *Sug.*: M. was to kiss Mlle. H. Delbœuf at the expiration of 700 m. *Res.*: Twenty-five m. before the suggestion fell due M. looked for Mlle. H. Delbœuf in order to kiss her, but could not find her.

Exp. 5.—Subject M.; time 10.4 P.M. *Sug.*: In 900 m. M. was to kiss Mlle. C. Delbœuf. *Res.*: At the time indicated, i.e. 1.4 on Tuesday afternoon, M. was having her lunch with the other servants when she

---

[1] *Exp.* = Experiment. *Sug.* = Suggestion. *Res.* = Result. d. = days. h. = hours. m. = minutes.

suddenly got up from the table, sought and found Mlle. C. Delbœuf and carried out the suggestion.

Exp. 6.—Tues. ; subject J.; time 6.30 A.M. *Sug.:* At the expiration of 1600 m. J. was to pull the cook's nose. *Res.* : Suggestion carried out 60 m. too soon.

Exp. 7.—Subject M. ; time 6.45 A.M. *Sug.:* At the expiration of 1150 m. (Wed., 1.55 A.M.) she was to go into the cook's bedroom and pull her by the ear. The cook was told what was likely to happen. *Res.:* At the exact hour the subject had a strong impulse to carry out the suggestion, but resisted this until 4.15 A.M., when she gave in and went to the cook's room. The cook laughed, whereupon M. said : " If you laugh I shall pull your ear."

Exp. 8—Wed. ; subject J. ; time 9.55 A.M. *Sug.:* At the expiration of 1300 m. (Th., 7.35 A.M.) J. was to ask Madame Delbœuf if she would like to have her hair dressed. *Res.:* Suggestion carried out 69 m. too soon.

Exp. 9.—Subject M. ; time 6.55 A.M. *Sug.:* At the expiration of 1500 m. (Th., 7.55 A.M.) M. was to ask Madame Delbœuf if she required anything. *Res.:* Suggestion carried out with absolute accuracy.

Exp. 10.—Friday ; subject M. ; time 6.30 A.M. *Sug.:* M. was to feel sleepy at 10 P.M. ; go to bed and sleep profoundly. *Res.:* Correct.

*Exp.*11.—Subject J. ; time 9.15 A.M. *Sug.:* At 11 P.M. J. was to go into M.'s room, and give her a complicated suggestion to be carried out at 5.30 next morning. *Res.:* J. went to bed at 10 P.M. in her own room and quickly fell asleep. At 10.50 P.M. (10 m. too early) she went to her sister as suggested, but could not afterwards recall what she had said or done.

Exp. 12.—Subject M. *Sug.:* M. to execute the orders just referred to at 5.30 A.M. *Res.:* She did nothing, however, beyond carrying out the first part of the suggestion, *i.e.* that she should go to bed and sleep profoundly, and was unable to remember whether her sister had said anything to her or not.

Exp. 13.—Sat. ; subject J. ; time 9.30 A.M. *Sug.:* At the expiration of 3300 m., J. was to ask Delbœuf if she should carry a small ladder to the pear tree. *Res.:* The impulse to ask the question arose 90 m. too late, but J. did not give way to it.

Exp. 14.—Subject M. ; time 10 A.M. *Sug.:* Similar to the last, to be executed after a like interval. *Res.:* Identical with the above, but 90 m. too soon.

Summary.—There were in all fourteen experiments. The suggestions, to be carried out after the lapse of 350, 700, 900, 1500, 1600, 1150, 1300 and 3300 minutes respectively, were made at varying hours of the day and night, while some fell due at night after the lapse of several days.

Results.—Three of the suggestions were fulfilled at the moment they fell due ; four were carried out, but not at the exact time. In three an impulse to carry out the suggestion arose at the right moment. In one of these, the subject successfully resisted the suggestion, in another, she was accidentally prevented from executing it, while in the third, she struggled

against it for two hours and twenty minutes, and then carried it
out. In three, the impulse to carry out the suggestion arose, but
not at the correct time. In one of these cases, accidental circumstances alone prevented the suggestion from being carried out,
but, in the two others, the subject successfully resisted it. One
alone, No. 12, failed completely, but this may have been due to
the fact that No. 11 was not fulfilled in its entirety, *i.e.* it is
uncertain whether J. gave the requisite orders to M. As, however,
the essential fact in the experiments was not the actual carrying
out of trivial and sometimes absurd suggestions, but the subject's
recognition of the terminal time, the cases in which an impulse
arose at the correct moment must be classed amongst the successes.
The number of these is thus raised to six, while of the eight
remaining experiments seven were partially successful. Of the
latter, four were carried out and an impulse to execute the suggestion arose in the other three, but in none was the time accurate;
the error varied from a tenth to a thirty-seventh of the interval.

Remarks.—J. and M. were strong, healthy peasant girls, who
had frequently been hypnotised and were both good somnambules.
At an earlier date, J. was the subject of the two symmetrical
burns already referred to [1]; later she married and her first child
was born painlessly during hypnotic trance.[2]

J. and M. were very imperfectly educated, and could with
difficulty tell the time by the clock. It was impossible for them
to at once reduce such a large number of minutes as 400 into
hours, and they were obliged to proceed by successive additions,
thus:—1 hour = 60 minutes; 1 hour and 1 hour makes
$60 + 60 = 120$; $120 +$ another hour makes 180, and so on.
Before reaching 360 they had often made mistakes, and, no
matter what method they adopted, were absolutely incapable of
reducing such numbers as 1600 and 1150 minutes into hours.
Further, supposing they recalled the suggestion on the termination
of hypnosis and noted what o'clock it was—which they neither
did nor could do—they would still, for example, have to determine
by mental calculation the hour which corresponded to 6.45 P.M.,
increased by 1150 minutes, a feat entirely beyond their powers.

Later, in order to discover whether J.'s hypnotic arithmetical
powers exceeded her normal ones, Delbœuf put the following
problems to her during hypnosis:—(1) "Turn 350 minutes into

[1] P. 84.   [2] P. 171.

hours." Answer: "Six hours. No, five and a half hours." (2) "Turn 1200 minutes into hours." Answer: "Fifteen hours. No, twelve and a half hours." (3) "Turn 150 minutes into hours." Answer: "Two and a half hours." (4) "Turn 240 minutes into hours." Answer: "Two hours." (5) "Turn 300 minutes into hours." Answer, after five seconds' calculation: "Four and a half hours." Then, after a further calculation: "Five and a half hours." Finally: "Five and three-quarter hours." Delbœuf asked J. to explain the last calculation to him. She replied: "This makes five and a half hours plus 3 times 10, which makes five and a half hours exactly." Delbœuf tried to help J. as follows: "How much is $60 + 60$?" Answer: "120 minutes." "$120 + 60$?" Answer: "180 minutes." "$180 + 60$?" Answer, after a long hesitation: "240 minutes." "$240 + 60$?" Answer: "290 minutes." J. had spent ten minutes over attempting to solve the last problem and showed great signs of fatigue. Delbœuf did not consider it necessary to push the question further. It is to be noted that M. was a somewhat better arithmetician than J., and that, in the experiments referred to, her results were more accurate than J.'s.

Further Time Experiments.—The following were inspired by Delbœuf's, and the results were so remarkable that I feel justified in giving as many details as possible, in order to present a fairly complete picture of the subject of the experiments, and of the circumstances under which they were carried out.

Miss D., aged 19, was sent to me by Dr. de Watteville for hypnotic treatment, on Sept. 2, 1895, and her medical history is fully given on page 183.

Hypnosis was induced at the first attempt; and at the seventh sitting Miss D. reached the stage of somnambulism, i.e. she was unable in the normal state to recall the events of hypnotic life. From that date she could at once be made analgesic or anæsthetic by suggestion: touching the cornea or tickling the back of the throat with a feather produced no reflex, and the passing of a needle deeply into the flesh was unattended by pain.

During treatment suggestions had been made fixing the hour at which Miss D. was to fall asleep at night, and the moment at which she was to awake in the morning. As these were remarkably successful, it occurred to me that she might prove a good subject for experiments similar to those of Delbœuf. Miss D.

was an intelligent girl who had received an ordinary Board-school education, and her arithmetical powers were in keeping with this; she could do ordinary sums in multiplication and subtraction with the aid of a pencil and paper; but failed, unless they were extremely simple, to solve them mentally. Notwithstanding this, she asserted that she had been the best in her class at mental arithmetic. She possessed no particular aptitude for appreciating the passage of time. The following experiments were made after her recovery, and with the consent of her parents :—

Exp. 1.—Nov. 5, 1895 ; time 4 P.M. Suggestion giving during hypnosis : At the expiration of 5 h. and 20 m. Miss D. was to make a cross on a piece of paper, and write down the time she believed it to be without looking at clock or watch.

Result.—The suggestion was carried out the minute it fell due.

Remarks.—On this occasion I did not say anything to Miss D. about the experiment, either before or after hypnosis; and, being a somnambule, she retained in her waking consciousness no recollection of the suggestion. I told her mother its nature, but not the time at which it should be fulfilled. At 9.15 the same evening her mother noticed that Miss D. was restless and asked her what was the matter. She replied: "I feel I must do something, but cannot tell what." At 9.20 P.M. she rapidly made a cross with a pencil, and wrote "20 minutes past 9" on a piece of paper, at the same time saying: "It's all silliness." There was no clock in the room; but her mother went into the next room where there was one, and found that the time was 9.20. When I again saw Miss D., I explained the nature of the experiments I proposed making, and instructed her to carry a pencil and paper during the day, and to put them by her bedside at night. I did not describe the experiments as anything extraordinary, but simply told her that hypnotised subjects were often able to appreciate time, and that I wished to see whether she could do so. No pecuniary or other reward was promised or given. I told her I should make these suggestions from time to time, but not on each occasion she visited me. I neither told her in the waking condition that suggestions had been made, nor informed her relatives when I made them, nor what they were. They knew that suggestions of this nature were given frequently, but only became acquainted with them by seeing Miss D. carry them out, or by hearing from her that she had done so. Before making the suggestions, I wrote them down in my case-book and, when Miss D. again visited me, I copied into it what she had written on the different pieces of paper. In many instances, I did not calculate when the suggestions fell due, and in others the calculations I made at the time were proved to be erroneous, the results of the experiments in these cases being only determined when the series was completed.

The experiments which followed were all of the same character, *i.e.* during hypnosis Miss D. was told that, at the expiration of a certain number of minutes, she was to make a cross and write down the hour she believed it to be without consulting the clock, an interval of waking life always intervening between the suggestion and its fulfilment. The simple and uniform character of my experiments was due to the consideration that Delbœuf's subjects resisted suggestions that were distasteful to them. The idea of making a cross on a piece of paper excited no opposition in Miss D.'s mind ; while the fact that she recorded in writing the time at which the suggestion was fulfilled, especially when this was witnessed by others, put me in possession of evidence of a certain value. The arithmetical problems involved in the first one or two of the following experiments were comparatively simple. In No. 3, for example, as Miss D. could easily tell when 24 hours fell due, the suggestion practically resolved itself into one to be fulfilled in 100 minutes. Soon, however, the experiments became complicated and involved much more difficult problems in arithmetic.

Exp. 2.—Nov. 28, 1895 ; 2 P.M. *Sug.:* To be fulfilled in 320 m.[1]

Result.—Correct.

Remarks.—The suggestion was carried out at 7.20 P.M. when the subject was in a friend's house. She had no watch with her and the clock in the room was wrong.

Exp. 3.—Dec. 4 ; 3.15 P.M. *Sug.:* In 24 h. and 100 m.

Result.—Correct.

Remarks.—When in a friend's house the following afternoon she carried out the suggestion at 4.55. She then asked the time. Her friend looked at her watch and told her, whereupon she

---

[1] In this and all the following experiments, Miss D. was to make the cross referred to, and write down the time corresponding to the terminal minute of the series involved in the suggestion.

remarked : " Your watch is 3 minutes fast." This was the case.

Exp. 4.—Dec. 12 ; 3.20 P.M. *Sug.:* In 24 h. 1440 m.

Result.—3.20 P.M., Sat., Dec. 14 : Correct.

Exp. 5.—Wed., Dec. 18 ; 3.45 P.M. *Sug.:* In 24 h. 2880 m.

Result.—3.45 P.M., Sat., Dec. 21 : Correct.

Exp. 6.—Tues., Dec. 24 ; 2.55 P.M. *Sug.:* In 30 h. 50 m.

Result.—9.45 P.M., Wed., Dec. 25 : Correct.

Exp. 7.—Tues., Dec. 24 ; 3.10 P.M. *Sug.:* In 7200 m.

Result.—3.10 P.M., Sun., Dec. 29 : Correct.

Remarks.—When No. 7 was fulfilled Miss D. was teaching a Sunday-school class, when she suddenly felt an impulse to make a cross and mark the time. It was only after doing so that she looked at the clock, which was behind her.

Exp. 8.—Tues., Dec. 31 ; 3.45 P.M. *Sug.:* In 4335 m.

Result.—4 P.M., Fri., Jan. 3, 1896 : Correct.

Exp. 9.—Dec. 31, 1895 ; 4 P.M. *Sug.:* In 11,525 m.

Result.—11.5 A.M., Wed., Jan. 8 : Wrong.

Remarks.—The result ought to have been 4.5 P.M., Jan. 8. I rehypnotised Miss D. on that day, and asked her to recall the suggestion I had made on Dec. 31. She said it was to be executed in 11,225 m.; it is possible that I had made a mistake, but not at all likely, as I read the suggestion to her with the figures before my eyes. The supposed suggestion of 11,225 m. had been carried out correctly.

I now attempted to find out during hypnosis the subject's mental condition in reference to these suggestions. In reply to my questions she informed me :—(1) That when the suggestions were made in hypnosis she did not calculate when they fell due. (2) That she did not calculate them at any time afterwards during hypnosis. (3) That she had no recollection of them when hypnosis terminated. (4) That no memory of them ever afterwards arose in the waking state. (5) That shortly before their fulfilment she always experienced a motor impulse, *i.e.* her fingers moved as if to grasp a pencil and to perform the act of writing. (6) That this impulse was immediately followed by the idea of making a cross and writing certain figures. (7) That she

At the time I made the suggestions I also calculated when they would fall due, thus:—No. 24, Feb. 14, 5 A.M. Wrong; half an hour too late. No. 25, Feb. 14, 6.5 A.M. Wrong; half an hour too late. No. 26, Feb. 19, 3.35 P.M. Right. No. 27, Feb. 19, 4.10 P.M. Right. No. 28, Feb. 26, 4.25 P.M. Wrong; 5 m. too soon.

Results.—No. 24, Fri., Feb. 14, 4.30 A.M. Correct. No. 25, Fri., Feb. 14, 5.35 A.M. Correct. No. 26, Wed., Feb. 19, 3.35 P.M. Correct. No 27, Wed., Feb. 19, 4.10 P.M. Correct. No. 28, Wed., Feb. 26, 4.30 P.M. Correct.

Remarks.—Nos. 24 and 25 were fulfilled during sleep. On the 14th, Miss D., on awaking, found papers by her bedside with 4.30 and 5.35 written on them. On the 19th, she was hypnotised in my room at 3 P.M., and carried out Nos. 26 and 27 while in hypnosis. On both occasions she wrote the time in my notebook, and this was witnessed. I asked her during hypnosis if she remembered my last suggestion (No. 28), made the previous week. She said she did, and repeated it correctly; but stated she had never thought of it since, and did not know when it would fall due, or the number of minutes that had elapsed since it was given. She had apparently forgotten that, when the suggestion was given, she had calculated when it would fall due. No. 28 was executed correctly during hypnosis on Feb. 26.

Experiments, Wed., Feb. 19.—No. 29, 3.30 P.M. *Sug.:* In 720 m. No. 30, 3.30 P.M. *Sug.:* In 780 m. No. 31, 3.30 P.M. *Sug.:* In 2160 m. No. 32, 3 P.M. *Sug.:* In 10,135 m. No. 33, 3 P.M. *Sug.:* In 20,210 m.

Miss D.'s calculations in hypnosis :—These, with the exception of No. 32, were all correct, and her replies were almost instantaneous. No. 32 was said to be due at 2.5 P.M. on Wed., Feb. 26. This was 1 h. 50 m. too early, and represented an interval of 7 d. less 55 m., instead of 7 d. plus 55 m.

Results.—No. 29, Thur., Feb. 20, 3.30 A.M. Correct. No. 30, Thur., Feb. 20, 4.30 A.M. Correct. No. 31, Fri., Feb. 21, 3.30 A.M. Correct. No. 32, Wed., Feb. 26, 3.55 P.M. Correct. No. 33, Wed., Mar. 4, 3.50 P.M., was written down at 3.48. The calculation, therefore, was correct, but the time appreciation 2 m. too early.

Remarks.—On awaking at 7 o'clock on the morning of the 20th, Miss D. found a piece of paper with 3.30 marked on it,

and another with 4.30. On the morning of the 21st, she found
a piece of paper with 3.30 marked on it. She had no recollection of waking during the night, and, as usual, questioning in
hypnosis failed to revive any memory of what she had done. The
other suggestions were fulfilled in my room and witnessed by
others.

Experiments, Wed., Feb. 26, 3.30 P.M.—No. 34. *Sug.*: In 2140 m.
No. 35. *Sug.*: In 3590 m. No. 36. *Sug.*: In 5030 m. No. 37. *Sug.*: In
10,125 m. No. 38. *Sug.*: In 10,100 m. No. 39. *Sug.*: In 20,180 m.

Results.—No. 34, Fri., Feb. 28, 3.10 A.M. Correct. No.
35, Sat., Feb. 29, 3.20 A.M. Correct. No. 36, Sun., Mar. 1,
3.20 A.M. Correct. No. 37, due Wed., Mar. 4, at 4.15 P.M.,
was not recorded. No. 38, Wed., Mar. 4, 3.50 P.M., was written
down at 3.48. Calculation therefore correct, but time appreciation 2 m. too early. No. 39, Wed., Mar. 11, 3.50 P.M., was
written down at 3.51½. Calculation, therefore, correct, but
time appreciation 1½ m. too late.

Remarks.—These suggestions were only read to Miss D.
once ; she was then asked to repeat them, and did so correctly,
with the exception of No. 37. She was told not to make any
calculations. Nos. 34, 35 and 36 were executed during sleep,
and the papers, as usual, were found at Miss D.'s bedside in the
morning. It is to be noted that 3.50, March 4, the terminal
time of No. 38, was also the time at which another suggestion,
made a fortnight before, fell due, and which has already been
recorded in its proper place. Miss D. stated at 3.48 that she
had to make two crosses and to put down 3.50 twice. No.
37, due at 4.15 P.M., Wednesday, March 4, I have no record of.
I am not certain whether this is my fault or Miss D.'s ; I was
hypnotising another patient when the suggestions were fulfilled,
and I might well have omitted to enter this one ; on the other
hand, Miss D. might have failed to carry it out. Three
suggestions fell due very quickly, and one of them, as we have
seen, belonged to another series. When suggestions were made to
fall due in a fortnight, and I saw the subject in the week between,
I sometimes questioned her in hypnosis as to the unfulfilled
ones : she always assured me that she had never thought of
them, did not know how much of the time had elapsed, nor when
they fell due.

Experiments, Wed., Mar. 4, 3.45 P.M.—No. 40. *Sug.:* In 10,080 m. No. 41. *Sug.:* In 10,055 m. No. 42. *Sug.:* In 10,040 m. No. 43 *Sug.:* In 750 m. No. 44. *Sug.:* In 2160 m. No. 45. *Sug.:* In 2195 m.

Results.—No. 40, Wed., Mar. 11, 3.45 P.M., was written down at 3.44. Calculation correct; time appreciation 1 m. too soon. No. 41, Wed., Mar. 11, 3.20 P.M., was written down at 3.22. Calculation correct; time appreciation 2 m. too late. No. 42 Wed., Mar. 11, 3.5 P.M. Correct. No. 43, Thur., Mar. 5, 4.15 A.M., during sleep. Correct. No. 44, Fri., Mar. 6, 3.45 A.M., during sleep. Correct. No. 45, Fri., Mar. 6, 4.20 A.M., during sleep. Correct.

Remarks.—When these suggestions were given Miss D. was not asked to calculate when they would fall due. Mr. Barkworth, a member of the Society for Psychical Research, and Dr. Barclay, of South Canterbury, N.Z., were present when Nos. 40, 41 and 42 were fulfilled.

At this sitting, March 11, fresh suggestions were made under the following conditions. Mr. Barkworth and Dr. Barclay were both put *en rapport* with Miss D., and it was agreed that they should each make two time suggestions, arranged so as to fall due at the next sitting, when they promised to be present. These were given when I was out of the room, and I was not told what they were until after their fulfilment. The suggestions were as follows:—

Experiments, Wed., Mar. 11, 4 P.M.—No. 46. *Sug.:* In 21,400 m. No. 47. *Sug.:* In 21,420 m. No. 48. *Sug.:* In 21,428 m. No. 49. *Sug.:* In 21,434 m.

Results.—No. 46, Thur., Mar. 26, 12.40 P.M., was written down at 12.38. Calculation correct; time appreciation 2 m. too early. No. 47, Thur., Mar. 26, 1 P.M., was written down at 12.59. Calculation correct; time appreciation 1 m. too early. No. 48, Thur., Mar. 26, 1.8 P.M. Correct. No. 49, Thur., Mar. 26, 1.14 P.M. Correct.

Remarks.—Miss D. was hypnotised at 12.30 P.M. on Thursday, March 26, and carried out the suggestions while in that condition. Mr. Barkworth and Dr. Barclay were both present and checked the records. None of us, however, had any idea whether the experiments were carried out correctly or

K

not, as Mr. Barkworth and Dr. Barclay had mislaid their notes,
and were unable to recall the suggestions they had given.
Miss D. was roused from the hypnotic state, and, as usual,
remembered nothing of the suggestions. She was then rehypnotised, asked to recall them, and replied as follows : " They
were made at 4 P.M. last Wednesday week, and were to be
fulfilled in 21,400, 21,420, 21,428 and 21,434 minutes.
Mr. Barkworth and Dr. Barclay gave two suggestions each."
Miss D. stated that she had made no calculation at the time
and had not thought of the suggestions afterwards. On April
22, Dr. Barclay sent me the lost memorandum of his two
suggestions, viz. 21,428 and 21,434 minutes from 4 P.M. on
the day already mentioned. On April 27, Mr. Barkworth wrote
to tell me that he also had found his lost memorandum and
that the suggestions were 21,400, 21,420, 21,428 and 21,434
minutes, the first two having been made by himself, the two
latter by Dr. Barclay. This agreed with Miss D.'s account.

A fresh series of suggestions was made on April 8, some to
fall due during the night, others the following week in my
presence. The subject lost her papers recording the former, and
I was too busy to enter the latter. These are the only experiments in the whole series which are not recorded, and they are
omitted for the above reasons. Later Miss D. found the records
of the suggestions, which had been carried out during natural
sleep. They were correct.

Experiments, Thur., May 7, 3 P.M.—No. 50. *Sug.* : In 8650 m. No.
51. *Sug.* : In 8680 m. No. 52. *Sug.* : In 8700 m.

I still further complicated these by suggesting as follows : " No. 50 is
to be fulfilled in the waking state. Five minutes before No. 51 falls due
you are to pass into the hypnotic condition. No. 51 is to be fulfilled during hypnosis, but five minutes afterwards you are to pass into the normal
waking state, and continue in that until after the execution of No. 52.
Eight minutes after No. 52 is carried out hypnosis will again appear."

Results.—No. 50. (*a*) Suggestion fulfilled, Wed., May 13,
3.10. Correct. (*b*) Hypnosis appeared at 3.31 P.M. This
ought to have been 3.35 P.M., and was therefore 4 minutes too
early.

No. 51, Wed., May 13, 3.40 P.M. (*a*) Suggestion fulfilled
during hypnosis. Correct. (*b*) Miss D. passed spontaneously
into the normal state at 3.45. Correct.

No. 52, 4 P.M. (*a*) Suggestion fulfilled in the waking state. Correct. (*b*) Hypnosis appeared exactly at 4.8. Correct.

Remarks.—On May 13, Miss D. came into my consulting-room at 3.5 P.M., and almost immediately fainted. She had recently met with a severe accident and was in acute suffering. Immediately on regaining consciousness, she said she had to make a cross at 3.10 and did so in my case-book: others were present in the room when all the suggestions were fulfilled, with the exception of the first.

Experiments, Wed., May 13, 4.30 P.M.—The suggestions were given in the following general terms: " You are to repeat all the experiments made last Thursday, but to-day you are to start from 2.55 instead of 3 P.M., and to each suggestion you are to add 1440 minutes." The original suggestions were not cited, nor any other information given. The experiments, therefore, were as follows :—

No. 53, Wed., May 13, 4.30 P.M. *Sug.* : In 8650 min. from 3 P.M., plus 1440 m., minus 5 m. from starting point. No. 54, Wed., May 13, 4.30 P.M. *Sug.* : In 8680 m. from 3 P.M., plus 1440 m., minus 5 m. from starting-point. No. 55, Wed., May 13, 4.30 P.M. *Sug.* : In 8700 m. plus 1440 m., minus 5 m. from starting-point.

Results.—No. 53, Wed., May 20, 3.5 P.M. Fulfilled in the waking state. Correct. Hypnosis appeared at 3.30. Correct. No. 54, Wed., May 20, 3.35 P.M. In hypnosis. Correct.

Miss D. passed spóntaneously into the normal state at 3.40. Correct.

According to the original suggestions, Miss D. was to remain in the normal state until the fulfilment of the next experiment, but, as she had a severe headache, I hypnotised her, made curative suggestions, and told her hypnosis would terminate one minute before the next experiment fell due. She passed into the normal waking state at 3.49, 6 minutes too soon. No. 55, Wed., May 20, 3.55 P.M., was written down at 3.50. Calculation, therefore, correct, but time appreciation 5 minutes too early.

I rehypnotised Miss D. immediately the above experiment was fulfilled. At 4.3 P.M., while still in the hypnotic state, she said it was 3 minutes past 4, and that I had suggested hypnosis would appear at that hour. This was correct.

Remarks.—It is to be noted that hypnosis appeared at 3.30 P.M., the exact time suggested. This is particularly interesting, as the experiment, correctly executed at 3.30 on May 20, was the erroneously carried out experiment of May 13, complicated by five minutes having been deducted from its starting-point, and 1440 added to its interval.

No. 55 was the last experiment of the series. A few others, similar in character, were made in October, 1896. These were successful, but presented no fresh features, and as Miss D. had to cease her visits, owing to her approaching marriage, further experiment was impossible.

Summary.—Fifty-five experiments are cited; of these one, apparently, was either not carried out by Miss D., or unrecorded by me, while in another (No. 9) she mistook the original suggestion, but fulfilled it correctly in accordance with what she thought it had been. Forty-five were completely successful, *i.e.* not only did Miss D. write down the correct terminal time, but this was done, also, at the moment the experiment fell due. Eight (Nos. 33, 38, 39, 40, 41, 46, 47, 55) were partially successful. In these the terminal time was correctly recorded in every instance, but there were minute differences, never exceeding five minutes, between the subject's correct estimate of when the suggestion fell due, and the moment at which she carried it out. The proportion which these errors bear to their respective intervals varies between 1 to 2028 and 1 to 21,420. The following table gives an analysis of the conditions under which the experiments were carried out and their results :—

EXPERIMENT	EXPERIMENTS	WITNESSED BY				RESULTS			REMARKS
		Friends or Relatives	Bralwell and Others	Bralwell Alone	Unwitnessed	Correct	Wrong	Unrecorded	
Fulfilled in the waking state	26	14	11	1	0	20	6	0	1 mistaken suggestion. 1 fulfilled 2 minutes too soon. 1 ,, 2 ,, ,, 1 ,, 1 ,, ,, 1 ,, 2 ,, ,, 1 ,, 5 ,, ,,
Fulfilled in hypnosis	15	0	15	0	0	12	3	0	1 fulfilled 1½ minutes too soon. 1 ,, 2 ,, ,, 1 ,, 1 ,, ,,
Fulfilled in natural sleep	13	0	0	0	13	13	0	0	In each instance figures which correctly represented the terminal time of the experiment were found at the subject's bedside in the morning; but there is no evidence to show whether this was done at the moment the suggestion fell due—i.e. the subject's calculations were correct, but evidence as to the time appreciation is wanting.
Unfulfilled	1	0	0	0	1	0	0	1	It is doubtful whether this experiment was carried out by the subject. It is, however, possible that I omitted to record it, as it fell due when I was engaged with another patient.
TOTAL	55	14	26	1	14	45	9	1	

Similar experiments, more or less successful, were made with other somnambules, but in none were the results so striking as with Miss D. In those about to be cited the subject was Miss O., aged 20, an intelligent, well-educated girl, who had received some scientific training. Her arithmetical powers were superior to Miss D.'s, but she possessed no particular aptitude for appreciating the passage of time. She was a somnambule, could be rendered anæsthetic and analgesic by suggestion, and had been the subject of several painless minor surgical operations. Her health, from the commencement of the experiments up to the last report (January 1903) has been good.

The first experiments consisted in determining by suggestion the time of waking from normal sleep. The hours selected varied widely; but the results were almost uniformly successful, and the greatest error recorded did not exceed five minutes. Others similar to Miss D.'s followed, thus:—

Exp. 1, Nov. 25, 1895, 3.55 P.M. *Sug.*: In 24 h. and 50 m. *Res.*: Correct. *Remarks*: In reply to questioning in hypnosis, Miss O. stated that when the suggestion was given she calculated when it would fall due and determined to carry it out at that hour. *Exp.* 2, Nov. 27, 1.20 P.M. *Sug.*: In 1445 m. *Res.*: 10 m. too early. *Exp.* 3, Dec. 6.3 P.M. *Sug.*: In 1440 m. *Res.*: Correct. *Exp.* 4, Dec. 9, 3.15 P.M. *Sug.*: In 2880 m. *Res.*: Correct. *Exp.* 5, Dec. 12, 3.30 P.M. *Sug.*: In 1540 m. *Res.*: 7 m. too late. *Exp.* 6, Dec. 16, 3.30 P.M. *Sug.*: In 1620 m. *Res.*: 13 m. too late. *Exp.* 7, Dec. 20, 3 P.M. *Sug.*: In 1380 m. *Res.*: Correct. *Exp.* 8, Dec. 31, 3.15 P.M. *Sug.*: In 24 h. 1200 m. *Res.*: Correct. *Exp.* 9, Jan. 2, 1896, 3.10 P.M. *Sug.*: In 24 h. 1430 m. Miss O.'s calculation, made in hypnosis, was 40 m. too early. *Res.*: 5 m. too late. *Exp.* 10, Jan. 6, 3.15 P.M. *Sug.*: In 24 h. 100 m. Miss O.'s calculation in hypnosis was correct. *Res.*: 8 m. too late. *Exp.* 11, Jan. 27, 3.10 P.M. *Sug.*: In 24 h. 150 m. Miss O.'s calculation in hypnosis was correct. *Res.*: 10 m. too soon. *Exp.* 12, Mar. 27, 3.10 P.M. *Sug.*: In 24 h. 240 m. Miss O.'s calculation in hypnosis was correct. *Res.*: Correct.

Time experiments more or less closely resembling those cited were repeated occasionally with Miss O. up to August, 1900, and with practically identical results.

Before considering theoretical explanations of hypnotic and post-hypnotic appreciation of time, I propose to discuss (A) the possibilities of mal-observation or deception, and (B) to draw attention to certain other points which appear worthy of notice.

(A) THE QUESTION OF MAL-OBSERVATION OR DECEPTION.

(1) The subjects of all my time experiments were either former patients or personal friends. None of them were trained hypnotic subjects, and in no single instance was a pecuniary reward promised or given. All this, however, does not in itself exclude the possibility of mal-observation or deception, and I would rather base my arguments in favour of the genuineness of the results on post-hypnotic amnesia, and the fact that some of the problems involved were beyond the subjects' waking powers.

(2) While, however, all observers recognise post-hypnotic amnesia, it must still be admitted that loss of memory might be assumed for purposes of deception. Fortunately, there are other hypnotic phenomena impossible of imitation; amongst these may be cited: (a) the absence of certain organic changes following injury (Delbœuf's case of two symmetrical burns), and (b) the absence of physiological signs of pain during severe and prolonged operation. The latter fact was clearly demonstrated in the operations on my patients at Goole and Leeds (*Journal of Dental Science*, March 30, 1890,[1] and *Lancet*, April 5, 1890).[2] Several of these patients were afterwards the subjects of my time experiments, and all who were employed for this purpose, including Miss D. and Miss O., could be easily rendered anæsthetic or analgesic by suggestion.

(3) Post-hypnotic amnesia alone, even when it is undoubtedly genuine, does not exclude possible error, as the subject might receive information from the operator or spectators. It is, however, difficult to say how this could have happened in Miss D.'s case. Thus, twenty-seven experiments were fulfilled in my absence, and no information regarding these—excluding of course the suggestions made to Miss D. during hypnosis—was given to any one until some time after the whole series was completed. I did not calculate when any of these twenty-seven suggestions would fall due, and did not know, until after their fulfilment, whether they had been carried out correctly or not. Twenty-seven further experiments were fulfilled in my presence; these, with one exception, were also witnessed by others. In four of them suggestions were made by Mr. Barkworth and Dr. Barclay; and I did not know what they were until afterwards. These

[1] Pp. 162-3   [2] Pp. 164-7.

two operators, however, could not assist the subject, as they had
lost the memoranda of their suggestions and were unable to recall
the figures.   In the remaining twenty-three, none of the spectators
knew what the suggestions were.   Indeed, in most instances they
did not know that any experiments were being carried on until
they saw them executed and were asked to witness the figures,
their ignorance being purposely arranged.

(4) In the twenty-three cases just cited, before giving the
suggestions I calculated when they would fall due.   Could Miss
D. have learnt anything about this through telepathy or muscle-
reading ?   During the last . twelve years, I have searched for
evidence of telepathy, and also taken part in the experiments of
other observers ; the results, however, have invariably been
negative.   If, for argument's sake, we conceded the possibility of
telepathy, recognising also that somnambules possess hyperæsthesia
of the special senses, it would still be difficult to see what information Miss D. could have obtained from me.   In the majority
of the experiments I did not work out when the experiments
would fall due ; and, even when I did, many of my calculations
were only approximately correct, although I was not aware of
this until after all the experiments were completed.   Moreover,
I have an unusually bad memory for figures, and never, either
before or during the execution of the suggestions, recalled my
calculations as to the time at which they were supposed to fall
due.   Further, when the experiments were carried out, I was
nearly always busily engaged with other patients, and so placed
that Miss D. could not see my face.

(5) Again, even supposing post-hypnotic amnesia had not
existed in Miss D.'s case, the retention in the waking state of
the memories of hypnotic life would not in itself explain her
feats in calculation and time appreciation.   Miss D.'s memory,
knowledge of arithmetic and power of appreciating time, in no
way exceeded that of other imperfectly educated girls in her
station of life.   Her normal memory was incapable of retaining
complicated series of figures, and she was unable to make even
much simpler mental calculations than those involved.   After
the suggestions were made, she remained in the hypnotic state
for an hour or more and could not consult the clock.   During
this period, it was absolutely impossible for her to record the
suggestion in any way other than mentally.

(B) OTHER POINTS OF INTEREST.

(1) Five minutes before the first experiment was fulfilled, Miss D. became restless and felt she must do something. This preliminary state of restlessness was absent in all the subsequent ones. In them, when the time for carrying out the suggestions arrived, Miss D. had a sudden twitching of the fingers of her right hand, immediately followed by the idea of writing down certain figures. The abruptness of this invasion of the normal consciousness, by a message from the subliminal one, was particularly noticeable when Miss D. was actively engaged in conversation at the time.

(2) On the twenty-four occasions Miss D. was asked to calculate when the suggestions fell due, she was wrong in the first nine instances, but in the remaining fifteen right in eleven and wrong in four. As the experiments advanced, not only the frequency, but also the extent, of Miss D.'s errors in calculation decreased, and the answers were given much more rapidly. Sometimes the correct replies were almost instantaneous, and in these instances no conscious calculation could be traced. It is to be noted that Miss D.'s mistaken calculations had no effect on the correctness of her results.

(3) *Memory.*—Once only did Miss D. spontaneously recall in hypnosis that a time suggestion—yet unfulfilled—had been given. This was Experiment No. 3, where the suggestion was an easily remembered one, viz. 24 hours and 100 minutes. On other occasions, when Miss D. was questioned in hypnosis as to the unfulfilled suggestions, she invariably recalled the fact that these had been made, but rarely remembered their exact terms. She always asserted that she had never thought of them, did not know how much time had elapsed since they had been given, nor when they were due. This was so even in cases where she had correctly calculated the terminal time. At first Miss D. forgot all about the suggestions immediately after they were fulfilled: she did not know she had made a cross or written down the figures, and could not recall what they meant. This condition of memory was identical with what is almost universally associated with post-hypnotic acts. Later, for convenience' sake, it was suggested to Miss D. during hypnosis that she should remember having executed the experiments. She then knew in the waking

state that she had made a cross, and written down certain figures, but recalled nothing of the original suggestion of which these acts were the fulfilment. When Miss D. was questioned in hypnosis, *after the execution of the suggestions*, her memory, on certain points, was very clear. She could recall in every detail the terms of all experiments that had recently been carried out, *i.e.* she remembered the hours at which they had been made, the number of minutes suggested, her own calculations, if any, and the moment and circumstances under which the suggestions had been fulfilled. Putting aside the calculations she made at the time in response to suggestion, she was unable to recall having made any others, or to give any information as to the methods by means of which she had correctly fulfilled the experiments. When a second series of suggestions was given, before the first had been fulfilled, after all had been carried out, she could recall both series and place each member of them in its proper order. This memory, however, was not persistent. A fortnight after the experiments had been executed, although Miss D. still remembered in hypnosis that they had taken place, she was unable to recall the details. When experiments were fulfilled in normal sleep she remembered their terms in hypnosis, and when they had been given, but not when they had been executed.

(4) The experiments had no prejudicial effect on Miss D.'s health. On the contrary, this steadily improved. She is now a strong, healthy, well-developed woman, the mother of two children, and has had no return of her nervous symptoms.

In no single instance did any bad effect, even of the most trivial description, follow these or other hypnotic experiments.

(5) The results of the experiments were only estimated after the series was completed, when a friend, Mr. Bartrum, B.Sc., kindly checked them for me. He discovered that some of my calculations made at the time had been erroneous. I am also indebted to him for a critical examination of the calculations the patient was asked to make when the suggestions were given.

(6) With the following exception, the phenomena observed in the cases of Miss D. and Miss O. differed little. When a simple suggestion was given, Miss O. sometimes spontaneously calculated when it would fall due. Miss D., on the other hand, never made any spontaneous calculations at all. Apparently Miss O. did not spontaneously calculate the more complicated

arithmetical problems. When she did so, in response to suggestion, her results were invariably correct; but, despite this, the
experiments were not always fulfilled at their appropriate time.
Miss D., on the contrary, was often wrong in her calculations,
while the suggestions themselves were carried out with phenomenal
accuracy.

(7) In some later experiments Miss O. apparently made no
spontaneous calculations, despite the fact that the arithmetical
problems involved were extremely simple. For example, I
suggested that she should shake hands with me forty minutes
after I aroused her from hypnosis. At the moment indicated, in
the midst of an animated conversation, she suddenly asked me to
shake hands with her. In reply to my questions, she said she
had felt impelled to do this, but could not tell why. A few
minutes later she had entirely forgotten the incident. I rehypnotised her; she then recalled the suggestion and the impulse
she had experienced, but could not remember having made any
calculation or having in any way marked the passage of time.

(G) Automatic Writing in Hypnosis.

Most of the time appreciation experiments just referred to
involved a certain amount of " automatic writing." In the experiments about to be cited automatic writing was the main feature;
and its occurrence, while the normal consciousness was otherwise
actively engaged, the chief point of interest.

In choosing a subject for this form of experiment two things
are essential, viz. (1) he must be a somnambule, *i.e.* retain no
memory on awaking of what has passed in the hypnotic state,
and (2) hypnosis must be capable of being induced and terminated
instantaneously. Thus, when hypnosis is terminated immediately
after the suggestion has been given, it follows that the problem
must be solved by the secondary consciousness, while the subject
is in the waking state, and his normal consciousness purposely
actively engaged.

I have often made the following and similar experiments. I
ask a subject while awake to write down a few verses: these I
take charge of and do not show him again. I then make him
read aloud from some book previously unknown to him: this

being chosen in order to engage his entire attention. While reading, I hypnotise him suddenly, place pencil and paper near his right hand and suggest: "On waking you will go on reading where you left off, and at the same time write down how often "b" (or any other letter selected) occurs in the verses you gave me. Wake up." He awakes, resumes reading, and at the same time writes down the answer to the problem suggested. This, almost invariably correct, is often done so rapidly that I have not had time to count the letters, even with the verses before me. I now tell the subject to stop reading, and ask him what he has written. He replies: "Nothing," and when I show him the paper, is astonished and declares he does not know what it means. I then rehypnotise him, whereupon the lost memory returns, and he not only recalls the suggestion, but also the fact that he has carried it out.

Thus, the primary waking consciousness retains no recollection of the hypnotic suggestions. It does not know that the secondary consciousness, after the hypnotic state has been terminated, first solves the problems and then directs the motor acts which record the solutions. It is also unconscious of the motor acts themselves.

Gurney made many interesting experiments, with healthy, non-hysterical men, which illustrate the severance of the normal or primary, from the latent or secondary, consciousness. Of these the following are examples:—

(1) The first were simple cases which involved memory, but not independent thought. Thus, Gurney showed P., one of his subjects, a planchette and made him write his name with it. P. was then hypnotised, told that it had been as dark as night in London on the previous day, and that he would record this fact in writing. On awaking he remembered nothing. His hand was then placed on the planchette—a large screen being held in front of his face, so that it was impossible for him to see the paper or the instrument—and in less than a minute he wrote: "It was a dark day in London yesterday."

(2) In the next experiments statements were impressed on the subjects, but nothing was said as to subsequently recording them. After waking, however, the writing was executed as before.

(3) Gurney made more complicated experiments with another subject. During hypnosis, questions were asked about his past life, or arithmetical problems were suggested. He was then awakened

immediately, before he had time to think of a reply, and, to engross his attention, told to count backwards from a hundred ; meanwhile the planchette wrote the correct answers to the different questions.

(4) Further experiments involved the reckoning of time. These, however, were not confined to the execution of an order at a given moment, but involved, in addition, other calculations made in the waking state *at a suddenly selected moment*, regarding which nothing had been previously said to the subject. For instance, during hypnosis he was told that he had to do something at a given date, and also that, before this time arrived, he would be required to write down the number of minutes that had passed since the suggestion was given, as well as the number that had still to elapse before its fulfilment. In the interval, when his hand was placed upon the planchette he generally wrote the answers to the problems. The results, allowing for the time occupied in writing, were remarkably accurate.

The mental states involved in these various experiments will be discussed in the chapter on " Theory."

(H) Telepathy, Clairvoyance, etc.

Many of the mesmerists, including Elliotson and Esdaile, believed in the existence of telepathy, clairvoyance, and other so-called "higher" or "occult" phenomena. In telepathy, thought was supposed to be conveyed directly from the brain of one person to that of another, without the intervention of any of the usual media of transmission ; in clairvoyance, the subject was supposed to see, as in a mirror or picture, events which were taking place at a distance. Braid, as we shall see in discussing his theories, showed that the belief in telepathy and clairvoyance was the result of mal-observation and self-deception. Within recent times, however, there has been a revival in the belief as to the existence of telepathy and clairvoyance, particularly the former. To confine ourselves for the moment to telepathy, we find its existence asserted by two classes of observers :—

(1) A small group—mainly comprised of men who had distinguished themselves in one or more branches of science— who

claimed to have investigated the alleged phenomena by scientific methods.   Amongst these may be cited the late Professor Henry Sidgwick, Frederick Myers, Edmund Gurney and Dr. A. T. Myers. Although their experiments were carefully conducted, it is doubtful whether all possible sources of error were excluded; and I am unable to accept them as conclusive.

(2) The second group—who boldly assert that telepathy is an accepted scientific fact, a phenomenon which any expert can produce at will—belong to a totally different class.   Thus, Hudson, in his book, *The Law of Psychic Phenomena*, talks of telepathy as a recognised commonplace, and describes it as the basis of the most successful branch of Christian Science, namely "the Absence Treatment."   Here the physician sits dreamily in his consulting-room at home, and sends mental curative suggestions to his different patients.   Or, better still, he just thinks of them a moment before going to sleep at night; and then his "subconscious mind" works on their "subconscious minds" while all of them are sleeping.   The patients are not aware of receiving any impression from the operator, but that is easily explained—their normal consciousness does not know what is happening to their "subconscious mind."   For these extraordinary statements Mr. Hudson has no evidence of value to offer; but, despite this, the merits of the absence treatment must be obvious to the hard-worked general practitioner.

After many years' hypnotic work, and frequent opportunities of investigating the experiments of others, I have seen nothing, absolutely nothing, which might be fairly considered as affording even the slightest evidence for the existence of telepathy, or any of the so-called "occult" phenomena.

For several years a Committee of the Society for Psychical Research, of which I was a member, devoted itself mainly to telepathic experiments.   Our methods were simple and effective, and yet placed no unnecessary barrier in the way of the appearance of the phenomenon.   The subject, generally hypnotised, was placed in an armchair, and told that the operator would select different cards from a pack and that he, the subject, was to try to guess the cards in turn.   The operator, who was so placed that the subject could not see what he was doing, drew the cards from the pack at random, told the subject that he had selected one, that he was looking hard at it, and that he, the subject, would see or know what it was. Meanwhile the operator stared fixedly at the card for several minutes, and concentrated his attention entirely on it. In these experiments, as well as in a long series of private ones, the percentage of correct guesses fell below the number which ought to have been reached according to the laws of chance. Despite all this, it would be unphilosophic to deny the possibility of telepathy; and I am quite ready to be convinced of its existence, if any one can divine even as few as six out of every dozen cards selected by the operator under circumstances similar to those described.

In all the cases of alleged clairvoyance that I have seen, the operator—either consciously or unconsciously—so aided the subject by suggestions as to render the experiments absolutely valueless. In some instances, of which an example will be cited later, the so-called clairvoyant not only pretends to see what is passing at the time, at some more or less distant place, but also claims to be able to foretell what will happen in the future.

(I) Volition in Hypnosis—Suggested Crimes—Automatism.

The question, whether the hypnotised subject is an automaton or still retains the power of exercising his volition, is the most important one with which we have to deal. In this chapter I ought to cite the cases which illustrate the mental condition in hypnosis, but, as these are conflicting, some apparently showing evidence of the existence of automatism, others of an opposite state, I shall defer doing so until discussing hypnotic Theories, when, for convenience' sake, the phenomena and their varying explanations will be dealt with together.

CHAPTER VI.

BRAID successfully demonstrated that many of the alleged phenomena of mesmerism owed their origin to defective methods of observation. He drew out a list of the more important sources of error which, he said, ought always to be kept in mind by the operator. These, which I now give, should be placed in a prominent position in every hypnotic laboratory :—

(1) The hyperæsthesia of the organs of special sense, which enabled impressions to be perceived through the ordinary media that would have passed unrecognised in the waking condition.

(2) The docility and sympathy of the subjects, which tended to make them imitate the actions of others.

(3) The extraordinary revival of memory by which they could recall things long forgotten in the waking state.

(4) The remarkable effect of contact in arousing memory, i.e. by acting as the signal for the production of a fresh hypnosis.

(5) The condition of double consciousness or double personality.

(6) The vivid state of the imagination in hypnosis, which instantly invested every suggested idea, or remembrance of past impressions, with the attributes of present realities.

(7) Deductions rapidly drawn by the subject from unintentional suggestions given by the operator.

(8) The tendency of the human mind, in those with a great love of the marvellous, erroneously to interpret the subject's replies in accordance with their own desires.

Braid considered that belief in thought transference arose from failure to guard against the sources of error similar to those just described, and stated that he had never met with any case where the subjects could correctly interpret his unexpressed desires, without some sensible indication of them. Braid was also absolutely incredulous as to the existence of clairvoyance; and, although he made numerous experiments, not only upon his own subjects, but also upon many of the renowned clairvoyants of the day, he never found anything but hypnotic exaggeration of natural powers. In reference to the alleged intuitive powers of mesmeric subjects he held that, whereas with animals instinct was usually right, with somnambules it was generally wrong. It was true that certain patients could successfully predict their own hysterical attacks, but here the prophecy produced its own fulfilment by self-suggestion.

The following may also be noted as possible sources of error in hypnotic experiment:—

(1) *Operator and subject may both voluntarily try to deceive the spectator.* For example, the stage performer frequently asserts that he can produce telepathic phenomena at will. The following are examples of the way in which this is done:—

(*a*) The operator leaves the room : his accomplice then arranges a number of cards face upwards upon the table, asks the spectators to select one, without altering their position, and to tell him which is chosen. The operator is then recalled : he asks the spectators to think of the card selected, and quickly tells them which it was. The accomplice has indicated it by touching that part of his own face, which represents the card, according to the private code existing between him and the operator.

(*b*) Sometimes the spectators are requested to choose any number they like. The operator enters, puts his hands on the head of each spectator in turn, and asks him to think of the selected number. When he comes to his accomplice, the latter indicates the number by moving his jaws.

(*c*) The trick may be made more striking by means of an elaborate code. The subject is blindfolded, and placed at the opposite end of the platform from the operator. The latter asks the spectators to hand him coins, watches, and the like. While he holds these in his hands, the accomplice correctly cites the dates upon them, etc. The necessary information is conveyed by means of a sort of patter: thus, each time the operator receives an object he explains to the audience the impossibility of deception, etc. This gives the necessary information. certain words

L

or letters, according to previous arrangement, indicating certain figures, etc.

In instances similar to the above, although the operator generally pretends that the subject's occult powers are due to hypnotism, it is often obvious that the latter has never been hypnotised at all. Sometimes, however, it is only the operator who is consciously acting a fraud, and the subject may be a somnambule who shows real, but erroneously interpreted, post-hypnotic phenomena. Thus, the operator may suggest to the subject during hypnosis that he is to perform certain acts in the waking state at a given date, and then skilfully induce the spectators—who are ignorant of the post-hypnotic suggestions—to believe that they have had a voice in the time fixed for the appearance of the phenomena to be evoked.

(2) *The operator may be honest, while the subjects may try to deceive him.* The latter are of two classes: (*a*) Those who deceive for gain: paid subjects whose interest it is that the desired phenomena should appear. (*b*) Hysterical subjects, who wish to attract attention, and whose vanity is flattered if the experiments succeed. A dishonest subject, acquainted with the phenomena of hypnosis, can undoubtedly simulate many of them more or less exactly. He may even, by training, acquire a certain amount of the hyperæsthesia of the special senses that characterises deep hypnosis, and use this in the production of the alleged telepathic phenomena, etc. In the case of hysterical subjects it is difficult to determine how much is conscious fraud, how much unconscious self-deception. In some instances, the phenomena are alleged to owe their origin to a spirit who "controls" the subject, and uses him for conveying a message from the other world.

The following case came under my own observation:—Mrs. —— has convinced many people, some of them of scientific eminence, that she is a medium of communication between this and the unseen world. She is not a paid subject: beyond this I have nothing to say, one way or the other, either as to her good faith or the condition of her nervous system, but will simply relate what occurred. At the request of a friend, who believed in Mrs. ——'s powers, I accompanied him to her house. At first we sat and talked, waiting for the moment when Mrs. —— should be "controlled" by the spirit—that of a dead child. In about a quarter of an hour, Mrs. —— partially closed her eyes, and I was informed she had passed into a condition of hypnotic trance. A few minutes later she commenced to talk in a baby-voice, and carried on a conversation with my friend. This was of no particular interest. She then asked whether I had a letter in my pocket. I gave her one; when she at once proceeded to give me alleged spirit information, both as to the letter and its writer. She said: " The letter has come a long, long way. It has come from over the sea. It has had difficulty in finding you. The person who wrote it is living in a strange land ; high, high up in a house with many steps. There are crowds of people down below walking loudly; they have clogs on. The person who wrote the letter is a woman. She is worrying about money, but she need not; she is quite rich. She thinks she is ill, but she isn't; there is nothing the matter with her. She wants a good shaking; it would do her good if you threw her out of the window."

Some of this information was correct, but could have been equally well given by any one with ordinary intelligence. The medium's eyes were partially open: the envelope bore a foreign stamp, and, owing to my absence from town, had been readdressed. Further, the character of the handwriting was obviously feminine. It was, therefore, easy to guess that the letter had come from a foreign country—consequently from over the sea—and that it was from a woman. The remaining statements, however, did not give me a high opinion of spirit intelligence. Thus, the writer of the letter had a sufficient and assured income, but was neither wealthy nor troubled about money. She was not an imaginary invalid: on the contrary, she had had her breast amputated for cancer, and also several of her fingers and toes on account of Rénaud's disease.[1] This latter malady was still progressing and caused her severe suffering, which she bore with great patience. She wrote from Mustapha Superior, where the Arabs do not go about in clogs; and, on account of her lameness, had certainly not chosen her rooms on the top of a tower.

My experiences as to other alleged cases of spiritualistic phenomena, whether occurring in mediumistic, hysterical, or alleged hypnotic trance, have left me equally unconvinced of the truth of spiritualism. On the other hand, they have produced strong conviction as to several other things ; but what these are I may leave my readers to divine.

[1] Case No. 5, pp. 181-2.

(3) *The accuracy of the experiments may be destroyed by un-intentional errors on the part of the operator, the subject, or both.* These form by far the most frequent sources of fallacy. Thus, the assumption by the mesmerists, and by the hypnotists of the Salpêtrière school, that the subjects were unconscious during the lethargic stage, was the source of widespread error. All the phenomena supposed to be due to the action of metals, magnets, drugs in sealed tubes, etc., were really due to the verbal suggestions of the operator. The "control" experiments by which Braid demonstrated this source of fallacy are worthy of note. He showed (*a*) how the phenomena, supposed to be due to a magnet, for example, appeared in the presence of an imitation one, which the subject believed to be real. (*b*) Again, the phenomena did not appear in the presence of a real magnet, when the subject did not know it was near. (*c*) Finally, the phenomena could be evoked by verbal suggestion, without the presence of magnets, either real or imitation.

Undoubtedly one of the commonest sources of error is the hyperæsthesia of the organs of special sense, which is so characteristic of deep hypnosis. Nor is the hyperæsthesia confined to the hypnotised subject alone, for I have seen professional thought-readers, who by watching the faces of the spectators were able to divine their thoughts. Even if the bulk of the audience controlled the expression of their emotion, one amongst them, more enthusiastic or less well-balanced than his companions, was apt to give the necessary information. Thus, the Hypnotic Committee of the Society for Psychical Research found that a thought-reader could successfully exercise her art in the presence of a certain group of the members. She failed entirely, however, when Dr. A., who may be described as a believer in the occult, was eliminated. When each member of the group, with the exception of Dr. A., was experimented on individually the results were also negative: when, however, Dr. A. was taken alone the experiments were again successful. On another occasion, Dr. B., a foreign *savant*, who had recorded numerous successful telepathic experiments, was present. In his case the indications given, by voice and gesture, were so obvious as to be absurd; but, notwithstanding this, he undoubtedly believed he was carefully conducting a scientific experiment.

Although many errors may arise in hypnotic experiment,

they can be usually avoided by care and experience. The following rules should be adopted, viz. :—

(1) Never experiment with paid subjects.

(2) If possible, choose healthy men : they will not suffer from a hysterical desire to appear interesting.

(3) Whenever it can be done,· the operator should select subjects whom he knows and can trust.

(4) The hypnotised subject, no matter in what stage, should be regarded not only as *awake*, but also as possibly possessing *increased* activity of the special senses.

(5) All physiological experiments ought to be conducted in a laboratory, and tested with instruments of precision. The operator should confine himself to exciting the phenomena, which should invariably be recorded by an independent observer.

(6) Psychological experiments cannot be conducted in the same way as physiological ones. Amnesia, for example, can neither be weighed in a balance nor precipitated in a test-tube. Experiments of this kind should therefore not only be numerous, but be made on many different subjects, with every precaution taken to ensure their trustworthiness. Further, the results should be checked by independent observers, and everything done to prevent error arising through the operator's unconscious self-deception.

CHAPTER VII.

As we have seen, many and widely varying phenomena occur in hypnosis, and frequent attempts have been made to group these in such a way as to divide the condition itself into different stages. Thus, Braid employed the term "Hypnotism" to denote, not a single state, but a large number of widely varying stages or conditions. These he divided into three main groups :—

(1) **Slight Hypnosis.**—The subjects became more or less lethargic, but were conscious of what took place and suffered no subsequent loss of memory. This group comprised 90 per cent of those who responded to curative suggestions.

(2) **Deep Hypnosis.**—The subjects on awaking were unable to recall the events of hypnosis, but, on being rehypnotised, the lost memory could be revived. This condition Braid termed "double consciousness."

This latter condition he further subdivided into two others :—

(a) *Alert*, characterised by hyperæsthesia of the special senses and increased power of co-ordinate muscular movements.

(b) *Deep*, distinguished by general loss of sensibility.

(3) **Hypnotic Coma.**—The deepest stage of all. Here, not only were the events of hypnosis forgotten on awaking, but the lost memory could not be revived in subsequent hypnoses.[1]

Braid believed also in the existence of numerous intermediate stages, which passed into one another by insensible gradations. In all of them, however, the training which the subject received from the operator played an important part.

Many other attempts at classification have been made.

Thus, in the opinion of the Salpêtrière school, the hypnotic condition is divided into three clearly defined stages, viz.

---

[1] At a later date, Braid believed that the lost memory could be revived in subsequent hypnoses.

Lethargy, Catalepsy, and Somnambulism. These, they say, usually occur in fixed order and are induced, as well as the phenomena which characterise them, by definite physical stimuli.

(1) Lethargy, usually obtained by causing the subject to look steadily at an object placed at a short distance above the eyes, is characterised by what Charcot termed "neuro-muscular hyper-excitability," *i.e.* the muscles contract either singly or in groups, when a mechanical stimulus is applied to the muscles themselves, to their tendons, or to the nerves which supply them. This stage is changed into others by the action of certain physical stimuli. Thus :—

(2) Catalepsy is evoked by raising the subject's eyelids and is marked by muscular rigidity ; the limbs maintaining, for an abnormally lengthened period, any position in which they are placed.

(3) Somnambulism is produced by pressing or rubbing the top of the head, and is distinguished by purely "automatic phenomena" originating solely from the commands of the operator.

The classification of the Nancy school is by no means uniform. Thus, Liébeault gives six stages :—

(1) Drowsiness.

(2) Drowsiness : suggestive catalepsy possible.

(3) Light Sleep : automatic movements possible.

(4) Deep Sleep : here the subject ceases to be in relation with the outer world ; he hears what the operator says, but not what is said by others around him.

(5) Light Somnambulism : memory on awaking indistinct and hazy.

(6) Deep Somnambulism : entire loss of memory on awaking. All the phenomena of post-hypnotic suggestion possible.

Bernheim divides hypnosis into nine degrees :—

(1) Drowsiness : the subject is able to open his eyes, but does not exhibit catalepsy, anæsthesia, hallucinations, or sleep properly so called. He is, however, to a certain extent suggestible ; and distinct therapeutic effects may be obtained.

(2) This stage resembles the first, with the exception that the subject is unable to open his eyes.

(3) Here, whether the eyes are open or shut, and the subject drowsy or wakeful, catalepsy can be suggested : the position, however, can be changed by an effort of the subject's will.

(4) In this stage automatic movements may frequently be

induced, but the subject is unable voluntarily to terminate suggested catalepsy.

(5) In addition to the phenomena manifested in the previous stage, contractures can now be induced by suggestion and various muscular movements inhibited.

(6) The subject now exhibits a more or less automatic obedience : he is inert and passive if left to himself, but rises, stands, or walks at command.

(7) This stage is characterised by loss of memory on awaking, but hallucinations cannot be suggested.

(8) Here, in addition to loss of memory, hallucinations can be induced during hypnosis, but post-hypnotic hallucinations cannot be evoked.

(9) In this stage, in addition to the phenomena already enumerated, post-hypnotic hallucinations are possible.

Forel gives three stages :—

(1) Drowsiness : the subject can resist suggestions with an effort.

(2) Hypotaxy (Fascination): here, voluntary muscular movements can be inhibited and the subject is unable to open his eyes.

(3) Somnambulism : this is characterised by loss of memory on awaking, *i.e.* the subject has forgotten the events of hypnosis.

Delbœuf divided hypnotic phenomena as follows :—

(1) The stage in which pain is felt.

(2) The one in which analgesia can be produced.

Edmund Gurney gave two stages, closely resembling those of Braid already referred to, viz.: (1) Alert; (2) Deep.

Max Dessoir divides hypnotic phenomena into the following two large groups, which are separated from each other by the extent of the functional disturbances :—

(1) In this class the voluntary muscles alone are affected.

(2) Here, in addition, changes in the special senses occur.

Remarks.—The artificial character of the stages is the point most worthy of notice in all these attempts at classification. According to Braid, the phenomena of hypnotism only appeared after certain changes had been evoked in the central nervous system. They did not even then arise spontaneously, however, but owed their origin either to self-suggestions or to the training of the subject by the operator. These facts have been largely ignored by later writers. The Nancy school, while

pointing out the artificial nature of the stages of the Salpêtrière, fail to recognise that their own classification not only
possesses similar disadvantages, but is also still more complicated.
Thus, in the case of such phenomena as closure of the eyes and
rigidity of the limbs, Max Dessoir has drawn attention to the
fact that the closing of the eyes in hypnosis is a pure accident—
the result of a method which has become more or less stereotyped—and states that hypnosis is frequently induced while
the eyes remain open.   This criticism is a just one, for the
suggestion that the eyelids should close is usually the very first
that is made in practice.   Further, once the eyes have been
closed by suggestion, rigidity of the limbs does not follow as a
natural sequence, but requires to be suggested in its turn.
Thus, if during hypnosis I lift the arm of an untrained subject,
it will fall directly I release it.   If I suggest, however, that the
limb shall remain in the position in which I have placed it,
the phenomenon generally appears.   I can only recall one instance
in which muscular changes took place in an untrained subject
without direct suggestion.   Deep hypnosis was obtained at the
first attempt and the condition known as *flexibilitas cerea* appeared.
This subject, however, had seen others hypnotised in whom
muscular changes had been induced ; and probably, in her case,
the *flexibilitas cerea* was the result of self-suggestion.

Further, the phenomena that characterise the lethargic
stage or appear on its termination are suggested, either by the
operator or by the subjects themselves.   The latter almost invariably believe that hypnosis is identical with sleep : this to them
means forgetfulness on awaking, *i.e.* post-hypnotic amnesia.   This
self-suggestion is so ingrained that explanation is usually powerless to remove it ; and, unless amnesia has been induced, the
subject almost invariably asserts that he has not been hypnotised.   In many of my earlier cases, it is true, analgesia and
hypnosis appeared simultaneously, although I had given no suggestion to that effect.   Indirect suggestion, however, had certainly
not been excluded, as the fact that many painless hypnotic operations had been performed on my patients was well known.

Moll, from the objections he raises to the classification of
Forel, Liébeault and Bernheim, evidently believes that certain
hypnotic phenomena arise spontaneously.   He complains that
the writers referred to contrast the particular group of hypnotic

states followed by amnesia with others in which no loss of memory occurs; whereas it would be better to base classification on the phenomena that appeared during hypnosis, rather than on the forgetfulness which follows it. Memory after hypnosis, he says, is influenced by many factors, including suggestion, which have nothing to do with the depth of the hypnosis. The same objection, however, as we have seen, may be applied with equal justice to all the phenomena which are usually selected as characteristic of the different stages. In nearly every instance the presence of direct or indirect suggestion can be easily demonstrated, while it would be difficult to find a single case in which it is possible to prove that suggestions have been entirely excluded. Another point to which I propose referring more fully is the question of volition. Bernheim's stages are largely based upon the so-called "automatism" of the subject, and his alleged inability to resist suggestions; but, as I hope to show, neither of these phenomena characterises hypnosis.

With so much evidence in favour of the artificial character both of hypnotic phenomena and of their sequence, I do not consider that one is justified in speaking of various phenomena as "occurring in," and being "characteristic of" certain stages. It would be more correct to state that one can induce different phenomena which vary according to the depth of the hypnosis, the personality of the subject, and his hypnotic training.

While admitting the artificial origin of hypnotic phenomena, we may still with advantage attempt to classify them. Among the various groupings of hypnotic stages, which we have just been considering, Max Dessoir's appears to be the best, and forms a distinct advance upon the numerous and misleading subdivisions of Bernheim. Exception might be taken to it, however, on the ground that on the one hand it takes no account of certain slight but important hypnotic states, and on the other omits all reference to Somnambulism, *i.e.* that hypnotic condition which is followed by amnesia. Under the first class, I include those cases in which patients are influenced by curative suggestions at a stage when alterations neither in the voluntary movements nor in the special senses can be induced. Now, although in some instances curative suggestions are not responded to until deep hypnosis is reached, in others this response forms the first and only evidence of its existence. Further, the therapeutic phenomena are the only ones to which the ordinary medical man attaches much importance; and to him a classification, which includes, as " hypnotic," cases where there is slight difficulty in opening the eyes, and excludes others where grave and long-standing disease has almost immediately vanished under the influence of suggestion, must appear faulty.

As regards somnambulism, the remarkable changes of memory which take place in this stage surely render it worthy of special mention. The fact that some of Wetterstrand's patients remained for months in a condition resembling sleep, and others passed lengthened periods in apparently active mental life, without the waking consciousness retaining any recollection of either of these conditions, is surely as striking a phenomenon as the alterations in the voluntary muscles, chosen by Max Dessoir as characteristic of one of his two great groups.

Again, many medical men are careful to avoid all merely experimental suggestions when employing hypnotism for curative purposes. This adds another difficulty to classification. In such instances, the patients voluntarily close their eyes and rest quietly while curative suggestions are made. As the muscular and sensorial conditions are not tested in any way, the only evidence of the existence of hypnosis is to be found in the response to the curative suggestions, and the amnesia which sometimes, though not always, follows awaking. These patients, therefore, do not fall under Max Dessoir's classification, as neither amnesia nor response to curative suggestions is included in his two groups. In some such cases, amongst my own patients, deep hypnosis had undoubtedly been induced, as it was readily evoked at a later date in response to a single suggestion. Putting these cases on one side, and confining ourselves to experimental phenomena alone, the most convenient classification is possibly Max Dessoir's, with the addition of the stage of somnambulism. Thus :—

(1) Slight Hypnosis : changes in the voluntary muscles can be induced.

(2) Deep Hypnosis : here, in addition, changes in the special senses can be evoked.

(3) Somnambulism : in this condition, while a large variety of hypnotic reactions (many of them characteristic of the " alert " stage) can be evoked, the waking consciousness is unable spontaneously to revive what has occurred.

CHAPTER VIII.

MANY observers, from Schwenter and Kircher onwards, have stated that they have succeeded in hypnotising guinea-pigs, rabbits, frogs, birds, crayfish and other animals. The principal argument in favour of this is drawn from the fact that some of these animals, after certain physical stimuli had been applied to them, presented the phenomenon of catalepsy. Is this catalepsy invariably a genuine one? I am inclined to think that in many instances it is a conscious simulation of death, adopted by the animals from the instinctive knowledge of the fact that certain birds and beasts of prey, except under pressure of extreme hunger, will not attack what is dead. If, for example, you turn a beetle on its back it will remain motionless and apparently cataleptic, with its legs sticking rigidly in the air. The moment you go away, however, it scrambles to its feet and resumes its journey. Here death, or catalepsy, was only shammed, and doubtless the insect was keenly watching your every movement and anxiously waiting for your departure.

Granting, however, that the catalepsy is a genuine one, important differences exist between it and hypnosis in general, thus:

(1) Physical means alone will not induce hypnosis in the human subject: he must also know what is expected of him. We have no evidence, however, that a crayfish becomes cataleptic from a clear idea that the operator has suggested that condition. On the contrary, it can be induced in vertebrate animals deprived of their cerebral hemispheres, and solely by the maintenance of the body in an abnormal position by means of an external force.

(2) The phenomenon is explained in varying, and even opposite, ways by different observers. Thus, Heubel and Wundt con-

sider the so-called hypnosis of animals a true sleep, resulting from the cessation of external stimuli. Preyer, on the other hand, believed the condition to be one of paralysis from fright, or catalepsy produced by sudden peripheral stimulus.

(3) Catalepsy is only one, and a comparatively unimportant, phenomenon of hypnosis. One of the main characteristics of the hypnotic state is the rapidity with which one phenomenon can be changed into its opposite: we have, however, no like condition in the so-called hypnosis of animals.

The most valuable observations on the subject are those of Verworn on Vertebrates. According to him, there exists in the so-called hypnosis of animals a special form of activity in the muscles, which is invariably associated with a peculiar condition of inactivity of the cerebral cortex. A persistent tonic contraction of the muscles exists, and is determined by excitation of the nervous elements of the mid-brain. During the immobile state, sensation, peripheral and central, is unaltered; and the animal appears to be conscious of sensations produced by external impressions. Further, if these are sufficiently intense to evoke an efficient discharge from the cerebral cortex, the condition of immobility and muscular contracture terminates. Reflex muscular excitability is not lowered: it only appears to be so because the muscles, owing to contracture, are incapable of responding properly to the central nervous discharge. There is no inhibition of the lower neuro-muscular mechanisms: on the contrary, the lower centres are released from cerebral control and discharge a continuous stream of nervous impulses. Finally, the cessation of the discharge of impulses from the cerebral cortex is complete. This was obviously so when the cerebral hemispheres had been previously removed. In the intact animal, Verworn believes that the sudden cessation of cerebral discharge is the result of an inhibition, due to the activity of other parts of the nervous system or to special conditions of the centres themselves. The more one appreciates the complexity of the hypnotic state—the fact that it is essentially distinguished by an increased power of controlling the organism, without diminished consciousness or volition—the more one must recognise that it finds no analogy in an animal deprived of its cerebral hemispheres, and discharging a continuous stream of nervous motor impulses from its lower centres.

CHAPTER IX.

In Elliotson's time, as we have seen, mesmerism was frequently employed as an anæsthetic in surgical operations, and a full account of many of these is to be found in *The Zoist*. In his day, too, the announcement of a birth in the daily papers was sometimes also followed by the statement: "painlessly during mesmeric trance."

ESDAILE'S SURGICAL CASES.

The most remarkable series of painless mesmeric operations, however, were those performed by Esdaile in India. Records of these are to be found in the Government reports, in Esdaile's published works, and in the pages of *The Zoist*. They comprised, as already stated, nearly 300 capital operations, and many thousand minor ones.

The following is Esdaile's own description of two typical cases :—

No. 1. "S., aged 27, came to the Native Hospital with an immense scrotal tumour as heavy as his whole body. He was mesmerised for the first time on October 10th, 1846, then on the 11th and 13th, on which latter day he was ready for operation. The operation was performed on the 14th. The tumour was tied up in a sheet to which a rope was attached, and passed through a pulley in the rafter. The colis was dissected out, and the mattress then hauled down to the end of the bed; his legs were held asunder, and the pulley put in motion to support the mass and develop its neck. It was transfixed with the longest two-edged knife, which was found to be too short, as I had to dig the haft in the mass to make the point appear below it, and it was removed by two semicircular incisions right and left. The flow of venous blood was prodigious, but soon moderated under pressure of the hand; the vessels being picked up as fast as possible. The tumour, after half an hour, weighed 103 pounds, and was as heavy as the man's body. During the whole operation, I was not sensible of a quiver of his flesh. The patient made a good recovery."

No. 2. "Two years before, the patient, a peasant, aged 40, began to suffer from a tumour in the antrum maxillare; the tumour had pushed up the orbit of the eye, filled up the nose, passed into the throat, and caused an enlargement of the glands of the neck." An assistant having failed to mesmerise this man in a fortnight, Esdaile took him in hand himself, and thus describes the result: "In half an hour he was cataleptic, and a quarter of an hour later I performed one of the most severe and protracted operations in surgery; the man was totally unconscious. I put a long knife in at the corner of his mouth, and brought the point out over the cheek-bone, dividing the parts between; from this I pushed it through the skin at the inner corner of the eye, and dissected the cheek-bone to the nose. The pressure of the tumour had caused absorption of the anterior wall of the antrum, and on pressing my fingers between it and the bone it burst, and a shocking gush of blood and matter followed. The tumour extended as far as my fingers could reach under the orbit and the cheek-bone, and passed into the gullet—having destroyed the bones and partition of the nose. No one touched the man, and I turned his head in any position I desired, without resistance, and there it remained until I wished to move it again; when the blood accumulated, I bent his head forward, and it ran from his mouth as if from a spout. The man never moved, nor showed any signs of life, except an occasional indistinct moan; but when I threw back his head, and passed my fingers into his throat to detach the mass in that direction, the stream of blood was directed into his windpipe, and some instinctive effort became necessary for existence; he therefore coughed, and leaned forward to get rid of the blood, and I suppose that he then awoke. The operation was finished, and he was laid on the floor to have his face sewed up, and while this was being done, he for the first time opened his eyes."

The patient afterwards informed Esdaile that he did not know he had coughed, and was quite unconscious up to the termination of the operation. The dressings were removed three days afterwards, when it was found that the wounds in the face had healed by first intention. The recovery was satisfactory.

The following cases of amputation of the leg were reported by "Visitors" to the Hospital:—

No. 3. "The patient was sinking: she had been attacked with fever, and Dr. Esdaile, though he was not satisfied that she had been mesmerised sufficiently, determined to operate at once, as further delay endangered her life. The leg was taken off a little below the knee. . . . The thigh and knee from which the leg had been taken were perfectly motionless, and the only evidence of life was her respiration. She was not held or tied down in any way, and, during the whole operation, not the least movement or change in her limbs, body, or countenance took place. Dr. Esdaile left her to awake naturally, which she did in about a quarter of an hour. She then told us that she had had a good and undisturbed sleep, without dreams or pain, and that she was ready to have her leg amputated. Upon receiving ocular demonstration that the operation had been performed her countenance expressed surprise and pleasure, and, as if doubtful of the fact, we observed her pass her hand over the stump apparently to test the reality of what she saw. Shortly afterwards we quitted the hospital, leaving her composedly waving a punkah over her face."

No. 4. "The patient had not been previously mesmerised, and Dr. Esdaile was doubtful whether this could be done deeply enough for operative purposes. He instructed a Native assistant to commence the process, and the patient quickly passed into a state of deep coma. Esdaile then amputated the leg six inches above the knee; not a muscle moved, the pulse was steady and regular, there was no perspiration on the forehead, no paleness of the countenance; in fact the patient was as motionless as a corpse. Shortly after the operation he awoke in the most natural manner, stretching out his arms, yawning and rubbing his eyes. He said, in reply to questions, that he had had a good sleep and felt all the better for it. He was intensely surprised when told that the operation was over; and showed his gratitude in the usual Native manner, by placing his hands on his breast and muttering blessings on the doctor."

From amongst many other interesting cases the following are cited:—A case of compound fracture of the leg, in which a

portion of bone was sawn off, and the fracture set during mesmeric trance. Several cases of strangulated hernia, which had
resisted all attempts at reduction : during mesmeric sleep, there
was complete relaxation of the abdominal muscles ; and in every
instance the hernia was easily reduced. Esdaile also recorded
cases of stricture of the urethra, with retention of urine, successfully treated by the induction of mesmeric trance ; and also a case
of labour which took place painlessly during the same condition.

BRAID'S SURGICAL CASES.

Braid's surgical operations were neither numerous nor varied,
and consisted mainly of dental extractions, opening of abscesses,
and the like. He claimed, however, to have cured several cases
of spinal curvature by suggestion, and asserted that the use of
mechanical appliances, except in cases of caries of the vertebræ,
was worse than useless. The following is an illustrative case :—

No. 5. The patient, a girl aged 16, suffering from spinal
curvature, had been treated by various specialists for six years.
At first she was kept in bed for sixteen months, and treated by
extension, counter-extension, and various gymnastic exercises.
Afterwards she wore a complicated mechanical apparatus for four
years, growing meanwhile steadily worse. Braid easily hypnotised
her at the first attempt, removed all mechanical apparatus, and
rendered the morbidly weak muscles cataleptic by suggestion.
After a week of this treatment, there was a marked increase of
muscular strength ; and the patient could walk for half an hour
without the support of stays or other mechanical apparatus. She
made a good recovery, as did also her younger sister, who had
been under treatment for the same complaint for three years
before Braid hypnotised her.

PERSONAL CASES.

Shortly after commencing hypnotic work I found I could
sometimes induce anæsthesia by suggestion, and from that time
occasionally performed surgical operations during hypnosis. In
most of the following illustrative cases, however, I hypnotised
while others operated :—

No. 6. Miss ——, aged 20, was operated on for double
strabismus by Mr. Bendelack Hewetson, of Leeds, November 4th,
1889 ; hypnotic suggestion being the only anæsthetic employed.
She obeyed all his commands ; kept her eyes in the required

position, or turned them so as to put the muscular fibres on the stretch. Anæsthesia was perfect; when awakened she would not believe that the operation had been performed, until shown her eyes in a looking-glass. There was no subsequent pain.

On December 26th, 1889, she fractured her nose; hypnotic anæsthesia was induced, and the bones moulded into position.

These operations were followed by others, and early in March, 1890, the late Mr. Arthur Turner, of Leeds, came to Goole to test my methods. The following account of his observations appeared in the *Journal of the British Dental Association* for March 15th, 1890 :—

" Being a firm believer in the advantages of the use of nitrous oxide over other methods of producing narcosis for the requirements of our specialty, I was by no means ready to believe that there existed any other means of inducing total insensibility to pain comparable, as regards safety and efficiency, with our justly valued anæsthetic. Within the last few days, however, I have been surprised to find that hypnotism properly applied is of the greatest value, not only in rendering a patient insensible, but also in preventing after-suffering. I do not here propose to enter into any lengthy detail, but merely desire to state some of the facts observed by me. I was recently invited by Dr. Bramwell, of Goole, to see some of his patients whom he was treating hypnotically, and to test the value of hypnotism in relieving or preventing pain during the removal of teeth.

" I had a large choice of patients, and selected those which I considered would afford a severe trial of this method. One upper molar, which another dentist had on three occasions failed to remove, I extracted without difficulty, and with no signs of pain from the patient. She then, without awakening, rinsed her mouth, and I extracted the fellow-tooth on the opposite side. The hypnosis was induced and removed almost instantaneously. She stated emphatically that she had no recollection of the operation being performed, that she had felt no pain, and there was no resulting tenderness of the gums.

" Another case, that of a young girl suffering from valvular disease, a weak anæmic subject, whom one would expect to find ' deepen ' considerably under nitrous oxide, and remain in a state of collapse for a whole day after ether, was quickly and quietly rendered unconscious. I then extracted two left lower molars, which were decayed down to a level with the alveolus, with pulps exposed; also two right lower molar stumps, and a lower bicuspid: all difficult teeth. There were slight muscular twitchings, such as one often finds under an anæsthetic, but there was no complaint of pain after the operation, and the patient was quickly restored to her normal condition. I extracted in all about forty teeth, tried my best to discover defects, and questioned the patients myself, but the results were most satisfactory. Three typical cases are here appended:—

"Miss A., age 15. Teeth extracted: right upper molar, left upper molar, *caries;* left lower molar, *abscess;* temporary canine, *persistent.*

"*Remarks.*—No conjunctival reflex, dilated pupils, no pain.

"Mrs. B., age 36. Teeth extracted: upper molar right, first and second lower molars right, left lower wisdom, and right lower bicuspid—stump forceps used in each case.

"*Remarks.*—Conjunctival reflex absent, no sign of pain.

"Miss C., age 24. This patient was sent to me from another room with a note from Dr. Bramwell, stating that he would not be present during the operation, and enclosing a written and signed order for her to sleep, and submit herself to my control. Upon presenting this the patient at once fell asleep.

"I extracted two upper bicuspid stumps, quite buried by congested gums and very tender to the touch. I then awakened the patient, and found that she was quite free from pain.

"This is important as showing that patients may be sent from a distance, without necessitating the personal attendance of the hypnotiser.

"A great advantage of hypnosis over narcosis is that no gag is required in the former, as the patient is entirely under the control of the operator, opening the mouth at command or altering position as suggested.

"I hope to get Dr. Bramwell to give a demonstration to a meeting of the Society, when those interested will be able to judge for themselves.   W. ARTHUR TURNER, L.D.S. Eng."
LEEDS.

The demonstration referred to was given at Leeds shortly afterwards, a report of it being sent without my knowledge to both the *British Medical Journal* and the *Lancet;* the following account appeared in the latter:—

" Demonstration of Hypnotism as an Anæsthetic during the Performance of Dental and Surgical Operations.

" A correspondent, on whom we can rely, kindly furnishes us with the following remarkable report :—

" A number of the leading medical men and dentists of Leeds and district were brought together on March 28th, through the kind invitation issued by Messrs. Carter Brothers and Turner, dental surgeons, of Park Square, Leeds, to witness a series of surgical and dental operations performed in their rooms by Dr. Milne Bramwell, of Goole, Yorkshire. Great interest was evinced in the meeting. . . . Upwards of sixty medical men and dental surgeons accepted the invitation. Amongst the gentlemen present were the following :—Mr. Thomas Scattergood, Prof. Wardrop Griffith, Mr. Pridgin Teale, Prof. Eddison, Dr. Jacob, Dr. Churton, Mr. Mayo Robson, Mr. H. Bendelack Hewetson, Mr. Henderson Nicol, Mr. Moyniham, Mr. Littlewood, Mr. Henry Gott, Mr. Churton, Mr. Edmund Robinson, Mr. William Hall, Dr. Braithwaite, Mr. Wood, Dr. Light, Dr. Trevellyan, Dr. Caddy, Prof. M'Gill, Dr. Turner (Menston Asylum), Dr. Hartley, Dr. Hellier, Mr. W. H. Brown, Dr. Bruce (Goole), Mr. Dennison, Mr. Edward Ward, Mr. H. Robson, Mr. King, Mr. Glaisby, Mr. Sherburn, and Mr. Wayles. A letter expressing regret at his inability to be present was read from Dr. Clifford Allbutt, in which he reminded the meeting that he remembered the time—thirty-five years ago —when Liston performed several serious operations, using hypnotism as the anæsthetic, at the hands of a scientific lay friend in Lincolnshire. Mr. Jessop was also prevented at the last moment from being present. The object of the meeting was to show the power of hypnotism to produce absolute anæsthesia in very painful and severe operations.

" The first case brought into the room was a woman of 25. She was hypnotised at a word by Dr. Bramwell, and told she was to submit to three teeth being extracted without pain at the hands of Mr. T. Carter, and further that she was to do anything that Mr. Carter asked her—such as to open her mouth, spit out, and the like. This was perfectly successful. There was no expression of pain in the face, no cry, and when told to awake she said she had not the least pain in the gums, nor had she felt the operation. Dr. Bramwell then rehypnotised her, and ordered her to leave the room and go upstairs to the waiting-room. This she did as a complete somnambulist.

"The next case was that of a servant girl, aged 19, on whom, under the hypnotic influence induced by Dr. Bramwell, a large lacrymal abscess extending into the cheek had a fortnight previously been opened, and scraped freely, without knowledge or pain. Furthermore, the dressing had been daily performed, and the cavity freely syringed out under hypnotic anæsthesia. To the ' healing suggestions,' daily given to the patient, Dr. Bramwell in a great measure attributes the very rapid healing, which took place in ten days—a remarkably short space of time in a girl affected by inherited syphilis, and in a by no means good state of health. She was put to sleep by the following letter from Dr. Bramwell addressed to Mr. Turner, the operating dentist in the case :—

"BURLINGTON CRESCENT, GOOLE, YORKS.

"DEAR MR. TURNER—I send you a patient with enclosed order. When you give it to her, she will fall asleep at once and obey your commands.   J. MILNE BRAMWELL.

"Go to sleep by order of Dr. Bramwell, and obey Mr. Turner's commands.   J. MILNE BRAMWELL.

"This experiment answered perfectly. Sleep was induced at once by reading the note, and was so profound that at the end of a lengthy operation, in which sixteen stumps were removed, she awoke smiling, and insisted that she had felt no pain ; and, what was remarkable, there was no pain in her mouth. She was found after some time, when unobserved, reading the *Graphic* in the waiting-room as if nothing had happened. During the whole time she did everything which Mr. Turner suggested, but it was observed that there was a diminished flow of saliva, and that the corneal reflexes were absent: the breathing was more noisy than ordinary and the pulse slower. Dr. Bramwell took occasion to explain that the next case, a boy of 8, was a severe test, and would not probably succeed ; partly because the patient was so young, and chiefly because he had not attempted to produce hypnotic anæsthesia earlier than two days before. He also explained that patients require training in this form of anæsthesia ; the time of training or preparation varying with each individual.

However, he was so far hypnotised that he allowed Mr. Mayo
Robson to operate on the great toe, removing a bony growth and
part of the first phalanx, with no more than a few cries towards
the close of the operation; and with the result that when
questioned afterwards he appeared to know very little of what
had been done. It was necessary in his case for Dr. Bramwell
to repeat the hypnotic suggestions. Dr. Bramwell remarked that
he wished to show a case that was less likely to be perfectly
successful than the others, so as to enable those present to see
the difficult as well as the apparently straightforward cases.

"The next case was a girl of 15, highly sensitive, requiring
the removal of enlarged tonsils. At the request of Dr. Bramwell,
Mr. Bendelack Hewetson was enabled, whilst the patient was in
the hypnotic state, to extract each tonsil with ease, the girl, by
suggestion of the hypnotiser, obeying each request of the operator,
though in a state of perfect anæsthesia. In the same way, Mr.
Hewetson removed a cyst, of the size of a horse-bean, from the
side of the nose of a young woman who was perfectly anæsthetic,
and breathing deeply; and who, on coming round by order,
protested 'that the operation had not been commenced.'

"Mr. Turner then extracted two large molar teeth from a
man with equal success; after which Dr. Bramwell explained
how this patient had been completely cured of drunkenness by
hypnotic suggestion. To prove this to those present, and to show
the interesting psychological results, the man was hypnotised,
and in that state he was shown a glass of water, which he was
told by Dr. Bramwell was 'bad beer.' He was then told to
awake, and the glass of water was offered him by Dr. Bramwell.
He put it to his lips, and at once spat out the 'offensive liquid.'
Other interesting phenomena were illustrated and explained by
means of this patient, who was a hale, strong working-man.

"Mr. Tom Carter next extracted a very difficult impacted
stump from a railway navvy, as successfully as in the previous
case. Dr. Bramwell described how this man had been completely
cured of very obstinate facial neuralgia by hypnotism. The
malady had been produced by working in a wet railway cutting,
and had previously defied all medical treatment. After the third
hypnotic treatment—some weeks previously—the neuralgia had
entirely disappeared, and had not returned. The man had also
obtained refreshing hypnotic sleep at night, being put to sleep

by a written order from Dr. Bramwell, and on one occasion by a telegram, both methods succeeding perfectly.

" At the conclusion of this most interesting and successful series of hypnotic experiments, a vote of thanks to Dr. Bramwell, for his kindness in giving the demonstration, was proposed by Mr. Scattergood, Dean of the Yorkshire College, and seconded by Mr. Pridgin Teale, F.R.S., who remarked 'that the experiments were deeply interesting, and had been marvellously successful.' The latter also said 'he felt sure that the time had now come when we should have to recognise hypnotism as a necessary part of our study.' The vote was carried by loud acclamations.

" Messrs. Carter Brothers and Turner were cordially thanked for the great scientific treat, which they had so kindly prepared for the many to whom hypnotism had been first introduced that day, and for the further opportunity, afforded to the few who had seen Dr. Bramwell's work previously, of studying its application as an anæsthetic. Mr. Henry Carter replied for the firm, and the meeting closed ; the patients looking as little like patients as persons well could, giving neither by their manners nor expression the slightest suggestion (except when external dressings were visible) that they had suffered, or were suffering from, extensive surgical interference."—*The Lancet*, April 5th, 1890, page 771.

The above account, with the exception of a few details, is correct. The removal of the exostosis was rendered a more severe operation, by a preliminary evulsion of the great toe nail, and, although the patient showed slight signs of pain, he was afterwards unable to recall what had happened. The after-condition of the patients was remarkable ; and the unpleasant symptoms which sometimes follow the use of anæsthetics were absent. They all made a hearty meal ; and then returned to Goole, a journey of over an hour by train. The nurse in charge told me she might have been conducting a party home from a fair, as they passed the time in laughing and singing. With the exception of the boy whose toe had been operated on, and who was unable to put on his boot, none of them kept the house ; while in every case the healing process was remarkably rapid, and unaccompanied by pain.

From that date I employed hypnotic anæsthesia in a number of minor operations ; but, with the exception of the two following, few are worthy of special note.

No. 7. Mr. ——, aged 40, was run over by a loaded railway waggon, and sustained severe comminuted fractures of the right clavicle, scapula, humerus, radius and ulna. The elbow joint was opened, and gangrene of the lower arm followed. The patient ultimately recovered; but all the joints of the right arm, shoulder, elbow, wrist, and fingers, were ankylosed. On several occasions he was put under chloroform, and the adhesions broken down; this was always followed by swelling, inflammation and return of the immobility. Later, he would neither take an anæsthetic, nor allow any attempt at passive movement to be made without one. He was easily hypnotised at the first attempt and analgesia induced. For some weeks this was repeated frequently, and on each occasion the adhesions were broken down, and the mobility of the joints increased. He ultimately returned to his employment, with a strong and useful, though somewhat deformed arm. This case was seen by Mr. Mayo Robson, both before and after hypnotic treatment.

No. 8. Mrs. ——, aged 41, a weak nervous woman, abnormally sensitive to pain, had her teeth extracted painlessly in what was apparently the waking state — the only anæsthetic being suggestion. This was regarded as an experiment which might possibly fail, and the patient made me promise to put her to sleep if she had pain. The operation was performed on July 21st, 1892, at Mr. Bendelack Hewetson's, Leeds, in the presence of a number of medical men, including Mr. H. Littlewood, F.R.C.S. The following account was given by Mr. Henderson Nicol, L.D.S. Eng., the numbers quoted showing the teeth extracted, according to Dr. Thompson's *Approved Record Plate*:—

"Nos. 21, 22, 24, 25 and 26 were removed without any interval, and entirely without pain, or any symptom of feeling, on the part of the patient. After an interval of a few minutes for rinsing out her mouth, Nos. 27 and 1 were removed without interval, and with some slight indication of pain in the case of No. 1, but none in the case of No. 27, which, in common with Nos. 21 and 22, was very firmly attached to the jaw. After a further interval of a few seconds, No. 16 was removed; it was much broken down, and there were symptoms of some pain. All the teeth were much diseased, and the extractions under ordinary conditions would have caused acute pain. . . . I think, considering the circumstances under which the operation was done, it was a remarkable success, and I am pleased to have seen it."

Remarks.—The patient was not prepared in any way for the operation, and the analgesia was not post-hypnotic, *i.e.* it was not suggested to her during a previous hypnosis that pain should be absent on this particular occasion. Without the employment of any mechanical methods, or verbal suggestion of hypnosis, she was simply told in the waking state that the operation should be painless. She lost much blood and felt faint, but this soon passed off, and she gave the following account of her sensations:—She had a little pain when No. 1 was extracted, but this was nothing to what she had felt when she had had teeth drawn previously, and not sufficient to make her remind me of my promise to hypnotise her. She had the fixed idea that this tooth would hurt her; a previous attempt to extract it having failed. She described the various steps of the operation, and asserted that all the extractions, except No. 1, were absolutely painless. The analgesia was still further tested by a powerful application of the faradic brush.

A few days later, under the same conditions, I extracted her remaining four teeth, and, despite the fact that they were all firmly attached to the jaw, this was accomplished without pain. Neither operation was followed by pain, and the gums healed rapidly; when the casts of the mouth were taken all unpleasant sensations were prevented by suggestion. It is to be noted that, in the above case, analgesia alone was suggested, and that this appeared unaccompanied by anæsthesia.[1]

SURGICAL CASES FROM OTHER AUTHORS.

(A) Confinements during Hypnosis.

No. 9 (Dr. Kingsbury, of Blackpool). V. S., aged 14 years and 7 months, was hypnotised twelve times before confinement, and deep anæsthesia induced. Dr. Kingsbury was called at 7.30 P.M.; the os was slightly dilated, and the pains occurred every 15 or 20 minutes. The patient was hypnotised, told to have no pain, and to bear down when the uterine contractions

---

[1] The medical history of this case is given later. (No. 20, pp. 191-4.)

occurred. At 11 P.M., she was delivered of a child weighing 8¼ lbs. The placenta followed in ten minutes; she still remained asleep and, when awakened, felt well, and remembered nothing of what had happened.

No. 10 (von Schrenck-Notzing). B., aged 25, primipara. Strong, healthy and well-nourished. First hypnotised, November 17th, 1891; this was repeated six times up to the 26th. At 2.45 A.M., on the 29th, she was hypnotised during labour. Notwithstanding that the uterine contractions were strong and very painful, she fell asleep in two or three minutes and her cries ceased. Rupture of the membranes took place at 3.5 A.M., and the labour continued rapidly till 3.30 A.M., when the head reached the vulva. At 3.58 A.M., the pains became very weak and no further progress was made. It was now suggested to the patient to bear down more forcibly; the pains at once became longer, and so strong that a rupture of the perineum was feared. These suggestions were then discontinued. At 4.12 A.M. the head was born, and at the next pain the body followed. At 4.15 A.M. the placenta was ejected. The patient was awakened by suggestion at 4.20 A.M.; she opened her eyes, gradually became conscious, and looked about her in a surprised manner. She declared that she had felt no pain from the moment she was first hypnotised. There was no rupture of the perineum. The os was fully dilated at 3 A.M., and the entire labour, including passage of the placenta, completed at 4.15 A.M.

No. 11 (Wetterstrand). Regina A., aged 25; married, four children. Previous confinements—followed by severe after-pains —lasted from 10 to 12 hours. The patient was hypnotised several times before this—her fifth—confinement. Wetterstrand was called on October 19th, 1887, at 2.45 P.M.: pains slight; os admitted three fingers. Hypnosis with deep anæsthesia was induced. At 3.15 P.M. the pains became stronger, and at 4.30 P.M. the child was born. Afterwards the patient could recall nothing: there were no after-pains and the recovery was rapid.

The same patient was again confined on April 8th, 1889. She was hypnotised at the commencement of the labour, and remained in a condition of somnambulism until after its completion. Again, awaking was followed by amnesia. The labour lasted two hours: there were no after-pains.

No. 12 (Dr. Pritzl, of Vienna). Mrs. S., aged 36, primipara. Admitted into hospital, September 10th, 1885, and easily hypnotised. On October 31st, 8 P.M., the os admitted three fingers and the pains were severe. Hypnosis was then reinduced : the birth took place at 11.15 P.M., and the placenta was expelled five minutes afterwards. The patient, awakened an hour later, was much surprised to find the confinement over ; she declared she had slept soundly from the moment she had been hypnotised.

No. 13 (Dr. Mesnet, of the Hôtel Dieu, Paris). Alice D., aged 22, primipara. Hypnotised previously to confinement. At midnight, on March 31st, 1887, the os was the size of a two-franc piece, and the pains violent. Hypnosis was then reinduced, and she ceased to suffer. The birth took place at 4.45 A.M., and the patient was not awakened until her linen had been changed, and the infant dressed. She was unable to recall anything.

No. 14 (Dr. Fraipont, Lecturer on Gynæcology at the University of Liège, Belgium). Mrs. ——, aged 29, primipara.[1] At 5 P.M. the os was the size of a five-franc piece, and the pains regular and severe. Hypnosis was induced by Professor Delbœuf and her sufferings ceased. At 8.45 A.M. Dr. Fraipont had to leave, and Delbœuf ceased to hypnotise her. Dr. Fraipont returned at 10.45 A.M., and hypnosis was again induced. The · child was born at 1 P.M., and was above the average weight. Although the patient appeared to suffer during Dr. Fraipont's absence, she was unable on awaking to recall anything that had occurred. Good recovery.

No. 15 (Dr. Fanton, Marseilles). L., aged 19, primipara. Hypnosis was first induced on December 19th, 1889, and somnambulism with anæsthesia obtained on January 4th, 1890. On February 8th, 10th, 15th, and 18th, Dr. Fanton induced uterine contractions by suggestion. On February 29th, at 6 P.M., labour commenced ; and at 10 P.M. the uterine contractions were strong and painful. The patient was then rehypnotised, and the suggestion given that the labour should be arrested from 11 P.M. till midnight. The suggestion was successful and the uterine contractions entirely ceased. At midnight they recommenced strongly and regularly, but were unattended by pain. At 1.30 A.M. they were again arrested by suggestion for two hours. From

[1] This patient had been the subject of several of Professor Delbœuf's experiments. See pp. 84, 116, 117, 118 and 119.

3.30 A.M. till 11 A.M., the labour progressed naturally, but without pain. At 11 A.M. the os was fully dilated, and the labour was again arrested by suggestion for three hours. Shortly after the expiration of this period the labour was completed painlessly. On being awakened, the patient did not know she had been confined, and could recall nothing of what had passed. She made a good recovery. The experiment took place in hospital, and Professors Mazaïl and Lojan, and Drs. Audiffrent, Jourdan, Rubino, Pourrière, Fournad and Lieutard were present.

No. 16. Dr. Dobrovolsky (Switzerland) reports eight cases of confinement during hypnosis, four of which were primiparæ. Three were hypnotised for the first time during labour; one once before labour; one twice; one three times; one four times; and one six times. The following is the most remarkable case :—

No. 17. M. L., aged 24, primipara, was hypnotised three times before confinement, the last occasion being on November 13th. During each sitting[1] it was suggested to her that her labour should be painless. In the evening of November 22nd, she felt uncomfortable and lay down for some hours. About 3 A.M. she found that she was wet, and got up and changed the linen on her bed. After this she could not sleep, and had from time to time a feeling of pressure in the body, but this hardly gave her any appreciable pain. At 7 A.M. she said to the patient in the next bed: "Fetch the nurse; I feel that something has passed from me." When the nurse arrived the child was born. In this instance, a practically painless confinement was the result of post-hypnotic analgesia suggested nine days earlier.

The anæsthesia, however, does not seem to have been complete in all Dr. Dobrovolsky's cases. One patient remembered her last three pains, while another was conscious of the application of forceps; but in all the suffering was undoubtedly diminished, and the results are especially remarkable considering how seldom hypnosis had been induced before labour.

(B) Other Operations.

No. 18 (Dr. Tillaux, Surgeon to the Hôtel Dieu, Paris). The patient, a young woman, suffered from cystocele, and the

---

[1] The word "sitting" is used for convenience' sake in all instances where patients have received hypnotic treatment with suggestion.

operation of colporrhaphy was performed. She was hypnotised in bed by the House Surgeon, M. Témoin, and passed into the stage of somnambulism. In obedience to suggestion, she then walked to the theatre and lay down upon the table. The operation lasted half an hour; she showed no symptoms of pain, and chatted continuously with the House Surgeon. She was carried back to bed while still asleep, and, on being aroused, was immensely surprised to find that the operation was over.

No. 19 (Dr. Bourdon, Méru). Mrs. D., aged 34, uterine fibroid. The tumour, which was about the size of the fist and sessile, was removed through the vagina by means of Grafe's *serre-nœud;* the operation was tedious, but the patient experienced no pain.

No. 20 (Dr. Schmeltz, Nice). M., aged 20. Enormous sarcomatous tumour of the breast. Hypnosis was induced on several occasions before the operation, which was performed in the presence of a number of medical men. The tumour was removed, the axilla thoroughly explored, five drainage tubes introduced, and the enormous wound closed with thirty-two wire sutures. The operation lasted about an hour. Dr. Schmeltz operated slowly, and quite at his ease. The patient was very merry, chatting brightly, and laughing heartily from time to time. She placed herself in different positions as requested, without the aid of an assistant, etc. She suffered pain neither during nor after the operation, and slept well the following night. Recovery was rapid, and the wound was only dressed once after the operation; the drainage tubes were removed on the third day, and the stitches on the fifteenth day, when union was complete. The tumour weighed over 4 lbs., and microscopical examination confirmed the diagnosis.

No. 21 (Schmeltz). Mlle. B., aged 18. Ectropion of the left lower eyelid since the age of 10 months. She had been twice operated on in 1889, but the condition had become worse. She consulted Dr. Schmeltz in November, 1890, and told him she had suffered so much from the after-effects of the anæsthetic that she would never take one again. Hypnosis was easily induced at the first attempt. On November 28th, 1890, in the presence of several medical men, Dr. Schmeltz successfully performed "Adams' operation"; this was neither attended nor followed by pain.

No. 22 (Dr. Edward Wood, America). Mr. ——, aged 17. Necrosis of the upper third of the humerus. The patient was hypnotised on the three days preceding the operation, which was performed in hospital on September 9th, 1889. An incision was made down to the bone, the diseased portion removed, drainage tubes inserted, etc. The operation was a tedious one, and, at its conclusion, it was suggested that the patient should continue to sleep for two hours. He did not awake until the time indicated, and then asked for food. No pain. Good recovery.

No. 23 (Dr. Grossmann, Berlin). Eight cases of fractures and dislocations reported in the *Zeitschrift für Hypnotismus*, March, 1894. In every instance, hypnosis appears to have been induced for the first time on the day of the operation, which was rendered painless by suggestion.

Numerous other operations during hypnotic anæsthesia have recently been reported. Amongst these the following may be mentioned:—Sandberg (Sweden), Dental operations; Forel (Switzerland), Cataract; Diaz (Cuba), Dental operations; van Eeden and van Renterghem (Holland), Dental operations.

HYPNOTIC ANÆSTHESIA. SUMMARY.

The chief objection to hypnotic anæsthesia is the difficulty and uncertainty of the induction of the necessary degree of hypnosis. Although recent statistics show that about 94 per cent of mankind can be hypnotised, with a considerable proportion many preliminary attempts are necessary, and generally hypnosis never becomes deep enough for operative purposes. Suggestive anæsthesia can only be induced, apparently, in about 10 per cent of those hypnotised. Under these circumstances, unless grave reasons existed for the non-employment of other anæsthetics, it would be waste of time to attempt to hypnotise a patient for operative purposes alone. Apart from this, hypnosis possesses many advantages as an anæsthetic. Thus:—

(1) Once deep hypnosis, with anæsthesia, has been obtained, it can be immediately reinduced at any time.

(2) No repetition of any hypnotic process is necessary; the verbal order to go to sleep is sufficient.

(3) The hypnotiser's presence is not essential. The patient

can be put *en rapport* with the operator by written order, or by other means previously suggested during hypnosis.

(4) No abstinence from food or other preparation is necessary.

(5) Nervous apprehension can be removed by suggestion.

(6) Hypnosis is pleasant, and absolutely devoid of danger.

(7) It can be maintained indefinitely, and terminated immediately at will.

(8) The patient can be placed in any position without risk— a not unimportant point in operations on the mouth and throat— and will alter that position at the command of the operator. Gags and other retentive apparatus are unnecessary.

(9) Analgesia alone can be suggested, and the patient left sensitive to other impressions—an advantage in throat operations.

(10) In labour cases, the influence of the voluntary muscles can be increased or diminished by suggestion.

(11) There is no tendency to sickness during or after operation—a distinct gain in abdominal cases.

(12) Pain after operation, or during subsequent dressings, can be entirely prevented.

(13) The rapidity of the healing process, possibly as the result of the absence of pain, is frequently very marked.

While Schrenck-Notzing and other observers state that hypnotic suggestion can render labour painless, and facilitate its course by regulating the position of the body and limbs, and increasing or diminishing the uterine contractions through the action of the voluntary muscles, Dr. Fanton claims other and more startling advantages. According to him, suggestion acts directly upon the uterus itself: the operator can thus cause its contractions to appear or disappear at will; and, in complicated cases, this may save the life of both mother and child. Further, uterine inertia may be successfully combated without the use of ergot, and the forceps frequently rendered unnecessary. The after-contraction of the uterus can be excited by suggestion, and post-partum hæmorrhage prevented. In cases of adherent placenta, turning, etc., the uterus can be relaxed by suggestion, and the necessary operations greatly facilitated. Finally, Dr. Fanton claims to have successfully excited premature labour by suggestion, and considers it criminal to have recourse to other means, such as dilatation of the cervix, perforation of the membranes, etc., without having first attempted this method.

Although Dr. Fanton founds his statements on numerous cases and experiments, many of them observed by other medical men, the results he claims are so startling that few are likely to accept them without further evidence. One must admit, however, that the involuntary contractions of the uterus are sometimes arrested by emotional states. An assistant, sent to a patient who expected to see his principal, often finds that the labour, which was progressing rapidly before his arrival, ceases the moment he enters the room.

It is possible that improvement in the method of inducing hypnosis may arise; but, until then, its usefulness in surgery will ever remain extremely restricted. Hypnotic anæsthesia, however, must always be of keen interest to both physiologist and psychologist. As will be pointed out later, it is a thing apart, and by no means an ordinary narcotic—not a fresh example of the methods for preventing pain by checking all conscious cerebration.

CHAPTER X.

To the physician, the chief interest of hypnotism depends upon its value in the treatment of disease. To illustrate this, I now propose to cite cases in which it has been employed for that purpose by myself and others.

Amongst the former are to be found a few drawn from my general practice at Goole. All of these cases, however, were seen by other medical men, generally before, during, and after hypnotic treatment; and most of them were shown at the meetings of one or more medical societies. The remainder—almost without exception sent to me by other medical men—have been treated since I came to London a little over ten years ago.

In most instances, sufficient time has elapsed to enable one to judge of the permanency of the results. In all the after-history of the case has been traced, and in many the last reports have been of quite recent date. Most of the cases drawn from other sources have neither been previously translated into English, nor published abroad in readily accessible form—the majority being taken from foreign medical journals, etc. Many of them are reported by well-known Continental medical men; and, again, in most instances, the after-histories of the patients have been carefully traced and recorded. This selection has been made in order to put fresh material before my readers, as accounts of many cases, treated by Bernheim, Wetterstrand, and others, have already been published in English translations. In each instance, the source from which the case is drawn will be given in the chapter of " References."

I do not propose to cite examples of all the different forms of disease in which hypnotism has been employed. The account

only claims to be an illustrative one : the majority of the diseases
selected, therefore, are those in which hypnotism has been most
frequently used as a curative agent. In some instances this rule
has been departed from, either because the employment of hypnotism in such other diseases has excited interest or controversy, or
because the cases themselves present points of special interest.

In the chapter of "References" many cases will be referred
to other than those about to be cited. Some of these are
additional examples of the various cases I propose to quote; the
remainder illustrate the use of hypnotism in diseases other than
those about to be reviewed. Successful cases have been chosen
purposely, and little reference made to those in which hypnotic
treatment failed. In my concluding chapter, however, I shall
again return to this point, and discuss—as far as the very
imperfect data permit—the value of hypnotic treatment as com-
pared with other methods.

For the present, in order to prevent misconception, it ought
to be clearly understood that those who employ hypnotism regard it only as an additional weapon by which disease may be
combated. They use it just as they would any other new
remedy, or fresh form of treatment that advancing science has
brought within their reach. If it sometimes succeeds where
other methods have failed, the opposite is equally true. Even
in the former case this implies no slur on "Medicine," regarded
in its widest sense ; on the contrary, if the therapeutic value of
hypnotism be proved, Medicine, as a whole, is so much the richer.

Hypnotism has undoubtedly given its best results in the
treatment of functional nervous disorders. Amongst these the
various forms of hysteria deserve the first place, and may be
grouped as follows :—

(1) Hysteria.

(A) *Grande Hystérie, or Hystero-Epilepsy, and the conditions
which sometimes persist after the convulsive attacks have
disappeared, e.g. paralyses, contractures, spasms, anæsthesiæ,
amauroses, etc.*

The following example is from my own practice :—

No. 1. Miss ——, aged 19, June, 1900. A tall, well-
developed Italian girl, educated and highly intelligent. Mother
suffered from hysteria. The patient had her first hysterical

attack in November, 1894, after overworking for an examination. This was preceded by headaches and boisterous laughter : then muscular twitchings, at first confined to the shoulders, appeared. Soon these movements became more violent and generalised, and alternated with various muscular contractures : the latter sometimes affected the jaws, and the teeth became firmly clenched. This condition lasted till May, 1895, then disappeared after a short hypnotic treatment.

In July, 1895, clonic spasms reappeared during sleep. In September, 1896, she came to England to teach in a High School ; and shortly afterwards began to have spasms in the daytime. At first these affected the left side only, then practically all the voluntary muscles. From the latter date, until December, 1899, the patient was hypnotised by Dr. —— at irregular intervals. At first the attacks ceased after one or two sittings, but the longest remission was only eleven weeks, and they frequently returned at the end of a few days. By degrees the treatment lost its influence : the spasms became more violent and severe, a contracture of the left leg appeared, and the patient could only limp a few steps. She suffered much from headache, was extremely emotional, often depressed, had morbid ideas and frequent attacks of hysterical laughter and weeping.

In December, 1899, hypnotic treatment was discontinued, and the patient consulted a well-known neurologist. At first she was placed in a medical man's house ; but, as her condition grew worse, she was removed in two months, and admitted as a contributing patient to the National Hospital, Queen's Square, Bloomsbury. There she was treated by isolation, rest in bed, and hot baths. Blisters were also applied in order to render the movements painful. Later, large doses of hyoscine, chloral, bromide, etc., were given, and the patient kept in a more or less narcotised condition for weeks. Despite this, the twitchings, convulsions, and contracture of the leg increased in severity, and she was discharged on June 18th, 1900, much worse than when she entered.

She was then brought to me by Dr. Sainsbury, and I began hypnotic treatment the following day. At that time, except during sleep, the patient had constant jerking movements of the left side, involving the face, arm, leg and trunk, while the head was drawn violently to the left. She had also frequent attacks— sometimes ten or twelve a day—of the true Salpêtrière type of *grande hystérie.* After violent generalised convulsions lasting several minutes, the head was drawn backwards towards the heels (*arc de cercle*), and the face became cyanosed; then, after much abdominal gurgling, the spasm relaxed, the attack ceased, and the unilateral muscular movements recommenced. She never lost consciousness, and the seizures were not followed by amnesia; there were no signs of organic disease.

For the first fortnight, every time I tried to hypnotise the patient she had a convulsive attack, but, despite this, I made suggestions in the usual way. She then gradually became quieter, and a week later the morbid symptoms disappeared. The treatment, however, was continued until July 31st; but neither during that time nor afterwards were any drugs given.

On September 20th, 1900, she returned to work, and from then up to the last report (May, 1903) there had been no relapse. She has gained in weight, is strong, and plays hockey and other outdoor games. She has become progressively less and less emotional; has lost the morbid ideas that used to haunt her, and ceased to worry over trifles. Since July, 1900, there has been no treatment, hypnotic or other.

In several other somewhat similar cases equally good results were obtained. In one of these, the patient had frequent attacks of generalised convulsions, invariably followed by amnesia. She also suffered from storms of neuralgic pain; these occurred several times a day, and were absolutely sudden in their appearance and termination.

In another case the patient had attacks of convulsions, followed by generalised catalepsy. During the latter condition, which frequently lasted for several hours, the patient was apparently unconscious, and insensible to external stimuli. In both cases recovery followed hypnotic treatment, and there was no relapse.

Successful cases were reported by the older writers, amongst the most interesting being one of Elliotson's :—The patient had suffered from convulsive attacks of hystero-epilepsy for nine years, and also during the same period from a contracture of one leg. She had passed twenty-two months in different hospitals without improvement, but recovered quickly under Elliotson's care, and had not relapsed three years later.

The following are more recent examples :—

No. 2 (Krafft-Ebing). Miss ——, aged 18, had always been nervous, excitable, and bad-tempered. From the age of six she had had hysterical symptoms, including nocturnal terrors, sleep-walking, etc. In July, 1890, she had an attack of hystero-epilepsy, which lasted three hours : then fourteen days' delirium, followed by amnesia. From that date the ordinary hysterical symptoms became worse ; the convulsive attacks soon averaged two a day, and consisted of generalised convulsions, *arc de cercle*, *grands mouvements*, etc., followed by delirium. Hypnotic treatment was begun about the middle of October, 1890, and in a month the patient was well. Two years later there had been no relapse.

No. 3 (Wetterstrand). Mrs. ——, aged 36, had suffered for eight years from attacks of hysterical convulsions, associated with dysmenorrhœa, menorrhagia, hæmatemesis, and hemi-anæsthesia. No organic disease had been detected. The patient improved under ordinary hypnotic treatment, and recovered completely after ten days' " prolonged sleep."

No. 4 (Dr. Tatzel, of Essen on the Ruhr, Germany[1]). Mrs. ——, aged 32, March 24th, 1894, was confined in July, 1892, and six weeks later began to suffer from hysterical convulsions. Her previous health had been good. The attacks always began with a loud scream, followed by muscular twitchings and convulsions : on awaking the patient remembered nothing, but felt ill and depressed all the following day. She had lost flesh, suffered from constipation, want of appetite, and palpitation ; she had also become sullen, indolent, parsimonious, and careless in dress and appearance. Complete recovery followed hypnotic treatment.

Equally successful cases are reported by Bernheim, Krafft-Ebing, Stembo and many other Continental observers. Bérillon, who for three years watched Dumontpallier's cases of *grande hystérie* at the Pitié Hospital, stated that most of the patients recovered completely and were then in good health — some married and mothers of families, others occupying responsible business positions.

(B) Monosymptomatic Hysteria ; Monoplegia, Mutism, Aphonia,
Hiccough, Blepharospasm, Discromatopsia, etc.

The following cases are from my own practice :—

No. 5. *Aphonia.*—Miss ——, aged 55, June, 1899, had suffered during childhood from " broken chilblains." In 1888, she showed

---

[1] Now of Munich.

unmistakable symptoms of Rénaud's disease: the third finger of
the right hand became contracted and gangrenous, and had to be
amputated. Later all the fingers and toes became more or less
contracted, rendering further amputations necessary—the last,
that of the left great toe, having taken place a few weeks before
she consulted me in 1899.

The patient had lost her voice early in 1897; but physical
examination revealed nothing abnormal, and galvanic and other
treatment had produced no result.

She was then sent to me by Mr. Stephen Paget, on account
of her aphonia, and first hypnotised on June 22nd, 1899: a
fortnight later the voice commenced to improve, and was normal
by the end of July, when treatment was discontinued. In January
1903, she reported that there had been no relapse, despite the fact
that she had been very ill from her other nervous trouble.

No. 6. *Singultus.*—Mrs. ——, aged 49, April 1895. Father
died insane. The patient had suffered for many years from
dyspepsia, constipation, depression, neurasthenic fears, etc. During
the last six years there had been frequent attacks of spinal
neuralgia, and she had rarely slept without narcotics. Severe
menorrhagia from 1890 to 1894, when the catamenia ceased.
In 1892, she was found to have a large uterine fibroid. In
August, 1892, violent attacks of hiccough commenced, and soon
only ceased during sleep. There were also frequent exacerbations
of a convulsive character, which sometimes lasted for hours and
left the patient exhausted.

After prolonged treatment by drugging, galvanism, etc., the
patient was sent to me by Dr. de Watteville. I first tried to
hypnotise her in April, 1895, but only succeeded in the following
December after eighty-five failures; my efforts till then being
frustrated by the constant attacks of hiccough which distracted
her attention. There was progressive improvement from the
latter date: at first the attacks only ceased while the patient was
being hypnotised; then they stopped when she came into the
consulting-room. Later the same thing happened when she came
into the waiting-room; then preparing to visit me would be the
signal for the hiccough to cease. The attacks entirely disappeared
a month after the first induction of hypnosis, and treatment was
abandoned. Up to the last report (1902) there had been no
relapse.

No. 7. *Muscular Tremor.*—Miss ——, aged 19, September, 1895. Good family history. The patient had suffered from obstinate constipation since infancy, and menstruation, which began at 11 years of age, had always been painful. With these exceptions her health had been good up to fifteen months previously, and she had had no hysterical symptoms of any kind. Then, after over-exertion and mental strain, violent muscular tremor of the right arm and hand commenced. This only ceased during sleep, and soon spread to the right leg, and then to the left arm and leg. Walking was difficult and painful, and latterly she could hardly cross a room: she also complained of constant diffused headache. From the beginning of her illness, if she looked at a bright object—especially anything blue—everything appeared of that colour. This impression persisted for about an hour, while its disappearance was always sudden and accompanied by a feeling of faintness. After electricity, massage, careful drugging, and change of air had been tried—all with negative results—the patient was sent to me by Dr. de Watteville.

Hypnosis was induced at the first attempt on September 2nd, 1895, and followed by immediate improvement; in a month the patient was well and returned to work. Three months later there had been no relapse; the bowels were regular, and menstruation painless. On several occasions, she had ridden over fifty miles a day on a heavy tricycle without undue fatigue, and had gained over a stone in weight. She married shortly afterwards, and, at the date of the last report (1901), was a strong, healthy, well-developed woman and the mother of two children. There had been no relapse.

No. 8. *Catalepsy.*—Miss ——, aged 28, dressmaker, was admitted to the National Hospital, Queen's Square, August 5th, 1896 (Dr. Gowers' Wards), and I am indebted to Dr. Stewart, House Physician, for the following notes :—

" For the last ten years the patient had suffered from sickness after food, and pain in the abdomen. Used to spit up blood in small quantities, but no cough, wasting, or night sweats. Said she had coffee-ground vomit followed by tarry motions. Since January, 1896, she had also had pain in back and attacks of stiffness.

" *On admission.*—A well-nourished, but pale, anæmic girl. Intelligent. No motor or sensory paralysis. No anæsthesia. Organic reflexes normal — plantars present, erector spinæ in-

creased. Jaw, biceps, and wrist jerks present. No ankle clonus.
Cranial nerves normal.   Some ovarian and epigastric tenderness.   Chest normal.   Visual fields, pupils, and discs normal.
Has had attacks of rigidity ; several a day, sometimes lasting
twelve hours.   These come on suddenly, painlessly, and without
warning.   Spasm first affects legs and feet.   Legs become stiff,
knees extended ; ankles extended and toes stiffly flexed.   Spasm
is most marked in extensor and adductor muscles of leg ; but all
muscles are rigid.   Pulling on one foot pulls the other over too,
as if glued to it.   When trunk becomes rigid, the whole body is
like a bar of iron and can be lifted up by one foot.   Abdominal
muscles hard, respiration shallow and back muscles rigid.   When
the arms are affected, they are stiffly extended parallel to the
body ; the fingers flexed at metacarpo-phalangeal joints, but
extended at others ; the thumbs adducted and wrists stiffly flexed.
Face sometimes stiff, jaws firmly clenched and unable to be
separated : speech impossible ; no risus sardonicus ; expression
impassive.   Eyes not affected.   Neck stiff and extended.

"November 23rd, 1896. Numerous observations have shown
that there are two hysterogenetic spots—(1) Interscapular region
of spine : (2) Lumbar spine :—pressure on these induces an attack.
Attacks can be relieved by application of faradic brush to external
malleoli in turn ; first one leg and then the other becoming
relaxed.   The duration of the attack varies from a few minutes
to several hours ; afterwards the patient perspires a good deal
about the hands and feet, and feels tired.   After a severe attack,
when the face has been involved, she usually vomits also.

"December 8th, 1896.   Patient has had several attacks of
urgent vomiting, apparently causeless, with severe pain, necessitating rectal feeding by peptonised enemata.

"January 20th, 1897.   Patient has been getting steadily
worse ; attacks have increased in frequency and severity ; she is
rigid nearly all day and occasionally wakes up rigid during the
night.

"Yesterday I (Dr. Stewart) induced stiffness of legs experimentally by rubbing lumbar region, and stiffness of shoulders and
arms by rubbing interscapular region.   Patient lay with trunk,
legs, and thighs rigidly extended ; toes pointed and arms parallel
to body.   She could be lifted by head and heels like a log ; the
face was rigid ; and she could neither speak, smile, protude her

tongue, nor move her facial muscles. The eyes, however, could be moved freely in all directions, and the eyelids could be opened and closed. Temperature before, during, and after this attack was 98·2. Rigidity of arms, neck, and face passed off when hands were rubbed, but that of the trunk and lower extremities required application of faradic brush to external malleoli one after the other.

"On January 26th, Dr. Bramwell saw the patient and commenced hypnotic treatment."

On March 4th, Dr. Stewart, in forwarding me the above notes, congratulated me on the result, which he said had been very satisfactory.

Remarks.—I saw the patient on sixteen occasions from January 26th to March 4th, 1897. At first I visited her at the hospital: she was suspicious and evidently dreaded some disagreeable experiment, and I failed to influence her, despite the fact that on several occasions suggestions were made during chloroform narcosis. Later she was brought regularly to my house, where I showed her others who had been hypnotised, and thus gained her confidence. From that time she improved rapidly, and before the treatment ceased the attacks had disappeared. Her recovery was confirmed by a later report.

No. 9. *Muscular Spasm.*—Miss ——, aged 26, July 3rd, 1900, although always nervous and never very strong, had fair health up to 1897, when, after a severe mental shock, she began to have muscular spasms in the arms. These soon spread to the legs, and a few weeks later practically all the voluntary muscles of the body became affected—the movements hardly ceasing a moment while the patient was awake. The attacks were very irregular in character: at one moment the flexors and extensors of the arm were affected, when the patient struck out with startling rapidity—hitting those near her, or any inanimate object that happened to be within range of the blow. A moment afterwards the legs would be similarly affected; the head violently jerked, or the muscles of the face convulsively twitched. She was cut and bruised from her involuntary violence, complained greatly of headache, and was anæmic and feeble. She could not walk without assistance, and was unable to dress or feed herself. Attacks of muscular spasm frequently occurred during sleep, and invariably awoke her.

The patient was sent to me by Dr. Bold Williams, of

Llandudno, on July 3rd, 1900. Hypnosis was induced at the first attempt and she began to improve; but a week later, although the hypnosis had become profound, the attacks still continued. For a few minutes she would rest quietly as if asleep, and then convulsive movements appeared : if slight they did not arouse her, but if severe, she came out of the hypnotic state with a start and looked confused. When this happened I rehypnotised her, repeating the process until she had had at least half an hour's continuous rest. At the end of three weeks the attacks ceased, and treatment was abandoned. She walked and slept well, had no difficulty in dressing or feeding herself, and her general health had greatly improved. Up to the last report (April, 1903) there had been no relapse.

No. 10. Mr. ——, aged 39, May, 1902, had done twelve years' service in the Royal Navy. No bad marks; all entries " very good." Good service medal. In June, 1893, he was Ship's Corporal on H.M.S. *Victoria* under Admiral Tryon, when she was rammed and sunk by the *Camperdown*.

When the ship was sinking it was his duty to go below and release the prisoners. This he did, then went down to the battery-deck to see if the ports were closed. While there the ship sank and carried him with her.

He thinks the subsequent explosion blew him to the surface. He was picked up unconscious by one of the boats, and taken on board H.M.S. *Nile*. After prolonged artificial respiration, he had an attack of noisy delirium, followed by seventeen hours' further unconsciousness. Immediately afterwards violent generalised muscular tremor appeared. This was constant, except during sleep, and was aggravated if any one approached him. He could do nothing for himself, and had to be fed through a bent tube, which extended from the back of his head to his mouth. The attendant, who had to stand behind so as not to be seen, poured liquid nourishment into one end of the tube, while the patient, with much difficulty, took it from the other end.

Three days later he entered Malta Hospital, where he stayed a month. He was then sent to the Naval Hospital at Haslar, where he remained until October 3rd, 1893, when he was invalided and sent home. During the first year after his accident he was stated to have had four " epileptic fits," but from the description I have been able to obtain, it seems probable that these were attacks of catalepsy. Marked muscular tremor continued for a year, then gradually became less violent and finally almost ceased. The most striking and persistent feature in the case was difficulty in walking. This showed itself from the beginning : at first the patient could walk a step or two alone, but if any one came near him, he fell suddenly on his back. After leaving hospital this symptom became more pronounced, and he only left his bed to be helped into a chair. He could stand, however, and move about a little, by holding the chair and pushing it in front of him. After being kept on as invalided, from year to year for four years, he was finally pensioned off as incurable.

On May 8th, 1902, he was sent to me by Dr. Roome of Southsea. The patient told me that he had never known what sickness was until his accident. He now complained of nothing but his inability to walk : his general health was excellent, and he never felt ill or depressed. He was powerfully built and strong in the arms, but the muscles of the lower extremities were markedly wasted and flabby, and the pulse weak. Reflexes much exaggerated : the slightest touch over the patella produced a violent convulsive kick. Further, any muscular stimulus, particularly if unexpected, produced an immediate response. For example, if his foot touched an inequality in the bedclothes, he would be almost thrown out of bed by the violence of the muscular start.

His walking was still limited to moving a little about his room, with the aid of a chair. Anything beyond this was followed by a fall. At first the exciting cause was mainly emotional : he fell if any one came near him. Later, he fell if he attempted to walk with the assistance of another person : if he encountered the slightest inequality in the ground he tumbled, and dragged his companion with him. This did not occur because his legs failed him ; his fall seemed always due to a distorted or exaggerated reflex. The slightest unexpected stimulus to the soles of the feet was followed by a convulsive response, when he fell rigidly and violently on the back of his head. Beyond this I could discover nothing abnormal. There was no paralysis, no loss of consciousness, and no alterations in sensation other than those just described.

I began hypnotic treatment on May 8th, and continued it five times a week until July 24th, 1902, when the patient returned to Portsmouth. Hypnosis, in the sense in which I understand it, was never induced. Apparently nothing was done beyond making " curative suggestions," while the patient rested quietly in an arm-chair : he never even became drowsy. Despite this, the result was striking. In a week he could cross his room ; and, after the first month, he spent hours at a time walking about the streets and parks. He even went into crowds without fear or tremor, and saw the various military reviews, etc., which were held at that time.

After returning home he wrote to complain that he felt nervous and depressed ; he also stated that he had fallen while walking. On February 2nd, 1903, he returned for four days' further treatment. He told me that his nervousness had passed off, and that he had several times walked as much as fourteen miles in one day. He had tumbled down on four occasions : the character of these accidents, however, differed from the earlier ones. Now, instead of falling rigidly backwards, his legs gave. way and he slipped down—somewhat in a sitting fashion. There had been no return of muscular tremor, but there was still a certain amount of timidity and difficulty in walking. This, however, was confined almost solely to mounting steps, and such-like obstacles. On February 5th, I took the patient to see Dr. de Watteville, who thought that, from the absence of emotional symptoms, one might almost call the case one of *muscular* hysteria. As the patellar reflex was now distinctly *below normal*, and the muscles of the lower extremities still flabby, he suggested giving glycerophosphates, with 5-drop doses of liqour strychninæ. This was done and the patient returned home. Later reports satisfactory.

It is of interest to note that, although the patient responded to suggestion in this instance, ordinary medical treatment associated with self-suggestion had entirely failed. He had had the fixed idea that a certain medical man could cure him, and, as soon as he left hospital, had placed himself under his care ; but despite his faith, he had received no benefit. From that date he had been almost continuously under treatment, and had consulted in all nineteen different medical men.

Many other successful cases, including all the various forms of hysteria comprised in this section, have been reported by Continental observers. Of these the following are examples :—

No. 11 (Dr. A. Gros, France). *Hysterical Paralysis.*—Miss ——, aged 30, had always been emotional, but hysterical symptoms only commenced at the age of 16. At 18, convulsive attacks appeared; these soon became frequent and severe, and were associated with boulimia and persistent spinal neuralgia. In October, 1894, the patient suddenly fell while walking and had to be carried home. Despite baths, electricity, and careful drugging, the paralysis and other hysterical symptoms were still unrelieved in September, 1897. The patient was then hypnotised and recovered in a week. No relapse.

No. 12 (Bérillon). *Hysterical Paralysis.*—Miss ——, aged 40, May, 1890, had an attack of hysterical convulsions at the age of 31 : this was followed by paralysis of the lower extremities, and she had been confined to her bed ever since—a period of nine years. Recovered after a short hypnotic treatment.

No. 13 (Bérillon). *Aphonia, etc.*—Miss ——, aged 22. Previous health good; no family history of hysteria. In July, 1886, after having spoken louder than usual when teaching, her voice became hoarse, then disappeared; a few days later the aphonia passed into mutism. Physical examination gave negative results, and there was no improvement from galvanism of the chords and other treatment. She recovered after the first hypnotic sitting, but relapsed five months later. The voice returned, however, after a single rehypnotisation; and two years later there had been no further relapse.

No. 14 (Dr. Burot, of Rochefort). *Singultus.*—Mrs. ——, aged 58, September, 1888, had suffered for many years from migraine, and hysterical weeping accompanied by muscular tremor. In April, 1888, she had her first attack of hiccough, followed a fortnight later by another at the same hour. Soon the attacks became continuous, were accompanied by retching and vomiting, and only ceased during sleep. Recovered after two hypnotic sittings : nine months later there had been no relapse.

No. 15 (Bérillon). *Blepharospasm.*—Miss ——, aged 20, March, 1889. Family history of phthisis and hysteria. In February, 1888, after mental shock, incessant convulsive twitching of the left eyelid appeared, followed three days later by complete blepharospasm : this had remained unrelieved ever since, despite constant and varied treatment. The spasm disappeared after the first hypnotic sitting, and a year later there had been no relapse.

No. 16 (Dr. Lemoine, of Lille). *Hysterical Tremor simulating Paralysis agitans.*—Mr. ——, aged 57, began to have muscular tremor of the right arm after a mental shock at the age of 36. This soon spread to the right leg, and later the left side was also affected; the tremor continued during repose and was increased by every attempt at voluntary movement. He also suffered from frequent headaches, and had anæsthetic patches on the right arm. After six days' hypnotic treatment, the tremor, which had lasted twenty-one years, entirely disappeared. No relapse.

No. 17 (Tatzel). *Clonic Torticollis.*—Mr. ——, aged 44, May, 1894, government official, had good health up to 1890, when he commenced to have pain in the right side of the neck. This was soon followed by constant clonic spasm of the muscles of the right side of the face and neck. The head was constantly drawn backwards, with such force that the resulting friction against the collar had rubbed off much of his hair. He was unable to dress or undress himself: breathing was difficult and eating painful. As he did not improve, he went into the hospital at Bonn in May, 1891, and remained till September, when he was discharged as incurable. From that time, he passed through the hands of several medical men and many quacks, trying, amongst other things, the Kneipp cure. After having spent all his money in this way, he had to be supported by the parish; and when Tatzel first saw him (May, 1894) he was a broken-hearted, despondent man, who only ventured out after dark, and then tried to control the muscular spasms by holding the handle of his walking-stick between his teeth. Result: after several months' hypnotic treatment the spasms entirely ceased, and the patient had gained fifty pounds in weight. No relapse.

No. 18 (van Renterghem). *Clonic Muscular Spasm.*—Mr. ——, aged 42, October, 1896. Family history good. The patient was supposed to have had meningitis in 1875, and suffered during convalescence from clonic spasms of the neck. These soon ceased, however, and he continued in good health until November, 1895, when some of his cervical glands became inflamed. He recovered from this, but in February, 1896, began to have constant and violent spasms of the muscles of the right side of the neck. Careful drugging, massage, the continued and faradic current, and prolonged rest in bed produced no improvement. He entered the Burgerziekenhuis Hospital on May 28th,

1896, where hot douches, baths, massage, etc., were employed without improvement. On June 24th, the accessory nerve of Willis was stretched, and the operation repeated on July 1st, but without result. On August 11th, the head was fixed in a mechanical apparatus and the patient discharged. On October 4th, when the spasms were as violent as ever, hypnotic treatment was commenced: this was continued for five months and resulted in complete recovery. No relapse.

No. 19 (Dr. Scholz of Bremen). *Paramyoclonus multiplex.*— Miss ——, aged 19, healthy and well developed: no previous symptoms of hysteria. Suddenly, after a shock, she felt intensely cold and all her limbs trembled. The same evening the first paramyoclonic attack appeared: there were short rhythmic quiverings of the muscles of both upper arms and shoulders— about 120 to the minute, also rhythmic spasms of the muscles of the eyelid.

In another case, also reported by Dr. Scholz, there were clonic spasms of the muscles of the head, neck, trunk, and extremities, resembling violent shivering fits.

Both patients rapidly recovered under hypnotic treatment, and six years later there had been no relapse.

Dr. Stadelmann (Germany) records two cases of severe generalised muscular spasm, both of which recovered after one hypnotic sitting. No relapse. Dr. Curt Schmidt, of Dresden, reported a case of supposed ulcer of the stomach, with sickness, loss of appetite, abdominal pain, hysterical twitching, neuralgia, etc., which yielded at once to hypnotic suggestion. Dr. Stembo, of Wilna, published a case of frequent attacks of sleep, which occurred several times a day and sometimes lasted for hours; the patient quickly recovered under hypnotic treatment. Successful cases of this form of hysteria are also reported by Bernheim, Dumontpallier and many others.

(C) *The various Manifestations of ordinary Hysteria—Dyspepsia, Visceral and Menstrual Troubles, etc.*

The following cases are from my own practice:—

No. 20. Mrs. ——, aged 41, March 20th, 1892, had always been more or less delicate. Obstinate constipation since infancy; this had been worse during the last twelve years, the minimum interval between successive actions of the bowels being a week. Chronic dyspepsia, anæmia, and emaciation. Severe dysmenorrhœa since commencement of menstruation. Married twenty years : no children, sexual desire absent, marked dyspareunia. Frequent attacks of depression since 1882 : for two years the condition had practically been one of melancholia—she had shunned all society, neglected her domestic duties, and frequently shut herself alone in her bedroom for hours, and spent the time in crying. Insomnia since 1889. Sick-headache since childhood : for the last twelve years these attacks had been more frequent and severe, and latterly had averaged one a day—invariably followed by vomiting. As long as she could remember, she had been short-sighted ; and reading and working, especially by artificial light, soon produced headache.

On December 9th, 1889, I sent her to see the late Mr. Bendelack Hewetson (Ophthalmic Surgeon to the Leeds Infirmary), who afterwards supplied me with the following notes : " Mrs. —— complained of distressing and almost constant headaches, with frequent nerve-storms of migraine. She had persistent pain over the eyes and at the back of the head, extending down the neck ; the roots of the hair were tender. She read ' Snellen's ' $\frac{20}{50}$ with the right eye and $\frac{20}{70}$ with the left unaided, but required a $-\frac{1}{50}$ to enable her to read $\frac{20}{50}$ with either eye. Ophthalmoscopic examination showed that she was hypermetropic, and that this condition was over-corrected by ciliary spasm, rendering her virtually myopic and necessitating a minus glass."

Mr. Hewetson prescribed atropine for a month, and afterwards a $+\frac{1}{40}$ glass for reading. The headaches ceased while the atropine was used, but the patient said the glasses hurt her and would not persevere with them, and the headaches soon returned with increased violence.

She suffered greatly from her teeth, of which she had but twelve left, all decayed. She was anxious to have them extracted, but was afraid to face a dentist, and asked me to have the operation performed during hypnotic anæsthesia. I explained that patients suffering from hysteria rarely became hypnotised deeply enough for operative purposes, and tried to persuade her to take an ordinary anæsthetic. As she refused to do this, I consented to the experiment. To my surprise, before I had finished my usual preliminary explanations, profound hypnosis appeared. I then suggested that she should sleep well, be free from headache and depression; that her appetite and digestion should be good, the bowels regular, etc., etc. I also successfully suggested local and general anæsthesia. The curative suggestions were quickly responded to: she slept well, her headaches disappeared, the bowels acted regularly. Menstruation and connection became painless, digestion and appetite improved, and she rapidly gained in weight and strength.

The toothache entirely disappeared; and, owing to this and other reasons, she deferred the operation for some time. Meanwhile, I discovered that I could produce profound anæsthesia by simple suggestion in the apparently normal waking state. On these occasions, the patient recognised and talked with those around her, and afterwards remembered everything that had happened, except the sensations which had been specially inhibited. The teeth were ultimately extracted in this apparently waking state, and the account of the operation has been already given (pp. 168-9).

Afterwards Mr. Bendelack Hewetson saw the patient several times, and gave me the following notes:—

"Dr. Bramwell brought Mrs. —— to see me in July, 1892. She stated that she had had no headache since being hypnotised on March 20th, 1892. She was a new creature mentally and physically—bright, healthy-looking and well nourished; formerly she had been a burden to herself and her friends. On examination, I found her vision in every way as defective as on the first occasion I had seen her. Dr. Bramwell then suggested to her, in what was apparently the normal waking state, that she should be able to read the bottom line of 'Snellen's' unaided by glasses. This she did successfully, and immediately afterwards repeated the feat on a changed series of test types. Obviously Dr. Bramwell could induce his patient to relax her accommodation, and to produce the same improvement of vision as had resulted from a minus glass. Dr. Bramwell then suggested that the increased range of vision should be maintained, and that the patient should continue to be able to read 'Snellen's' $\frac{20}{40}$ unaided.

"I saw her again on October 26th, 1892, when she stated that she had remained entirely free from headache, and that the increased range of vision had been maintained. I found that Dr. Bramwell, by suggestion in the apparently normal waking

o

state, could enable the patient to reproduce the ciliary spasm
and the original condition of vision, and again to relax the
accommodation and gain the increased visual range."

On June 30th, 1893, Mr. Hewetson wrote me as follows :—
" As I am much interested in Mrs. ——'s case, I asked her to
visit me in order that I might make a further examination. She
came to-day looking bright and well nourished. She told me
that she felt well in every way, and had had no return of her
headaches or other nervous symptoms. There was no evidence
of ciliary spasm, although she had been using her eyes very much
of late for reading and fine work. She never wore glasses, and
could read ' Snellen's ' $\frac{20}{20}$ easily with either eye."

No. 21. Miss ——, aged 33, April, 1893, was anæmic and
emaciated, and had suffered all her life from insomnia : since an
attack of influenza in 1890, she had only averaged three hours'
sleep per night. Menstruation commenced at 13 years of age,
and had always been painful and excessive. Obstinate constipation since 1889. During the last three years she had had
several attacks of eczema and herpes, the latter followed by
intercostal neuralgia, which still persisted : she also suffered from
muscular rheumatism, was nervous, irritable, and intolerant of
all forms of noise.

She was sent to me by Dr. Roe, of Penryn, on April 15th,
1893. Deep hypnosis was easily induced at the first attempt,
and it was suggested that she should sleep all night. Two days
later, she told me that the night after she saw me she had slept
from the moment she had put her head upon the pillow till called
the following morning, a thing she had never done before. The
next night was equally good. I rehypnotised her, and suggested
the disappearance of all morbid symptoms ; but, as she was
obliged to leave London next day, I did not see her again until
March 5th, 1894. She looked well, was bright and cheerful,
and had gained over a stone in weight. She was entirely free
from dysmenorrhœa, constipation, rheumatism and insomnia. Up
to the last report (1903) there had been no relapse.

No. 22. Miss ——, aged 20, April 6th, 1894, had always
slept badly. The insomnia varied, but according to her mother's
account, she had not had a good night's sleep since birth. At
the age of 8, pains in the back, particularly in the lumbar region,
began ; these soon became constant, and were aggravated by the

slightest exertion. Since 1883, there had been frequent attacks of headache; pain usually frontal, sometimes occipital—rarely followed by sickness. Myopia corrected by glasses. Periods—always painful and excessive—lasted eight or nine days, and necessitated rest in bed. Latterly all the symptoms had been worse; she was never free from pain, always felt fatigued and depressed, while even a short walk was followed by acute suffering. She had had prolonged medical treatment without benefit. No organic lesion of any kind had been discovered : with the exception of a tendency to conical cervix, the uterus and ovaries were normal.

She was sent to me by Dr. Boulting, of Hampstead, on April 9th, 1894, and hypnosis was easily induced at the first attempt. This was repeated sixteen times up to June 26th; then abandoned, as all the morbid symptoms—menorrhagia excepted—had disappeared.

Miss —— again consulted me early in 1896. She now slept well, was free from headache and spinal pain, and capable of more than the average amount of exertion. The periods were painless; but, as the menorrhagia still persisted, she was hypnotised twice a week for three months. Result nil. I then decided to keep her in the hypnotic state during a period. On June 1st, 1896, she entered a nursing home, where she was hypnotised and put in charge of a nurse, who was placed *en rapport* with her. Hypnosis was maintained until the evening of June 3rd, when she was aroused, as the period had not begun. It did so, however, during the night of the 7th. She was rehypnotised on the morning of the 8th, and kept in the hypnotic trance until the 12th, when the period terminated some days earlier than usual. Before hypnosis the temperature was 98·8°. During hypnosis the morning and evening temperature was almost invariably 98°; on two occasions the evening temperature rose to 98·2°. Before hypnosis the pulse was 80; during hypnosis it varied from 60 to 65. The patient was fed by the nurse at stated intervals without being aroused, and the action of the bowels and bladder regulated by suggestion. Since then the periods have been normal in duration and amount; and, ·instead of keeping her bed, the patient has been able to cycle, &c. No relapse up to last report (1903).

No. 23. Miss ——, aged 28, July 1896. Father markedly

neurotic; two brothers and a sister had nervous breakdowns, and one brother, aged 38, had been paralysed for seven years. The patient had good health up to September 12th, 1891, when severe pain in the right hip and leg suddenly appeared. This lasted two years, then ceased, only to reappear almost immediately in the left leg. During the first two years of her illness she never walked more than a quarter of a mile; then even this was abandoned, and she took to a bath-chair. She became emaciated, suffered from insomnia, constipation and headache, lost all interest in life, and would not even read a novel.

Treatment.—Rest on her back in bed for two months, Weir Mitchell, careful drugging, massage, electricity, baths at Droitwich and Bath. Then, under the advice of a well-known neurologist, Paquelin's cautery to leg; 70 applications daily from July, 1895, to May, 1896, about 20,000 in all. Meanwhile, she grew steadily worse, and was finally pronounced incurable.

The patient then consulted Dr. Raymond Crawfurd, who brought her to me on July 18th, 1896. I at once began hypnotic treatment, and repeated it daily until July 31st. She slept well the night following the first sitting, and two days later her pains had disappeared, and she walked without difficulty. At the end of a week she exchanged her bath-chair for a bicycle, and, although she had never formerly mounted the latter, soon became a good rider. On July 31st, she started on a cycling tour, and on her return home at once commenced to lead an extremely active life. At the last report, December, 1902, she was in good health, and had been free from pain ever since the treatment.

No. 24. Mrs. ——, aged 25, February, 1894, had always been nervous and emotional; when a child, any excitement caused vomiting. Attacks of migraine since the age of 8: latterly these had been very frequent, and accompanied by feelings of giddiness and confusion. Catamenia appeared at 15; slight dysmenorrhœa. Married at 19: the succeeding period, an exceedingly painful one, was followed by pregnancy. After the periods recommenced they were regular, but invariably preceded by much uneasiness, and accompanied by attacks of severe spasmodic pain in the lower part of the body and back. This lasted from one to three days; and the patient, who kept her bed, was unable to lie down during the paroxysms, and had to get on her hands and knees, maintaining this position almost continuously for the first twenty-four hours. There was constant nausea with occasional vomiting. Discharge scanty. Uterus retroflexed; slight leucorrhœa. Depression; frequent attacks of hysterical weeping. Dyspareunia; no sexual desire.

After drugging, pessaries, and other local treatment had been tried without result, the patient was sent to me by Mrs. Dickinson Berry, M.D., in February, 1894.

Hypnosis was induced twenty-nine times up to May 5th, 1894, when the morbid symptoms had disappeared. In April, 1895, the patient reported that the periods were free from pain, lasted three days, instead of five as formerly, and that the discharge was more abundant. The interval was now four weeks instead of three. Marital relations normal. About a year later, the patient wrote to say that she had again become pregnant, and that the periods had been normal up to then.

No. 25. Miss ——, aged 19, November, 1889, was markedly anæmic and had suffered from attacks of frontal headache since the age of 7; these averaged two a week and were invariably followed by vomiting. Menstruation, always painful, commenced at 13. Early in 1887, the periods began to be scanty, with prolonged but irregular intervals, and ceased in May, 1888. After a short hypnotic treatment in November, 1889, somnambulism with anæsthesia was induced. The patient was the subject of the two painless operations reported, pp. 161-2. In February, 1889, her health was remarkably good, with the exception that the amenorrhœa still persisted. I rehypnotised her and suggested that, on March 13th, 1889, she should experience all the symptoms which had formerly preceded menstruation—pain in the back and thighs, sensation of weight and dragging in the abdomen, etc.—that these should last two hours, the catamenia then appear and all pain cease. During the six weeks which preceded the date fixed, I hypnotised the patient two or three times a week, and repeated the above suggestions. On the morning of March 13th, the symptoms indicated appeared, continued for two hours, and were followed by menstruation, which lasted five days. During the next fortnight, I hypnotised her on three occasions, and suggested that menstruation should appear on April 7th, and, on this and subsequent occasions, be free from pain. After this, menstruation was normal for over two years; the patient then married and became pregnant. She had no return of headache, and her general health remained good. Case shown at medical meetings in London, Leeds, and elsewhere.

No. 26. Mrs. ——, aged 34, December, 1901. Nervous temperament. Amenorrhœa since the birth of her youngest child two years previously. She was only able to suckle the child two days, owing to the scanty secretion of milk. Later, the secretion increased, but was never enough for nursing purposes; it persisted, however, despite both external and internal treatment. In September, 1901, she had had an attack of inflammation of the breast with threatened abscess; this was followed by two other attacks at monthly intervals.

The patient was sent to me by Dr. Swan, of Devonport Street, W., on December 31st, 1901, and was hypnotised on fifteen occasions from that date until March 6th, 1902. The secretion of milk ceased, and there was no return of the mammary inflammation. Menstruation appeared on January 21st, 1902, and was regular from then until pregnancy occurred some months later.

Braid found hypnotic treatment valuable in menstrual disorders, and his results have been confirmed by recent observers, thus :—

No. 27 (Bernheim). Mrs. ——, aged 35. Menstruation normal, with an interval of twenty-one days, up to her first pregnancy. Afterwards she suffered from menorrhagia and dysmenorrhœa: at first the interval between the periods was fifteen days, but for the last two years it had varied from eleven to thirteen. During hypnosis, Bernheim suggested a progressive retardation of the period—a definite time being fixed for its appearance, *i.e.* after 26, 27, 28 and 29 days—these suggestions were successful; an interval of 29 days was established, the dysmenorrhœa relieved, and the period reduced from six days to three.

No. 28 (Voisin). Miss —— suffered from amenorrhœa, with hysterical symptoms and abdominal neuralgia, which had resisted ordinary treatment. On October 16th, 1886, it was suggested during hypnosis that menstruation would appear on the evening of the 20th. This was successful: the patient was rehypnotised on the 21st, and told that the discharge would continue until the evening of the 23rd. This was also responded to. On

November 9th, it was successfully suggested that the menses would appear at the end of four weeks and last two days.

In two other cases of amenorrhœa cited by Voisin, the catamenia appeared in each instance in response to a single hypnotic suggestion.

The following table gives the results in some of the cases treated by Dr. Tyko Brunnberg, of Upsala:—

	Cases.	No Improvement.	Improved.	Cured.
Amenorrhœa	9	1	2	6
Menorrhagia	9	3	2	4
Menorrhagia and Dysmenorrhœa	5	1	1	3
Dysmenorrhœa . . .	3	1	1	1
Total .	26	6	6	14

One of the patients, a girl over 20 years of age, had never menstruated: the catamenia appeared after the second hypnosis. Several of the successful cases of dysmenorrhœa were severe and of long standing, the periods being much lengthened and the intervals shortened.

Gascard reported two cases of menorrhagia in which recovery almost immediately followed suggestion, while Bérillon, Burot and Dècle claimed to have succeeded in many cases similar to Bernheim's just cited.

Successful cases of amenorrhœa, dysmenorrhœa and menorrhagia are also recorded by Drs. Delius, Wetterstrand, Voisin, Bérillon, Gascard, Journée, Marandon de Monthyel, Burot, Dècle. Many of the cases had long resisted other methods of treatment, while their recovery was confirmed by later reports.

At the First International Congress of Hypnotism, Paris, 1889, Dr. Briand, Physician to the Asylum of Villejuif, showed a hypnotised subject to whom it had been suggested (1) that menstruation should commence the following morning at six o'clock, and (2) that a blister should appear on her right arm where a piece of cigarette-paper had been applied. The first suggestion was successful, but to the latter there was no response. The further suggestion that the catamenia should cease was at once fulfilled.

Dr. Bugney reported a case of menorrhagia, associated with uterine fibroid, which was successfully treated by suggestion: the menorrhagia disappeared and the tumour diminished.

Some of the patients above referred to were undoubtedly hysterical, but in others the only symptom of nervous disorder was the menstrual disturbance. The fact that this was un-associated with discoverable organic cause is the excuse for having included all the cases under " Hysteria."

Insomnia.—Insomnia is frequently present in hysteria and neurasthenia, and sometimes, as in the following cases from my own practice, forms the chief symptom of nervous trouble.

No. 29. Master ——, aged 16, April 24th, 1890, had not had a good night's sleep since birth. There had been no break in the insomnia, but it had varied in intensity, and had been worse since January, 1890. While in bed the patient recalled all the events of the day; he did not feel excited, ill, or tired, but his brain remained abnormally active and he lay awake till 4 or 5 A.M., when he would perhaps get two or three hours' sleep. Physical fatigue did not influence the insomnia, nor had it been relieved by various forms of medical treatment and prolonged travel. His education had been almost entirely aural, but one term at school had been tried with disastrous results: he became absolutely sleepless and prostrate.

He was hypnotised at the first attempt on April 24th, 1890, and slept well the following night. Hypnosis was repeated about forty times during the next two months, after which he started active mental and physical work. Since then there has been no relapse; and, in 1900, Dr. Oliver, of Harrogate, who had originally sent the patient to me, reported that he was then leading a useful, active, and successful life.

No. 30. Mr. ——, aged 60, May 1900, had always been a light sleeper, but this had never been a serious trouble to him. His health had been good up to 1895, when he gave up business, after having worked hard from boyhood. Immediately afterwards insomnia appeared; this grew worse, despite medical treatment and much exercise in the open air. For a time narcotics helped him, but afterwards they lost their effect, although changed fre-quently. From 1896, he had never had three consecutive good nights, and often passed many with an average of two hours' sleep. His dread of insomnia became an obsession; he feared going to bed, and would not retire to rest unless some one shared his room.

The patient was sent to me by Dr. Herbert Tilley, whom he had consulted for aural trouble. At first he was absolutely incredulous as to the possibility of his being helped by hypnotic treatment, and often interrupted the process to explain this. After a few sittings, however, although he did not become drowsy or even restful, the suggestions took effect and he began to sleep better. In a month he was well, and had abandoned all drugs. Up to the last report (1901) there had been no relapse.

The following case presents many points of interest. The patient, who describes his own condition, is a trained observer, well known by his contributions to more than one department of natural science. He was originally sent to me by Dr. Boulting, of Hampstead. The results obtained by the patient's self-suggestion are worthy of note, particularly considering the slight amount of hypnosis which had been induced.[1]

No. 31. "A professional man, aged 51; subject to migraine, heavy smoker, very abstemious from alcohol.

"Having suffered from sleeplessness and other nervous symptoms, I sought Dr. Bramwell's aid at Easter, 1900.

"I had tried various systems of counting myself to sleep, and each in turn, as it became more familiar and easy, had lost its effect. Dr. Bramwell asked me to sit down and compose myself to sleep in my usual way, and to pay as little attention as possible to him. His procedure was that which I understand he usually adopts; and during the sittings I tried to get drowsy by using my most recent method of counting (synchronous with respiration). I had three sittings, and during the second alone was I at all somnolent, and that very little. The following has been the result of the treatment:—

"(1) My sleeplessness has been completely removed, and my sleep has been more continuous and more restful than before. I have even slept when new business cares of a most acute kind presented themselves suddenly a quarter of an hour before bedtime.

"(2) Further, I have been able to influence myself in various ways by suggestion, which I employ in the following manner. I count, as I formerly did, when trying to get to sleep, and alternate this with self-suggestions. What I aim at is to produce a stage in which I am sleepy enough to be suggestible, and yet sufficiently awake to make suggestions to myself.

"The method is least efficacious when I go to bed sleepy. I then find it difficult to count, sometimes even impossible, a

[1] It is to be noted too that I did not teach the patient to hypnotise himself.

drowsy state intervening. A vigorous effort, however, to wake up completely and count afresh is usually successful.

"(3) I have been able to induce analgesia and sleep during toothache, whether the latter arose from periostitis or from inflamed pulp: in these cases the pain goes a few moments *before* sleep. I suggest that 'I shall sleep well and without pain.' Sometimes the pain comes on again and wakes me, but a few more suggestions will induce fresh analgesia and sleep. Similarly, being subject to sea-sickness, I send myself to sleep on embarkation without much difficulty, and sleep, usually very lightly, quite free from qualms: on awaking, even in rough water, I feel no tendency to sickness. I have had two failures to send myself to sleep on the boat by suggestion out of some twenty passages: the one was due to flies which kept alighting on my face; the other instance was when I was convalescent from influenza, and I attribute it to the lack of power of myself as operator.

"(4) Post-hypnotic suggestion has on the whole failed. I think that I have sometimes succeeded in relieving constipation: I know that I have sometimes been unable to do so. I have failed by suggestions going on every night for three weeks to escape sea-sickness without going to sleep. I have not succeeded in curing migraine. I have, however, stopped or prevented the simple congestive headache of coryza. I have been also much less irritable during migraine-fits, etc.

" I attribute my difficulty of post-hypnotic suggestion to the fact that here the operator is the subject, and that the former is least efficient at the time when the latter should be most impressionable.

" I am usually able next morning to remember at what stage of my 'count' I lost consciousness. This is generally almost sudden. However, the approach of sleep is usually preceded by hallucinations or idiotic questions which I all but hear,[1] or by twitchings, or by a combination of these. A moment of intense wakefulness now comes on, in which I *know* from recollection of past experience that I shall sleep very soon, improbable as it *feels*. Much more rare is the drowsy condition referred to above, which recalls the state of insomnic people, who 'have heard the clock strike every hour in the night,' but not heard a child wailing for half an hour in an adjoining room."

[1] "My thought is mostly verbal, auditive: I am a poor visualist."

(*D*) *Mental Troubles of a Hysterical Nature, Perversions of Senti-*
ment, Obsessions, Irresistible Impulses, Hallucinations, Melan-
cholia, Maniacal Excitement, etc.

The following cases are from my own practice :—

No. 32. Mrs. ——, aged 30, April 26th, 1897. Father, and
several brothers and sisters, markedly nervous. The patient had
always been nervous ; had bitten her nails since early childhood
and never slept well. After her first confinement, in 1891, she
became afraid of driving, and got into a panic during thunderstorms : on one occasion this was followed by a short attack of
aphonia.

Her second confinement took place on January 12th, 1897.
Almost immediately afterwards she became profoundly melancholic, suffered from insomnia, constipation, indigestion, and loss
of appetite, amounting to absolute disgust for food. She refused
to see her child ; and her home became wholly distasteful to her.
Careful medical treatment and change of scene were without
result. She was sent to me by Dr. Boulting, of Hampstead, on
April 26th, 1897. In addition to the symptoms just described,
she was haunted by the idea of suicide, and could think of nothing
else. She was extremely agitated, could not sit still or keep her
attention fixed, and had frequent attacks of uncontrollable weeping.
After a few weeks' hypnotic treatment she commenced to
improve, and before the end of July had recovered and returned
home. Not only did her morbid ideas and suicidal impulses
disappear, but she also lost many of the nervous symptoms which
had existed before her illness. There has been no relapse up to
the present date (1903).

No. 33. Mrs. ——, aged 46, June 22nd, 1900. Father and
an uncle on the mother's side committed suicide. Patient had
always been nervous, emotional, and a bad sleeper. Since 1897,
after influenza, the insomnia had been much worse, and she
rarely got more than three hours' sleep at night. She suffered
constantly from a peculiar sensation in the neck, with a feeling
that she must fall forward. She was very depressed, had fits
of uncontrollable weeping, and had lost interest in life. There
were also strong suicidal impulses, and the fixed idea that she
would commit suicide like her father and uncle. She was sent

to me by Dr. Seton, of Kensington, and completely recovered
after a month's hypnotic treatment: there had been no relapse
up to the last report (November, 1902).

No. 34. Mr. ——, aged 37, May, 1899.   Father insane
and under restraint.   Twelve months previously, the patient
began to suffer from constant pain at the back of the head and
neck, which was followed by marked decrease in his powers of
attention and work.   He then became profoundly depressed,
lost all affection for his wife and children, and had the fixed idea
that he would become insane.   Drugs, lengthy holidays with
plenty of exercise in the open air, and finally treatment in an
asylum, were tried without benefit.   Complete recovery, however,
took place after six weeks' hypnotic treatment.   On December
18th, 1902, the patient wrote to say that he was in good health,
and that there had been no return of any of his morbid symptoms,
despite the fact that he had had much family trouble.   He had
recently lost both parents, and one sister had become insane.   In
January, 1903, Dr. Wonnacott, of Wandsworth, who had originally
sent the case to me, wrote confirming this report.

No. 35. Miss ——, aged 38, November, 1900.   Mother
suffered from religious melancholia, and died in an asylum.
Maternal uncle weak-minded.   One of the patient's cousins
committed suicide, several are insane, and one suffers from
obsessions.   One sister has delusions, another obsessions.   The
patient had good health up to puberty, then became quiet and
depressed.   In 1892, she had an attack of acute melancholia,
which lasted several months; since then she has always been
depressed and peculiar.   In 1895, after a shock, she had a second
attack of acute melancholia, and a further one in July, 1900,
following a similar cause.   When I first saw her, in November,
1900, she hardly ever spoke, was profoundly depressed, had
morbid religious ideas, and was untidy and extremely eccentric.
She was never permitted to go out alone, as she was quite incapable of taking care of herself, or of avoiding the traffic.   After the
first sitting, on November 2nd, 1900, she commenced to talk
brightly, and told me next day of the various religious fears
which had been tormenting her, but which had now entirely
vanished.   Hypnosis was repeated on four subsequent occasions
up to November 14th, when all morbid symptoms had disappeared.   A few days later, she was well enough to go alone to

San Francisco to nurse a sister during her confinement. In November, 1902, Dr. Ozanne, of Harrogate, who had sent the case to me, reported that the patient was in good health and leading a useful life. There had been no relapse.

No. 36. Miss ——, aged 22, April 30th, 1901. Father very unstable mentally. One of the patient's brothers was insane, and a sister suffered from chorea. Six months previously the patient became depressed, and was tormented with religious doubts and fears : she believed she had committed the unpardonable sin, and felt she ought to punish herself in consequence. She gave up all pleasures, and finally refused to see her friends or write to them. There were strong suicidal impulses. Medical treatment, including residence in nursing homes and isolation from friends, had been without result.

The patient was brought to me by Dr. Shuldham, of Hampstead, and hypnotised on twenty occasions from April 30th to July 23rd, 1901. She rapidly improved, and was well before the treatment terminated. At the last report, May 15th, 1903, she was still in good health, both mentally and physically.

No. 37. Mrs. ——, aged 56, had a bad family history : her mother, sister, and two brothers having suffered from insanity. The patient had her first attack of melancholia fifteen years previously : this was followed by others, both prolonged and severe. Hypnotic treatment was begun on February 12th, 1902, at the request of Dr. Sainsbury. At that time the patient had kept her bed for several months : she was profoundly depressed, had frequent attacks of hysterical weeping, suicidal impulses, etc. Her physical health was good, but she asserted that she could not leave her bed, as her mind was gone, and she did not know what to do, or even what clothes to put on. She felt that nothing in life could ever interest her again. At the end of four months she was well, and at the last report (February, 1903) there had been no relapse. She was leading an active, happy life, without the slightest trace of any nervous trouble.

Another somewhat similar case, sent, about the same time, by Dr. Harrison, of East Grinstead, was equally successful ; and many of a like nature might be cited from my own practice and those of others. The two following cases are examples from the latter source :—

No. 38 (Voisin). Mrs. ——, aged 30, June, 1888, suffered

from muscular movements resembling chorea: these started in
1870, and had continued ever since. In 1881, she became
depressed and had suicidal impulses. Shortly afterwards marked
hysterical attacks appeared: these were characterised by pains in
the head, sensations of choking, hyperæsthetic and anæsthetic
points, amnesia, etc. Later she became profoundly melancholic:
suffered from severe insomnia, had constant suicidal ideas, and
twice tried to end her life. For eighteen years she had taken
iron, valerian, bromides, and other drugs: hydropathic treatment,
the actual cautery, etc., had also been tried, but without result.
Hypnosis was easily induced at the first attempt, and after three
sittings all morbid symptoms disappeared. The recovery was
confirmed by later reports.

No. 39 (Voisin). Miss ——, aged 24, March, 1887. Maternal
grandfather nervous, impressionable, and addicted to alcohol.
Father was highly nervous, and died of consumption at 39.
Mother living, aged 45; also very nervous. The patient had
good health up to 1885, when she became depressed, had attacks
of uncontrollable weeping, and was obliged to abandon work.
She was tormented with erotic thoughts, and dreaded becoming a
prostitute: she had also the fixed idea that she would become
insane, and felt that she ought to commit suicide in order to
prevent this dishonour to her family. She was hypnotised five
times during March, 1887; all morbid ideas disappeared, she
gained in health and strength, resumed work, and passed a
scholastic examination. Recovery confirmed by later reports.

(2) Neurasthenia.

The following examples are from my own practice :—

No. 40. Mr. ——, aged 32, May, 1895, although nervous
and highly strung, had been physically strong and athletic up to
1887, when he broke down, apparently from overwork and
under-feeding. His appetite became capricious, and he suffered
from constipation, dyspepsia, nervous trembling, and persistent
feelings of lassitude and weariness. The slightest physical exertion, such as walking a quarter of a mile, produced feelings of
collapse and utter exhaustion. He was constantly depressed,
and wished to end his life—according to his own account,

nothing but want of pluck prevented his committing suicide. He gave up smoking, dieted himself strictly, tried change of air, sea voyages, and prolonged medical and hydropathic treatment without benefit.

He was first hypnotised in May, 1895 : this was repeated almost daily for six weeks, when his morbid symptoms ·had disappeared, and he had gained eight pounds in weight and enjoyed exercise. In September, 1900, he stated that he had practically perfect health ; that he frequently bicycled over a hundred miles a day without undue fatigue ; sometimes danced the greater part of the night, and was fresh for his office next morning. There had been no return of any of the symptoms which had formerly troubled him. In December, 1902, Dr. Eric Pritchard, of Hampstead, who had sent the case to me, informed me that the patient was still in good health, although he had been living in the tropics for some considerable time.

No. 41. Major ——, aged 45, April, 1900, had good health up to 1890, when he began to suffer from insomnia, constipation, irritability, depression and morbid terrors. He constantly felt he was about to die, or that something dreadful was going to happen to him. Despite treatment, the symptoms persisted, and the patient left India and returned to England in 1898, with the intention of retiring from the Army. While at home his health improved, and he went back to India in 1899. Shortly afterwards, all the old symptoms returned with increasing violence : he never slept without narcotics and, despite them, frequently awoke during the night in abject terror, with a feeling of impending death. He dreaded going about alone, and felt that he would die before completing the shortest journey. The most trivial accident, such as a puncture of his bicycle tyre, plunged him into irritability and despair: he believed he was under a curse, etc. He habitually took too much alcohol, not because he had any craving for stimulants, but because they steadied him and relieved his neurasthenic fears. He was sent to me by Dr. Roe, I.M.S., for hypnotic treatment. This was begun in April, 1900, and continued for six weeks : before the end of that time the patient was well. He then returned to duty in India : later reports confirmed his recovery.

In 1893-94, Schrenck-Notzing published an account of 228 neurasthenics treated by himself, Brügelmann, Bérillon, Bourdon,

Voisin, Burckhardt, Forel, Ringier, Ritzmann, Bourru, Burot, Stadelmann, von Corval, Michael, Drozdoivski, von Kozuchoivski, Neilson, Tuckey, Bernheim, van Renterghem, and Wetterstrand. The following were the results :—

I. HYPNOTIC.

In 70 cases—equalling 31·8 per cent—slight hypnosis was induced.

In 134 cases—equalling 60·9 per cent—either deep hypnosis, or somnambulism, was obtained.

In 16 cases—equalling 7·3 per cent—there was no hypnosis.[1]

II. THERAPEUTIC.

72 cases—equalling 31·6 per cent—recovered.

84 cases—equalling 36·8 per cent—were much improved.

72 cases—equalling 31·6 per cent—showed no improvement.

The following are examples taken from the cases just referred to :—

No. 42 (Bérillon). Major ——, aged 40, had been healthy and athletic up to two years previously ; then, following anxious sedentary work, he became emaciated and anæmic, and suffered from headaches and generalised muscular pain. He almost entirely lost the power of walking ; complained of indigestion, insomnia, frequent attacks of giddiness, palpitation, and pseudo-angina. He became profoundly depressed, and had suicidal impulses, together with the fixed idea that he would never be able to work again. Dilatation of the stomach was diagnosed, and for two years he was treated for that and other symptoms without benefit. He was hypnotised regularly for three weeks : then recovered and returned to duty. No relapse.

No. 43 (Bourdon). Mlle. ——, aged 23, after an accident at 15, suffered from sickness, headache, constipation, vertigo, spinal neuralgia, muscular weakness, insomnia, nocturnal terrors, etc. Treatment : Drugging, electricity, washing out of stomach, etc. Result nil. Hypnotised : recovered. No relapse.

No. 44 (Brügelmann). Mr. ——, aged 44, clergyman, had long suffered from spasmodic attacks of asthma, which gradually became so frequent and severe that he had to abandon his profession ; finally he could neither walk nor talk. He also had various other nervous symptoms of a neurasthenic character. Treatment : Drugging, electricity, inhalations, local applications

---

[1] In this group 8, out of the total of 228 cases, are omitted. In 6 the stage is not given, and 2 were treated in the waking condition.

to throat and nose, etc. Result nil. After twenty hypnotic sittings the patient recovered and resumed work.

Bérillon has reported good results in many cases of neurasthenia : some of these were associated with profound melancholia, others with fixed ideas and sexual aberrations.

Successful cases are also reported by Bingswanger, Hirt, Valentin, Tatzel, Auguste Voisin, Delius, Mavroukakis, Wetterstrand, Forel, van Eeden and van Renterghem. The two last authorities have reported 99 cases, of which 35 were improved and 21 cured.

The following have also written in favour of the hypnotic treatment of neurasthenia :—Arndt, Beard, Lehr, Bouveret, Holst, Loewenfeld, Koch, Laufenauer, Rosenthal, Gerhardt, Romberg, Jolly, Maack, Mueller.

In Schrenck-Notzing's opinion, impotence of psychical origin is sometimes the only symptom of neurasthenia ; out of 18 cases which he reported, 10 were cured by suggestion.

I have seen several cases which tend to confirm this view. In the following one, sent to me by Dr. Raymond Crawfurd, if the patient suffered from neurasthenia, impotence was the only symptom of that disorder.

No. 45. Mr. ——, aged 35, healthy and athletic. Continent before marriage. No masturbation. The patient had been married over three years; he was completely impotent, and this condition had not been improved by medical treatment.

Hypnotic treatment was begun on November 28th, 1898, and continued for a month. Despite the fact that deep hypnosis was not induced, curative suggestions were responded to. From Christmas, 1898, his sexual life has been that of a vigorous, normal man. There has been no relapse, and he is now the father of a healthy child.

According to Schrenck-Notzing, onanism, sexual hyperæsthesia, paræsthesia, and perverted sexual instincts are frequently associated with neurasthenia. He asserts that the grossest sexual aberrations, even when they have become deeply rooted and have changed the entire personality, are frequently cured by suggestion; and that this forms one of its most important therapeutic applications. For an account of these disorders and their successful treatment by suggestion, the reader is referred to the writings of Krafft-Ebing and Schrenck-Notzing. Both these

P

authorities have not only been successful in cases of satyriasis and nymphomania, but have also had good results in "sexual inversion."

I have seen little of the grosser forms of sexual disorder, either because these conditions are rare in this country, or because those who suffer from them do not seek medical aid. The results, however, have been encouraging. In one case of "sexual inversion" in an adult male, all morbid habits were abandoned after hypnotic treatment; and the patient is now leading a normal life. Another similar case, sent to me by Dr. van Renterghem, of Amsterdam, also did well.

Several cases of nymphomania were also successful. In one of these, an unmarried woman, both ovaries were removed at her own urgent request. This, however, was only done after consultation with Dr. Savage, in order to ascertain that her mental condition entitled her to be listened to. The operation, apparently, had no effect upon the disease; but this yielded to hypnotic treatment. The patient is now leading a useful and respectable life.

(3) Insanity.

Personal Results.—I have only attempted to employ hypnotic suggestion in eight cases of *undoubted* insanity. In five I failed to induce hypnosis, while three were more or less deeply hypnotised, with the following results :—

In the first case, although suggestion produced sleep and relieved the pain of an organic malady, it left unaffected the delusions of persecution from which the patient had long suffered.

In the second, the treatment quieted excitement and produced sleep: while the third was as follows :—

No. 46. Mrs. ——, aged 35. Nervous family and personal history. On June 7th, 1898, the patient's husband informed me that she had made a determined attempt at suicide, during an attack of acute mania. She had then been certified, and sent to the Priory, Roehampton, on June 3rd. There she was violent, slept badly, never spoke, refused all nourishment, and had to be fed artificially. Her husband was anxious that I should hypnotise her, and had obtained the consent of Drs. Savage and Chambers to the experiment.

I visited the patient on June 8th, apparently succeeded in inducing slight hypnosis, and suggested that she should take her food naturally, sleep well, cease to be violent, etc. From that date she never required artificial feeding, and soon began to be quieter and to sleep better. One day, by a ruse, I succeeded in making her speak, and from that time she talked more and more freely. Hypnotic treatment was continued till the end of July, when she was practically convalescent. When last I heard of her, in 1901, there had been no relapse. How far the hypnotic treatment aided the patient's recovery it is difficult to say. The fact that she commenced to take food immediately after the first induction of hypnosis may have been a mere coincidence; and it must not be forgotten that she was also receiving careful medical treatment.

Remarks.—Although I have cited few personal examples of the use of hypnotism in insanity, it is to be noted that I have related, under other headings, several cases in which the patients showed more or less marked evidence of insanity. Thus, amongst the cases of obsession will be found several in which the fixed ideas had become true insane delusions, which influenced the patient's whole life and conduct. Some of these patients also suffered from hallucinations, and had been certified; while others had been voluntary boarders in asylums.

Amongst the cases of " hysterical " melancholia are to be found several as grave as those usually cited as " insane " by other authorities. Some of these had long suffered from attacks of profound melancholy; a large proportion had suicidal impulses, while several had made more or less determined attempts at suicide. In more than one successful case the patient had been certified before treatment was commenced.

In some of the cases of moral insanity, the condition was considered sufficiently grave to necessitate restraint, both for the sake of the patients themselves, and in order to prevent them from corrupting others: restraint, indeed, was only delayed until the result of hypnotic treatment could be ascertained.

Although Elliotson claimed to have obtained good results in insanity, Esdaile's was the first systematic work in that field with which I am acquainted. He employed mesmerism in the

Calcutta Asylum for six months, but admitted that the general results were disappointing. In excuse he stated that the majority of the patients suffered from grave and apparently hopeless insanity, and that little or nothing was known of their history: most of them had been brought in by the police, who had found them wandering alone and deserted. , Despite this, Esdaile claimed to have obtained good results in several instances: few details, however, are given. One patient who suffered from frequent attacks of epilepsy, invariably followed by eight or ten days of acute mania, was stated to have recovered. Another, who had cut his throat during an attack of mania, had the necessary surgical operation performed during mesmeric anæsthesia.

Later, Esdaile stated that Dr. Keen, of Berhampore, had employed mesmerism for several years in his large asylum, where he claimed to have obtained excellent therapeutic results, and also to have found it of great use in maintaining quiet and discipline.

Braid also recorded the successful treatment of several cases of delusional insanity, which in most instances were complicated by hallucinations. Many cases are also reported by more recent observers :—

No. 47 (Voisin). Miss ——, aged 22, 1880, was the first insane patient treated by Voisin. For seven months she had had sub-acute mania, with hallucinations; also frequent inter-current attacks of acute mania, with homicidal impulses. It was during one of the latter, when extremely violent and confined in a strait-jacket, that Voisin first tried to hypnotise her. He succeeded with difficulty at the end of three hours, and the patient fell into a profound sleep which lasted three hours and a half. At first, the treatment appeared to have no effect upon the recurrence of the acute maniacal conditions, and Voisin frequently found her violent and furious. On each occasion, however, he cut short the attack; and it was, he said, astonishing to see her fall into a profound and calm sleep, when a moment before she had been yelling, gesticulating and striking her attendants. He then commenced to prolong her sleep by suggestion, and kept her in the hypnotic state for ten or twelve hours a day. Notwith-standing this, as soon as she awoke her language and conduct were deplorable. She was then told during hypnosis to be obedient and well-behaved; these suggestions were quickly responded to : she became well conducted, careful of her person, and employed herself in sewing, &c.   Finally, she recovered completely, and became a nurse in one of the Paris hospitals, where her conduct has been irreproachable.

No. 48 (Voisin). Miss ——, aged 25, November, 1884. Grandmother epileptic.   Five years previously, the patient began to suffer from mania, with auditory and visual hallucinations. When Voisin first saw her she had frequent acute attacks of furious delirium, lasting from eight to fourteen days, during which she refused to eat or drink, spat at her attendants and tried to bite them.   Voisin succeeded in hypnotising her in one of the attacks, by holding her eyes forcibly open for three hours, and compelling her to look fixedly at a magnesium lamp.   He then successfully suggested that she should sleep twenty-three hours and a half, during which she took the food and drink she had refused in the waking state.   At first, she was only allowed to remain awake three hours and a half per week, but as she improved the duration of the hypnotic sleep was diminished. After four months' treatment, all morbid symptoms disappeared, and she became polite, sociable, and amiable.   Fifteen months later there had been no relapse, and she obtained the post of wardrobe maid at the Salpêtrière.

No. 49 (Voisin). Miss ——, aged 40, entered Voisin's wards on June 24th, 1886.   She was profoundly melancholic and almost completely mute; when she spoke, which was at rare intervals, she stated that she was accused of murder, and that the police had come to arrest her.   During the day she rarely moved; but she was restless at night, and, as she was continually trying to strangle herself (her neck was surrounded by an ecchymosed circle evidently produced by a cord), she was put in a strait-jacket.   She had refused to eat for a fortnight, and there was incontinence of urine and fæces.

On June 29th, the condition was unchanged.   She was then hypnotised, told to sleep all night, to drink the milk given her, etc.   These suggestions were successful; she commenced to improve from that date, and at the end of a month her recovery was complete.

No. 50 (Voisin). Miss ——, aged 20, had entered Voisin's wards a year previously; she was extremely violent, rolled on the ground, tore her clothes, would not work, and used filthy language   During menstruation, these symptoms were so

aggravated that she was kept in a strait-jacket. Voisin succeeded
in hypnotising her at the beginning of a menstrual period, and
made her sleep for a week: this was repeated on four subsequent
occasions with similar results. Not only did the patient sleep
quietly during the whole of each period, but she gradually became
calmer and more rational in the intervals, and then recovered
completely.

In 1889, Voisin reported, amongst others, the following cases
of which he had traced the after-history :—(1) Melancholia with
hallucinations, treated in 1885. (2) Melancholia with hallucinations, suicidal ideas, and attempted suicide, treated in 1885.
(3) Acute mania with convulsive attacks, treated 1886. (4)
Melancholia with refusal of food, treated in 1884. (5) Sub-
acute mania, treated 1885. (6) Sub-acute mania, treated 1888.
(7) Acute mania, treated 1885. (8) Melancholia, treated 1888.
(9) Melancholia, treated 1888. Cases (8) and (9) relapsed after
attacks of epilepsy; the remaining seven continued well.
Numerous other insane cases, many of them equally interesting
and successful, were reported by Voisin from time to time.

No. 51 (Dr. Brémaud, of Brest). Mrs. ——, aged 25, had good
health until after her third confinement, when she became melancholic, and developed an intense aversion for her husband and
children. This was associated with morbid religious ideas; she
believed that virgins alone could enter heaven, and that she was
damned eternally on account of her marriage and pregnancies. She
thought she could only save her soul by penance, and tried to
starve herself to death. She refused all food, suffered continuously
from insomnia, and rapidly became very feeble and emaciated.
She was hypnotised at the first attempt, and took food during
the hypnotic state. The disappearance of all morbid fears was
suggested; on waking these had vanished, and she asked for her
children. Hypnosis was repeated the next day, after which her
recovery was complete; two years later there had been no
relapse.

No. 52 (Velander, Sweden). Miss ——, aged 36, had good
health up to 25, when she suddenly commenced to be troubled
about her soul. From that date she became markedly melancholic,
and more and more silent; by the end of twelve months she was
absolutely mute, and remained so for *ten years*. Then hypnotic
treatment was commenced: at the first sitting, after repeated

suggestions, she spoke a few words indistinctly ; a fortnight later she was well.

No. 53 (Liébeault). Mrs. ——, aged 36, May, 1892. Her father worried about trifles, and, after losing some money, became melancholic and threatened to commit suicide : four months later he drowned himself. The patient's first husband was accidentally drowned twelve months after marriage, and her second husband died suddenly when she had been married three years. From that date, early in 1891, she became profoundly melancholic, avoided her friends, slept badly, neglected her work and person ; and had the fixed idea that she would commit suicide by drowning. She was hypnotised 52 times from May to July, 1892, when all morbid ideas entirely disappeared. In 1894, Liébeault told me that she was still well, both mentally and physically.

No. 54 (Burot). Mrs. ——, aged 29. Father died from congestion of the brain ; on the mother's side an aunt and cousin were insane, and another aunt was hysterical. At the age of 20, a year after her marriage, the patient had miliary fever. Up to that time, she had excellent health both mentally and physically, but after her illness she became emotional and irritable. Three years later, after mental shock, she began to sleep badly, and suffered from nightmares and nocturnal terrors. She complained of pains, flushings, dizziness, difficulty in breathing and walking, cough, palpitation, obstinate constipation, etc. She dreaded death, and became profoundly depressed. Two years later she began to hear noises and voices, and had the delusion that certain persons had combined to kill her and her family, etc. She became so excited and violent that she was placed in La Fond Asylum. At first the excitement continued, she suffered from insomnia, was dirty in her habits and refused food : gradually she became calmer, and finally passed into a semi-idiotic condition. . At the end of four months she was sent home, when she again became violent and difficult to manage ; she sometimes escaped and tried to drown herself, and always complained that she was pursued by voices.

The patient then had six weeks' hypnotic treatment ; this was followed by very marked improvement, which was still maintained six months later, when she was again brought to Dr. Burot, and had renewed treatment for six weeks. From that date all morbid symptoms entirely disappeared ; she had neither delusions nor hallucinations, became once more bright and cheerful, and resumed her former active and orderly habits. She slept well, the constipation disappeared, and her periods, formerly irregular and scanty, now became normal. Later reports confirmed the recovery.

Successful cases are also reported by other Continental authorities; amongst these may be mentioned Répoud (the Cantonal Asylum of Marsens, Fribourg), who claims to have obtained results similar to Voisin's, with insane patients who were not hysterical; Burckhardt (Préfargier Asylum), cases of delusional insanity and acute puerperal mania; de Jong, and Rubinovitch, cases of melancholia, etc.

Until recently few attempts have been made in this country to hypnotise the insane.

In 1890, Drs. Percy Smith and A. T. Myers published an account of the hypnotic treatment of 21 insane patients in Bethlem Hospital. Improvement followed in six instances, but the results appear to have been due more to increased personal attention than to hypnotic influence.

In 1893, similar experiments were conducted at Morningside Asylum by Dr. George Robertson. He did not succeed in curing any case of genuine insanity, but hypnotism enabled him to control the worst case of suicidal and homicidal mania that had been in Morningside for ten years. He also reported that a patient suffering from hypochondriacal melancholia recovered after six weeks' hypnotic treatment.

The following is his summary of the uses of hypnotism among the insane :—

(*I.*) *As a Direct Therapeutic Agent.*

(*a*) Hypnotism sometimes succeeds in intractable cases of insomnia where narcotics have failed, and thus ought to be of great service when the brain nutrition is bad, and depressing drugs specially undesirable.

(*b*) Where the brain is highly unstable, it may be of direct therapeutic value as a sedative, and thus prevent an outburst of excitement from passing into mania.

(*c*) It is useful in dispelling fleeting delusional states, and minor psychoses.

(*II.*) *For Purposes of Management.*

(*a*) Hypnotism may be used to overcome the morbid resistance of patients to the administration of food, medicine, etc.

(*b*) It may be employed in cases of excitement and violence, instead of mechanical, chemical, or physical means of restraint.

In 1897, Dr. Woods, Hoxton House Asylum, reported the following cases treated by hypnotism :—

10 cases of melancholia (in 8 there were delusions). Result : 6 recovered, 3 improved, and 1 uninfluenced.

1 case of puerperal mania. Recovered.

3 cases of mania. 1 recovered, 2 improved.

1 case of dementia. Result nil.

The following is an example :—

No. 55 (Woods). *Melancholia.*—Miss ——, aged 16, admitted December 20th, 1893. The patient was in great distress, cried continually, and had delusions. She fancied that she was lost, wished to die, was full of self-accusations of wickedness, slept badly, and refused food.

She had ordinary asylum treatment without improvement until the second week in January, 1894, when she was hypnotised three times, and curative suggestions were made. Distinct improvement followed.

Third week.—Hypnotised twice and continued to improve.

Fourth week.—Hypnotised twice. She now had good nights, took her food well, was stronger, and had not cried for some days.

From that time she was not again hypnotised, but continued to improve, and by April 3rd had recovered.

Remarks.—Voisin's claim to have been the first to employ hypnotism in the treatment of the insane is untenable, and was obviously made in ignorance of the work of Esdaile and others. It is also interesting to note that the observations of Dr. George Robertson, as to the advantages of hypnotism in procuring quiet and maintaining asylum discipline, had been forestalled by Dr. Keen more than forty years previously.

While most modern writers are agreed that minor psychoses can be dispelled by hypnotic treatment, few, save Voisin, have claimed to have cured true insanity by this means. Although no one denied the genuineness of Voisin's results—his patients were mostly treated in asylums, and open to the observation of his colleagues—the accuracy of his diagnosis was disputed by Forel.

In the opinion of the latter, Voisin's so-called insane patients simply suffered from hysteria; and this, together with analogous mental troubles of a fugitive character, could undoubtedly be cut short by hypnotism. Forel admitted that he had been able to induce sleep in the insane by suggestion, and to obtain a temporary cessation of hallucinations. In a case of dementia (with inactivity, vicious tendencies, and intercurrent submaniacal attacks) he succeeded in making the patient work, improved his mental condition, and arrested the maniacal attacks, which had not returned three years later. On the other hand, he had never cured genuine insanity by suggestion; and, even when he had succeeded in obtaining hypnosis, had entirely failed to produce any permanent influence upon the morbid mental condition. In true melancholia, he had only been able to induce sleep and hasten convalescence. The brain, he said, was the instrument we employed in suggestion; and, if the instrument itself were spoilt, we were no longer able to make use of it, or only to a very small extent, as a means of reacting upon itself, and influencing its functions in general.

In reply, Voisin admitted that hypnotism could do nothing in somatic mental affections, such as general paralysis, apoplectic affections, cerebral softening, etc.; but, on the other hand, he claimed to have cured many cases of genuine insanity by its means—for example, delusional insanity, in which the patients had the fixed belief that they were persecuted, and had marked suicidal impulses; also cases of true melancholia, as well as acute and sub-acute mania, etc. Further, he had also succeeded with other mental maladies, more or less closely connected with insanity, such as hysteria, epilepsy, and conditions of mania, etc., associated with them; also with morphinomania, dipsomania, moral insanity and perversity, as well as the various forms of obsession.

Finally, even if his patients had suffered from hysterical—not true—insanity, their recovery still marked a therapeutic advance of no little importance. Asylums, he said, contained a large number of the hysterically insane, who were violent and dangerous, and who inspired both disgust and pity by their tendency to drink and steal, their lies, dirtiness, and obscene and unnatural acts. Many of these, who had long been asylum inmates, were now—thanks to hypnotism—leading active and useful lives.

Répoud and others claim to have obtained results similar to Voisin's; but, despite their support, the question whether insanity in its graver forms can be cured by hypnotism is still under discussion. One must not forget, however, in endeavouring to estimate the value of this form of treatment, that the experiment practically dates from Voisin's first case in 1880, and that comparatively few attempts have been made by others to give the method a fair trial. This is partially explained by the amount of time and trouble the process frequently requires. At first Voisin only succeeded with 10 per cent of his insane patients, and this often only after prolonged and repeated sittings. Later, his percentage rose, and the time required was less; but the process was still usually difficult and tedious. Dr. George Robertson, it is true, states that between a third and a half of suitable cases may be hypnotised, and considers one attempt of fifteen minutes sufficient. It is to be regretted that this statement, confirmed by no other modern observer, is unaccompanied by a complete list of cases treated. The value of the Bethlem experiments is much lessened by the fact that in no instance did the number of attempts exceed nine, while in six cases only one was made.

Many of those who stated that they were unable to personally confirm Voisin's results, admitted that their experience had been extremely limited—some, for example, had only tried hypnotism in one or two cases of true insanity.

My own experiments, in cases of undoubted insanity, have been too few to be of value. I have, however, as already pointed out, had good results in many cases of melancholia, such as have been classed as insane in some other statistics.

On the one hand, then, we have negative or imperfect results cited by authorities who, as a rule, have only attempted to hypnotise a limited number of insane cases, and generally speaking not under the conditions Voisin found essential to success. Thus, (1) Frequently sufficient time was not given to the attempted induction of hypnosis. (2) The experiment was not repeated often enough. (3) After hypnosis was obtained, Voisin's methods—prolonged sleep, etc.—were rarely employed.

On the other hand, we have the strong positive evidence of Voisin's successful cases. These number several hundreds, and

represent eighteen years' work; while the after-history of many
of them was carefully traced, when it was found that the recovery
had been maintained.

The question, as raised by Forel, is really little more than
one of diagnosis as to the conditions—organic or functional—
associated with the mental disturbances.   To the ordinary
individual, patients who have been asylum inmates for years,
who are filthy in language, person, and conduct, who refuse food,
attack their friends and attendants, and suffer from delusions and
hallucinations, are insane enough for all practical purposes.   The
treatment which in Voisin's hands cured such patients, and
enabled them to return to work, is surely worthy of further
investigation and experiment.   Apart from this, it must also be
admitted that a certain proportion of the insane are cured or
recover; and it seems reasonable to suppose that a method of
treatment which—without drugs—can sometimes procure sleep,
remove excitement and other morbid mental conditions, may prove
a valuable remedial agent.

Further, at a later date, Forel himself reported successful
cases.   In one instance the patient, who believed himself to be
controlled by a spirit, which entirely regulated his life and forced
him to do the most absurd things, was easily hypnotised by Forel:
the hallucinations disappeared after the first sitting.   Another
patient, who suffered from paranoia with delusions of persecution,
also recovered after hypnotic treatment.   No relapse.

In conclusion, the following points as to Voisin's methods
deserve notice :—

(1) His first attempt to induce hypnosis was sometimes
continued for three hours, and the process repeated daily for
weeks.

(2) He did not give varied curative suggestions to begin with,
but frequently repeated one as to the relief of some prominent
symptom, and then left the patient in the hypnotic trance for an
hour or two.

(3) When patients did not respond readily to suggestion,
Voisin kept them continuously in the hypnotic state—often for
several weeks at a time.   He found this a therapeutic method of
great value; it was also of much use in preventing regularly
recurring attacks of mania, especially those associated with the
menstrual period.

(4) Voisin neither experimented with his patients nor suggested delusions, hallucinations, nor any act or thought that could be hurtful. He invariably suggested obedience and usefulness, good thoughts and actions, and the desire to be helpful, amiable, etc.

(4) Dipsomania and Chronic Alcoholism.

Since I came to London, about ten years ago, I have treated 76 cases of dipsomania and chronic alcoholism by means of hypnotic suggestion. I propose (I.) to draw attention to the general results; (II.) to cite illustrative cases; (III.) to discuss some points in reference to the morbid conditions involved, and to this particular method of treating them.

(I.) General Results.

(a) *Recoveries.*—28 cases recovered: by this I mean that the patients ceased drinking during treatment; and that, so far as I have been able to learn, they have remained total abstainers up to the present date, or to that of the last report received. Although the earliest of these cases has now passed ten years without relapse, I will not describe the patient as "cured," for it is possible that the disease may return: one of my patients relapsed after eight years' total abstinence.

Of the above 28 cases, 17 were males and 11 females. The average age was 40. Average number of hypnotic treatments, 30. Average length of time since recovery, 3 years.

All the patients in this, as well as in the two other groups, belonged to the educated classes.

(b) *Cases improved.*—These numbered 36—26 males and 10 females. Average age, 39. Average number of hypnotic treatments, 32. Average length of time since treatment, $3\frac{1}{2}$ years.

The results obtained in this class varied widely. The best case abstained for eight years, then relapsed, but has now—after further treatment—again abstained for eighteen months. In a considerable proportion of the remainder the improvement has been marked and valuable. Several of the patients, who formerly led lives of drunkenness, are now engaged in useful work and only drink at rare intervals.

(c) *Failures.*—These numbered 12—10 males and 2 females. Average age, 43.   Average number of hypnotic treatments, 20.

In the majority of the above cases it was impossible to get the patients to cease drinking during treatment, which, in 6 out of 12, was very short.   In more than one instance, however, although the treatment was prolonged, and carried out under favourable circumstances, no benefit was obtained.

As far as I have been able to learn, all the cases of failure that passed through my hands are now dead or still remain un-cured.   Several of them left me to go into retreats; but few, if any, derived lasting benefit there.

(II.) Illustrative Cases.

(a) *Recoveries.*

No. 56. Dr. ——, aged 32, February, 1893, began taking stimulants at college, and took them regularly afterwards, although rarely in excess till 1888.   At that date, he had been in practice for two years and was doing well, then had frequent drinking-bouts.   Despite continued and careful supervision, he drank rectified spirits in secret, sometimes several gallons a month. His health suffered greatly, he was often on the verge of delirium tremens, and on one occasion was supposed to have had slight cerebral hæmorrhage.   He complained of palpitation and angina pectoris, and asserted that it was the pain of the latter which made him drink.   As his bouts of drunkenness became more frequent and severe, he was compelled to abandon work and to return home.   There he became steadier, and his parents pur-chased another practice for him.   At first he did well, but soon began drinking again and often took narcotics.   I was told that, unless I could cure him, he would have to give up work and be kept by his parents.

He was hypnotised 44 times from February 21st to April 18th, 1893 : he then returned to his practice at a distance from town, and I have not seen him since.   Shortly after beginning treatment he entirely abandoned stimulants and narcotics, and soon lost all craving for them.   He rapidly improved in health and weight, and ceased to complain of palpitation or angina. After passing twelve months without relapse, he married.   On

February 27th, 1894, his mother wrote as follows:—"The treatment has been completely successful. My son is perfectly well, and quite like his old self—sound in mind and body, and without the slightest wish or need to take drugs or stimulants in any form whatever. His practice increases steadily. Could anything be more satisfactory?" About the same date Dr. —— wrote to say that he had never felt better in his life, and had no desire for stimulants. From then up to the present time (1903) I have heard occasionally from my patient or his wife. All the reports are of the same character: he is strong, well, happy, prosperous, and a total abstainer.

No. 57. Mr. ——, aged 35, with a family history of alcoholism, had taken stimulants in excess since the age of 18. Marked dipsomania during the last four years. Two attacks of delirium tremens. The patient was sent to me by Dr. Walker, of St. John's Wood; hypnotic treatment was begun in December, 1896, and continued for about two months. The patient abstained from alcohol from the beginning of treatment until his death from accident three years later.

No. 58. Mr. ——, aged 37, December, 1898, had a family history of alcoholism. With the exception of six months, which he spent in a doctor's house, the patient had drunk to excess for many years. He was not easily affected by stimulants, and rarely got into a state of obvious intoxication: he soaked, was sodden, dull, stupid, and listless. He had enough money to live on, and was without occupation, hobbies, or friends. After ordinary medical treatment had been abandoned, his relatives persuaded him to place himself under my care. Hypnotic treatment was begun in December, 1898: shortly afterwards all craving disappeared, and the patient became an abstainer. Up to the present date—February, 1903—there has been no relapse, and he leads a healthier, more interested, and active life.

No. 59. Mrs. ——, aged 44, November 23rd, 1894, was sent to me by Mr. Jessop, of Leeds. Family history of alcoholism. At the age of 20 the patient had frequent hysterical attacks, and for these stimulants were prescribed in rather large quantities. Two years later she began to drink in excess, but did not do so often, and rarely became intoxicated. From 32 to 36, she was an abstainer; she then commenced taking stimulants again, and attacks of genuine dipsomania soon appeared. From that time she suffered from an almost constant craving for alcohol. She was, however, a woman of culture, refinement and high principle—devoted to her husband and children—and the idea of giving way to drink was in every way abhorrent to her. She struggled with all her might against the temptation ; but, after fighting it successfully for a week or two, the craving became irresistible, and a drinking-bout invariably followed.

Hypnotic treatment was begun on November 23rd, 1894, and continued to February 14th, 1895. From the very first sitting she abstained from stimulants, but the craving, although much diminished, did not entirely disappear for some months. Up to the present date—April, 1903—there has been absolutely no relapse. It is to be noted that in this case, although the patient responded immediately to suggestion, there were no other indications of hypnosis.

(b) Cases Improved.

No. 60. Mr. ——, aged 40, October, 1891, had a family history of alcoholism and had long taken spirits too freely : for the last four years his drinking - bouts had been frequent and severe. He suffered from insomnia, digestive troubles, and lightning pains, and walked badly—his feet seemed encased in wool, and he had difficulty in feeling the pavement. A well-known specialist told him he had locomotor ataxy, and was incurable. He was then sent to me by Dr. Morier, of St. John's Wood, and hypnotised 15 times. Result : six months' abstention from alcohol, with marked improvement in general health and nervous symptoms. Insomnia then reappeared, and he took alcohol occasionally and narcotics — generally sulphonal—regularly. After six weeks' renewed treatment in the autumn of 1892, he remained an abstainer for three years, and the ataxic symptoms entirely disappeared. Later, he again took narcotics regularly and stimulants occasionally, and died suddenly from cardiac syncope.

No. 61. Mr. ——, aged 47, April, 1895. Father and mother drank to excess. The patient, who lived in Australia, commenced drinking when at Oxford, and had done so ever since. He married in 1876, and was frequently intoxicated during his honeymoon. In 1878, he had his first epileptic fit, followed by six others at distant intervals. There had been three attacks of delirium tremens, the first in 1879. He not only had frequent excessive drinking - bouts, but also took stimulants regularly, except when ill after an unusually bad attack. He always got drunk when he visited his farm, and only returned home sober four times out of a hundred and fifty. He came to England in 1895, and had an attack of delirium tremens just before beginning treatment in April, 1895. He was then sent to me by Dr. Allden, of Bridport, and easily hypnotised at the first attempt : he at once become a total abstainer, but treatment was continued for two months. He then went back to Australia, fought a keenly contested election without touching stimulants, and gained a seat in Parliament. There was no relapse until the autumn of 1898, when he began to take stimulants occasionally. He returned for further treatment on January 9th, 1901. He was again easily hypnotised, and at once gave up all stimulants. There has been no return of the epilepsy.

(c) Failures.

No. 62. Mrs. ——, aged 40, September, 1893, with a family history of alcoholism, had suffered from dipsomania for seven years. After a fortnight's treatment, during which time the patient took stimulants regularly, and became intoxicated on more than one occasion, the treatment was abandoned.

No. 63. Mr. ——, December, 1893, aged 32, with family history of alcoholism, had taken stimulants in excess since the age of 18. Well-marked dipsomania during the last five years. The patient was seen on four occasions, but, as each time he presented himself in an intoxicated condition, the treatment was abandoned.

Remarks.—In addition to cases reported by other observers in this country, successful ones have been published by Knory, Farez, Vlavianos, Bourdon, Bechterew, Ribokoff, Bushnell, Voisin, Ladame, Forel, Tatzel, Hirt, Nielson, de Jong, Bernheim, van Eeden, van Renterghem, Hamilton Osgood, Wetterstrand, Schrenck-Notzing, Krafft-Ebing, etc.

For example, de Jong reported that he had treated many cases, some of which had then remained over three years without

Q

relapse. Hirt claimed to have had eight complete recoveries out
of thirteen cases. Wetterstrand cited the case of a man who
for several years had drunk a bottle of brandy, and injected
30 centigrammes of morphia, daily. Recovery took place after
34 sittings, and there had been no relapse. Voisin published
numerous successful cases, some of them being women over 40
years of age. He traced the subsequent history of many of
them, and reported years later that there had been no relapse.
Ladame drew special attention to three cases treated by Forel :
all of them had suffered from chronic alcoholism and attacks of
delirium tremens, and had long been inmates of his asylum.
They were extremely difficult to manage, and expressed their
determination to resume drinking as soon as they were liberated ;
but, despite this, complete recovery followed hypnotic treatment.

(III.) SOME POINTS IN REFERENCE TO THE MORBID CONDITIONS
INVOLVED, AND THEIR TREATMENT BY HYPNOTIC SUGGESTION.

As the majority of my patients suffered from dipsomania, I
wish to say a word as to that condition, and the differences
between it and ordinary alcoholism. A typical case of the
former presents the following phenomena :—The patient, while
abstaining, begins to be haunted with ideas about drink. This
is soon followed by the desire for drink, but at first the impulse
is combated by the will. It soon, however, becomes irresistible ;
and, after the first glass is taken, the craving is increased, and
the struggle is abandoned in despair. The patient then drinks
for a varying period, after which the craving suddenly disappears ;
this stage is followed by one of physical weakness accompanied
by remorse. These conditions in their turn disappear, and the
patient enjoys a period of more or less complete health and comfort,
undisturbed by any morbid craving for stimulants. This passes, and
a new attack begins which follows the course of its predecessors.

The Exciting Causes of Dipsomania.—In many, but by no
means all my cases, there was a family history of alcoholism.
It is difficult to determine, however, what part this played in
the production of the dipsomania, as I have also known many
instances where drunkenness in the parents was followed by
total abstinence in the children. On the other hand, all the
dipsomaniacs I have observed showed symptoms of degeneracy;

most of them were impulsive, nervous, emotional, sensitive, and thus more or less ill-balanced mentally.

An accidental circumstance—usually some mental trouble—is generally the immediate exciting cause of the first attack. Similar causes may excite subsequent attacks ; but when the disease is fully developed, its manifestations occur at more or less regular intervals, and often without any discoverable immediate exciting cause. I do not know, however, of a single case in which dipsomania has been suddenly aroused, no matter by what cause, in those who till then had been total abstainers. In all there was a previous history of the use of alcohol.

Differences between Dipsomania and other Forms of Intemperance.—Many persons, who are strong both mentally and physically, habitually take too much alcohol—they do so on account of the physical or mental comfort it brings. Usually they do not struggle against their self-indulgence until it begins to endanger their health, pocket, or reputation. The dipsomaniac, on the other hand, drinks because he is impelled to do so against his will. Drink, though it may have been enjoyed previously, now gives him neither physical comfort nor mental pleasure, and he struggles through an attack like a felon working out his sentence.

The moral condition of the average inebriate differs widely from that of the ordinary dipsomaniac. Shame is often sadly lacking in the former, while the dipsomaniac, on the contrary, feels his degradation keenly. Finally, the drunken bouts of the dipsomaniac, unlike those of the ordinary inebriate, are rarely associated with other excesses.

Prognosis.

According to Ladame, the prognosis in dipsomania, especially where there is a family history of alcoholism, is an extremely grave one ; and prolonged retention in an asylum or a retreat rarely yields good results. He admitted that total abstinence societies did valuable work, but considered their method of treatment somewhat analogous to the hypnotic. When they succeeded, the patient was generally under the influence of religious ideas, propounded and received " *au moment psycho-logique*," while he was in a condition of remorse and despair. The solemn vow which he made to abstain from drink was also a powerful self-suggestion. If the subsequent circumstances

were favourable, and his friends rallied round him and encouraged
him in every way possible, there was a chance of his being
cured.   On the other hand, many dipsomaniacs were not
responsive to religious or ordinary moral influences : such cases
were not likely to receive benefit from total abstinence societies
and similar means, but often recovered under hypnotic treatment.

Hypnotic Treatment.

The following are the most important points :—

(1) The patient must be willing to be cured.   Difficulties as
to this are more frequently encountered in cases of chronic
alcoholism than in dipsomania.   Even the latter patients, however, sometimes dread treatment, as they think it may raise an
artificial barrier between them and drink, and yet leave them
fighting with the craving.   Probably also they have been told
that hypnotism is dangerous, and will rob them of their will-
power.   These fears are usually dispelled by means of a little
tact and explanation.   The patient must be made to understand
that the object of the treatment is to remove the craving ; that
the force of the volition is increased, not diminished, by hypnosis ;
and that the use of hypnotism for medical purposes, in skilled
hands, is absolutely devoid of danger.

(2) Susceptibility to hypnosis is a varying and important
factor.   Most authorities agree that all, except idiots and those
suffering from certain forms of mental disease, can be hypnotised.
On the other hand, the ill-balanced are usually difficult to
influence.   Time and trouble are often requisite ; and frequently
slight hypnosis alone can be induced.   Fortunately deep hypnosis
is not essential to the production of good therapeutic results.

(3) In dipsomania one ought to begin treatment at the
commencement of a period of quiescence, and aim at preventing,
or at all events retarding and weakening, the next attack.
When stimulants are taken continually, the patient must be
helped and encouraged to reduce them as speedily as possible,
and then stop them altogether.

(4) The management of the patient during the earlier part
of the treatment, before suggestion has taken effect, is important.
If possible, he should never be left alone, but always have
near him some trustworthy person, to whom he can confide his
temptations, and turn for aid in overcoming them.   As restraint

had proved useless in all the cases which came under my notice I never employed it. Doubtless it might have been a help at the commencement of the treatment, but its moral effect is invariably bad.

(5) The operator must be persevering and not easily discouraged : many persons, who ultimately do well, relapse more than once during treatment.

(6) A distaste for alcohol ought to be suggested, as well as the abolition of the craving for it. The patient must be made to understand that he can never look forward to being a moderate drinker, and that the only choice before him lies between total abstinence and the gutter.

(7) Even when the craving disappears quickly, the patients ought to be hypnotised regularly for a month. If they can be seen from time to time for the next six months, so much the better and safer.

(8) The object of the treatment is not only to cure the diseased craving, but also to strengthen the will of the patient, and help him to combat the temptations of social life. The latter point is important. Some patients forget what they have gone through, and, although they have no diseased craving, yield to ordinary temptation. If the patient has not gained the power of controlling himself, the treatment has failed in its object ; for self-control, not artificial restraint, is its essential feature.

In estimating the results, it must not be forgotten that the majority of my cases were extremely unfavourable ones.

(5) Morphinomania and other Drug Habits.

Patients suffering from hysteria and neurasthenia frequently acquire drug habits ; the latter, however, are usually abandoned as soon as the insomnia and other morbid symptoms disappear under treatment. This, however, is only true of ordinary hypnotic drugs, and does not apply to opium or morphia. The treatment of patients addicted to the latter, especially where the drug is administered subcutaneously, presents many difficulties, and relapses are frequent. My personal results have been so much less satisfactory than those of Wetterstrand, that I will only cite two cases from my own practice, and deal more fully with his statistics.

No. 64. Mr. ——, aged 25, February, 1899, suffered from chronic diarrhœa at the age of 16, for which a mixture containing laudanum was prescribed. This was the commencement of an opium habit which had continued ever since : it was difficult to ascertain the exact amount taken, as the patient tried to conceal this, but he admitted to a daily consumption of 6 drachms of laudanum. Latterly he had much changed in character, while his memory and general business capacity were markedly impaired. The patient was sent to me by Dr. Ware, of Hampstead, on February 24th, 1899, and hypnotised 40 times up to July 19th, 1899. Result : recovery, confirmed by later reports.

No. 65. Mrs. ——, aged 37, February, 1898. Twelve months previously, after an attack of influenza, the patient began to suffer from insomnia and severe depression. Sleep was never obtained without narcotics, and there was one attempt at suicide. Six months later, there were frequent attacks of intercostal neuralgia, and, to relieve these, morphia was injected subcutaneously. This had been continued ever since, and repeated several times daily. The amount taken varied, but it was never less than 3 grains. Hypnosis was induced at the first attempt in February, 1898, and the patient slept well the following night. After a fortnight's treatment the morphia was abandoned, and all morbid symptoms quickly disappeared. Up to the last report (1903) there had been no relapse.

The following table, published in 1896, gives Wetterstrand's results in 51 cases :—

	Men.	Women.	Total.	Died.	No effect.	Relapsed.	Cured.
Morphinism in which the morphia was injected subcutaneously .	16	22	38	2	5	3	28
Morphinism in which the morphia was taken internally . .	1	2	3	...	...	1	2
Morphinism and Alcoholism .	1	...	1	...	...	...	1
Morphinism and Cocainism .	2	1	3	1	1	...	1
Cocainism	1	...	1	...	...	...	1
Opium internally . . .	...	4	4	...	...	1	3
Chloralism	...	1	1	...	...	...	1
Total . .	21	30	51	3	6	5	37

Many of the cases were extremely grave and of long standing; and with several abstinence-treatment in a nursing home had been tried, sometimes more than once, without success. Amongst the successful ones was a medical man who had taken morphia for eighteen, and cocaine for four, years. Another patient, Dr. Landgren, published his own case five years after he had been successfully treated by Wetterstrand. He had taken morphia for nineteen years, with the exception of a few months spent in a retreat.

In many instances the morphia had been prescribed for the relief of some disease. When this was a functional nervous disorder it generally yielded to suggestion; but, even in organic and incurable maladies, Wetterstrand was often able to arrest pain, procure sleep, and break the narcotic habit. From this he concluded that suggestive treatment ought to be tried before narcotics were prescribed, even in diseases likely to end fatally.

All Wetterstrand's cases, with the exception of one, were treated in private houses, and he found residence in a retreat quite unnecessary. The following are the points which he considered the most important in order to ensure success :—(1) The patient should be placed under the care of an absolutely trustworthy nurse. (2) The doctor must gain the patient's confidence, treating him as an invalid deserving of sympathy, and not blame him for having given way to a bad habit. (3) The morphia should not be stopped at once, but rapidly decreased, and the patient constantly informed of the diminution. (4) Injections of water, instead of morphia, were wrong and ought to be scrupulously avoided. (5) The sittings should be held once or twice daily, and, if possible, profound hypnosis induced.

Latterly Wetterstrand has treated many of his drug cases by " prolonged sleep," and his results have been even more brilliant than those already cited. Successful cases are also reported by other observers. Thus :—

No. 66 (Fulda). Miss ——, aged 36, had suffered from hysteria for eleven years, and had injected morphia subcutaneously during the last ten, the average amount taken being 20 centigrammes daily. Insomnia, depression, and amenorrhœa— the latter of fifteen months' duration. After three months' hypnotic treatment all morbid symptoms had disappeared, and the morphia habit was abandoned. Two years later there had been no relapse.

﹀ No. 67 (Marot). Mrs. ——, aged 37, had suffered since the age of 26 from *grande hystérie* of the true Salpêtrière type—convulsions, anæsthesiæ, ovarian pain, restriction of the field of vision, etc. There were also marked gastric disturbances: the patient had kept her bed for nineteen months, and was much emaciated.

In August, 1883, her medical man gave her an injection of morphia, and this was repeated daily by herself or others until the end of July, 1889. It was impossible to determine the exact amount taken: her own chemist admitted that he supplied her with 10 to 20 centigrammes daily; but it was known that she also got it from others, but not to what extent. Finally, she could not pass more than an hour without an injection: her arms, legs, and abdomen were covered with numerous cicatrices, the result of abscesses, as well as subcutaneous nodules and the ordinary marks resulting from the use of the syringe.

In July, 1889, the patient was deeply hypnotised at the first attempt, and slept till nine o'clock the following morning in response to suggestion. The treatment was continued daily until the patient's recovery, which was rapid. Three and a half years later there had been no relapse, and the skin was absolutely normal.

According to Marot, the craving for morphia can only be removed by suggestion: ordinary treatment may get rid of the physical necessity for taking it, but there is always the danger that the craving will return.

Further successful cases are also reported by Voisin, Bérillon, Tanzi, Bauer, and many others.

(6) Vicious and Degenerate Children.

The following conclusions as to the value of hypnotism in the treatment of vicious and degenerate children were submitted by Bérillon to the International Congress of Hypnotism, Paris, 1889:—

(1) Many carefully observed facts prove the therapeutic value of suggestion in the following diseases of children: incon-

tinence of urine and fæces, nervous twitchings, nocturnal terrors, onanism, blepharospasm; and other disturbances of the nervous system of a functional character.

(2) So far, no appreciable results have been obtained in cretinism, idiocy, or deaf-mutism.

(3) Suggestion constitutes an excellent auxiliary in the education of vicious and degenerate children, especially where there are habits of lying, cruelty, inveterate idleness, or cowardice.

(4) Suggestion should be confined to cases where the usual methods of education have failed, and medical men alone should employ it. It is not necessary to hypnotise normal children: ordinary training ought to be sufficient for them. When, however, children are addicted to theft, and other vicious or repulsive habits, and are afflicted with disgusting infirmities, we ought to try to cure them by hypnotism, especially when their parents are in despair, owing to the failure of all other forms of treatment.

These conclusions were adopted unanimously by the Congress, and were transmitted to the Minister of Public Instruction and the Minister of the Interior.

The following are illustrative cases from my own practice :—

No. 68. Mr. ——, aged 19, February 26th, 1893. Family history bad ; mother highly nervous, father died insane. Up to the age of 14 the patient was lively and intelligent; he then commenced to masturbate, and his mental condition rapidly deteriorated. He lost interest in his studies, and frequently stole, generally in a purposeless manner. He had been expelled from school, and, when I first saw him, was under the care of Dr. Kingston, of Willesden, who sent him to me. I was informed that the patient was still guilty of theft, addicted to self-abuse, untruthful, absolutely untrustworthy, and strangely apathetic and lazy. There was little or nothing, even in the way of amusement, in which he took the least interest.

After two months' hypnotic treatment he began to improve : before the end of the year he had recovered, and learnt a business in which he took great interest. Later reports satisfactory.

✓ No. 69. Miss ——, aged 15, January 22nd, 1894. Her mother, who had a family history of insanity, was morally insane, and lived a vagabond, drunken life. Her father and uncle both drank, and died insane. I was informed that the patient was deceitful, rebellious, and mischief-making. She frequently complained of queer feelings in her head, but it was difficult to tell how much was real and how much pretence. She was quick and intelligent, and could do her lessons in about a quarter of the time most children took. She was very impatient of restraint: she had been sent to two or three families and one school, but in each instance had been dismissed, as she was so insubordinate and unmanageable.

I was also informed that the patient lied, stole, and had frequent outbursts of violent passion. I found her strong, muscular, and well-developed; palate normal, menstruation regular.

On January 22nd, 1894, after consultation with the late Dr. Hack Tuke, she was placed in a nursing home, and regularly hypnotised for a month. This was followed by marked improvement, and for the next three years the treatment was occasionally repeated, but at distant intervals. The patient finally grew into a bright, healthy, attractive woman, who now (1903), with the exception that she is still somewhat emotional, shows hardly a trace of her former defects.

No. 70. Miss ——, aged 13, March, 1894. Bad family history. Before the patient was born her mother suffered from melancholia. The child herself had been mentally peculiar from infancy; she was persistently untruthful, deceitful, insolent, and dirty in her habits. She had been addicted to self-abuse since the age of 7. On several occasions she had stolen money from servants and others—sometimes considerable amounts. She had been expelled from school, and had to be kept at home. She was strong, healthy, and well-grown, with nothing abnormal about the head or palate.

After consultation with Dr. Savage, the patient was hypnotised three times a week from March to May, 1894; this was followed by marked improvement, and the treatment was repeated at intervals during the next two years. Complete recovery took place, and up to the present date (1903) there has been no relapse.

No. 71. Miss ——, aged 22, April, 1895, had suffered from fits of violent passion since early childhood. She was so little able to control herself that her mother often feared she might kill her sister, and she still (1895) often came to blows with her younger brother. She had always been intensely selfish, and could not see why she should do anything for others. She admitted her defects of character without shame, and said she heartily enjoyed quarrelling and setting others by the ears. She consented in the waking state that I should try to alter her character, and I suggested during hypnosis that she should give up quarrelling, and take a pleasure in helping others. A complete change took place: she became affectionate, good-tempered and helpful. Even when ill there was no trace of her former irritability. Up to the present date (1903) there has been no relapse. This patient was originally sent by Dr. Boulting, of Hampstead, on account of spinal neuralgia and insomnia, and was successfully treated by hypnotism for these affections.[1]

No. 72. Miss ——, aged 13, February, 1900, had always been emotional and highly nervous. For several years she had walked in her sleep, and during the last four had been addicted to constant nail-biting. Wearing gloves at night and other careful treatment failed to check the habit, and the nails were always worn to the quick. This patient, who was sent to me by Professor William James, of Harvard University, was easily hypnotised at the first attempt, and neither bit her nails nor walked in her sleep after the second sitting. Later reports satisfactory.

Enuresis nocturna is of frequent occurrence in degenerate children, and, with one exception, in every case in which I induced genuine hypnosis the patient recovered. In 1890, for example, I had 18 cases, all successful. Of these, 12 were girls and 6 boys, their ages varying from 4 to 12 years. In every instance the recovery was confirmed by later reports.

The failure already referred to was a young lady, aged 23, who had suffered from *enuresis nocturna* from infancy. This had become progressively worse, and since the age of 16 had occurred every night. She was of a nervous temperament and somewhat irritable, but otherwise strong and healthy: there was nothing physically wrong with the bladder or urethra. Careful and varied medical treatment had been without result. Hypnosis was easily induced at the first attempt, and the incontinence disappeared as long as she remained under treatment. Shortly after returning home she relapsed; with renewed treatment the enuresis again ceased, but only to reappear later.

No. 73. Mr. ——, aged 27, April, 1900. When I first saw

---

[1] Case No. 22, pp. 194-5.

this patient I was informed that he never spoke, except when questioned, and that his replies were generally unintelligible. Nothing seemed to interest him, and he neither worked nor amused himself. He was heir to an entailed estate, a fact which added importance to his mental condition. The latter, in the opinion of a well-known alienist, was more likely to terminate in idiocy than improvement.

Apparently the patient had been backward in development, and in consequence had been the butt of his schoolfellows. As the result of this, he had progressively lost confidence in himself, and had become more and more self-conscious. Behind all this, however, he appeared to possess much more intelligence than he was credited with; and this view was shared by Dr. Fletcher Beach, who saw the patient in consultation with me.

Hypnotic treatment was begun on April 19th, 1900, and repeated on 44 occasions up to February, 1901. During that time the patient spoke more and more distinctly, and became less shy and self-conscious. Since then his life has become progressively more normal. He is now engaged in active work, and even speaks in public. The last report, in December, 1902, was thoroughly satisfactory.

The following are from the practice of others :—

No. 74 (Voisin). Miss ——, aged 11, December, 1886, lied persistently, and had masturbated since she was two years old. She could not be left alone for a moment during the day, and it was always necessary to tie her hands at night. Recovered after hypnotic treatment.

No. 75 (Voisin). Miss ——, aged 9½, July, 1887, was intelligent, but excessively idle. At the age of 7, while living with the children of peasants, she was taught to masturbate. Six months later she was dismissed from school on this account, and her mother frequently caught her renewing the practice. Hypnotised five times from July 25th to August 15th, 1887. Recovered.

No. 76 (Voisin). Master ——, aged 16, June 1888, had always been difficult to manage, but from the age of 6 had become more and more uncontrollable. He lied, stole, and masturbated: treatment and discipline produced no improvement, and he was expelled from every school he went to. He recovered after being hypnotised regularly for a month. A year later there had been no return of his vicious habits: his character was completely changed, he enjoyed work, was amiable and well-behaved, admired what was good, and sought every possible occasion to be useful and pleasing to others.

In 1889, Liébeault published 22 consecutive cases of more or less grave mental disturbance in children; of these 10 recovered, 8 were improved, and in 4 there was no result. The following are three examples:—

No. 77. Master ——, aged 18, collapsed after overwork, and had long been under medical treatment without benefit. He was dull, stupid, morose, and avoided everybody; he rarely did anything on his own account, was obstinately silent, and would hardly reply to questions. He suffered from general feebleness, diarrhœa, incontinence of urine, muscular tremor, profuse perspirations, and headaches. He recovered after a month's hypnotic treatment, and there was no relapse.

No. 78. Master ——, aged 17, began to suffer from headache some months previously when preparing for an examination. Shortly afterwards he became stupid, and then passed into a condition resembling melancholia with mutism. He recovered after two months' hypnotic treatment, and there was no relapse.

No. 79. Miss ——, aged 8, had always been stupid and had learnt with difficulty: she also masturbated and suffered from incontinence of urine. Complete recovery after short hypnotic treatment.

Bérillon has recorded numerous cases of nocturnal terror in children in which recovery took place after a few hypnotic treatments. Equally good results were obtained in various nervous " *tics* "; amongst these patients one constantly made a noise with his tongue, another suffered from involuntary winking of the right eyelid.

Bérillon has reported many cases of nail-biting which have been cured by hypnotic suggestion; in some this habit was the only symptom of degeneracy, in others it was associated or followed by other nervous symptoms.

Bérillon terms nail-biting *onychophagie*, and considers the condition a serious one for the following reasons:—

(1) It is a sign of degeneracy, and is frequently followed by other symptoms of this condition, *e.g.* onanism, nocturnal terrors, sleep-walking, nervous irritability, etc.

(2) It may be the means of introducing the germs of disease into the mouths of the patients.

(3) Nail-biters become clumsy in the use of their hands; and the condition is often associated with a certain amount of local anæsthesia.

(4) The habit is a common one: in one school 34 per cent of the children bit their nails, and 36 per cent bit their pen-holders; in another 20 per cent of the boys and 52 per cent of the girls were nail-biters.

In 1887, Liébeault published 77 cases of *enuresis nocturna*, of which 45 were boys and 32 girls; the average age was a little over 7; the youngest being 3 years old, the eldest 18. With all, except 9, the habit dated from birth.

Results.—56 recovered, 9 were improved, 8 showed no improvement, while 4 were only seen once, and of these there was no further news.

Cullerre has reported 24 cases of *enuresis nocturna*, with 21 recoveries.

Many other equally successful cases of the hypnotic treatment of vicious and degenerate children have been published by Voisin, Liébeault, Bérillon, Bourdon, Régis, de Jong, Schrenck-Notzing, Ladame, Forel, Teuscher, Bouffé, Bechterew, Wetterstrand, Cullerre, Bauer, Ringier, Lemoine, Joire, Farez, and others.

(7) Obsessions.

The following cases are from my own practice:—

No. 80. Mr. ——, aged 24, consulted me in May 1889. Some months previously he had had a number of diseased glands removed from the face and neck, and went up the Mediterranean to recruit. While crossing a plank he fell and injured his perineum: an abscess formed, which burst externally and into the urethra. When I saw him there was a large unhealthy wound through which the urine escaped. I instructed him to pass a soft catheter regularly, and the wound became more healthy. One day he was impelled to empty his bladder before he could pass the instrument, and the water again escaped from the wound. This happened more and more frequently; at last the idea of passing water caused him at once to empty his bladder, no matter where he was at the time. This appeared to be entirely independent of the physical condition of the bladder, which did not contract because it was full or uncomfortable, but because the idea of urination presented itself to the patient's mind, and was instantly translated into its physical equivalent. He now thought constantly about his condition, which thus became greatly aggravated. He began to sleep badly, and awoke frequently during the night : the instant he did so he thought of his bladder and was immediately compelled to empty it. Despite treatment, these symptoms continued for several months, and his state became a grave one. I had not previously employed hypnotism, but the mental element in this case seemed so marked that I determined, since other treatment had failed, to try what this would do. After explaining to my patient, an educated man, that I had no practical and only slight theoretical knowledge of the subject, I proceeded to hypnotise him by Braid's method. In a few minutes his eyeballs rolled upwards and inwards, and he became lethargic. I repeated this the two following days ; then suggested during hypnosis that he should cease to think about his bladder, should always be able to pass his catheter, retain his urine eight hours, and sleep well. These suggestions were immediately fulfilled ; from that day there was no return of his troublesome symptoms, and the wound healed without operation in about twelve months. At the present date (February, 1903) Mr. —— is in good health.

No. 81. Mr. ——, aged 25, first consulted me March, 1890. Formerly strong and athletic, distinguished football player, bicyclist, etc. Two years previously, after the death of his mother from cancer of the breast, he began to fear that he might contract the same disease. This idea grew stronger and stronger ; he became neurasthenic, and suffered from insomnia, depression, dyspepsia, etc. Finally the dread of cancer passed into the firm conviction that his left breast was infected by it. He now remained nearly always in one room, and would not go into another without muffling himself up and putting on an overcoat. For some months he complained of difficulty in moving the left arm, and carried it in a sling. I found nothing to justify his fears, but the muscles of the arm were distinctly wasted from disuse. He was easily hypnotised at the first attempt, and this was repeated nearly every day for a fortnight, when deep hypnosis with somnambulism was obtained. His morbid ideas at once disappeared; his general health speedily improved, and, a few days after the treatment was abandoned, I saw him driving a spirited horse. A week afterwards he told me he felt perfectly well, and was going to train a young horse to jump. Up to the last report (1901) there had been no relapse.

The two cases given above were drawn from my general practice at Goole.

No. 82. Mrs. ——, aged 46, March, 1894. The following notes of this case were supplied by Dr. ——, the patient's husband: "My wife suffered from myxœdema, following influenza; she had low temperature, loss of hair, dulness of intellect, slowness of movement, general irregular swelling of the body, facial disfigurement, alteration of voice, and muscular pains. I put her on thyroid extract in January, 1893, and although the symptoms peculiar to myxœdema disappeared, she became utterly sleepless, her limbs trembled after the least exertion and her digestion became very bad. I brought her to you on March 1st, 1894, to see whether suggestion would procure sleep. At the second attempt you succeeded in inducing very slight hypnosis, and she began to sleep fairly well. For more than a year she had never had more than three hours' unbroken sleep, and often far less. She soon began to sleep thoroughly well and uninterruptedly, and her indigestion, for which I had found drugs and careful dieting ineffective, disappeared after a few suggestions. Her legs became stronger, and her energies restored very much to what they were twenty years ago, when she was renowned amongst her acquaintances for her untiring energy. The fact, however, that strikes me most forcibly is this—several members of her family are sleep-walkers, and she also walked in her sleep in childhood and once or twice as a young woman, while the habit is transmitted to our youngest girl. When her first baby was born, sixteen years ago, the thought crossed my wife's mind: "What if I walk in my sleep and do an injury to my child?" I endeavoured to persuade her that she had grown out of the habit, but the attempt was wholly fruitless. The idea grew until it assumed the character of an *idée fixe*, and she always tied herself to the bedpost at night. All attempts to break herself of the habit were failures; and if she went to bed without fastening herself she was never able to go to sleep until she did so. When we moved into our present house, three and a half years ago, she became alarmed at the great height of the bedroom windows from the ground, and their lowness from the floor. She began to suggest that possibly she might undo her own knots during her sleep, and get out of the window. I pointed out how unlikely it was that she should walk in her sleep after a score of years' complete immunity. She granted my reasoning was just, but it did not dispel her fear; and she insisted upon my tying her to the bedpost each night in a very effective manner. In May, 1894, I told you of this persistent dread, and asked you to suggest that she should neither walk in her sleep, nor be apprehensive of so doing. During that sitting you repeated this suggestion two or three times, but have not done so since. The effect was magical. She has never asked me to tie her to her bed from that day, and tells me she has never once thought about it. To me it is all the more remarkable as the hypnosis in her case is so slight, and appears to pass into natural sleep if you leave her for a few seconds. She is of a nervous, excitable temperament, but by no means greedy of the marvellous or ready to accord belief to any doctrine. She had a healthy scepticism of the possibility of any one hypnotising her, but was anxious for the attempt to be made as she suffered so acutely." Recovery confirmed by later reports.

No. 83. Mr. ——, aged 28, first consulted me in April, 1894. His father was very nervous and passionate, and had suffered from "brain fever" and chorea. At the age of 14, the patient had many religious doubts and fears, and believed he had committed the unpardonable sin. At 16, while working in a cocoa manufactory, he began to fear that the red lead, which was used in fastening certain hot pipes, might get into the tins containing cocoa, and so poison people. This was the commencement of a *folie du doute* and *délire du toucher*, which had never since left him. Instead of going on with his work he was irresistibly impelled to clean and reclean the tins. The following is taken from the letter of a friend to whom he confided his troubles: "On October 1st, 1891, Mr. —— told me that he had attempted to commit suicide, as his life was so miserable (he had taken poison). He had read of a case of poisoning through eating chocolate, and connected himself with it, though it was five years since he had helped to manufacture any. He now

R

believed he might have been careless with the moulds, and thus have produced a poisoned chocolate, which years afterwards had caused the child's death! The grotesque absurdity of the story, as he related it to me, would have made me laugh, had I not felt how terribly real it was to him. His vivid imagination had pictured every incident of the tragedy: the child buying the chocolate, running home full of happiness, then becoming ill and gradually sickening in awful agony till released by death. The keenness of mind with which he sought to prove the reasonableness of his belief that he had poisoned the child was extraordinary. He wrote: 'Yesterday I was unscrewing some gas burners in a provision shop and got some white lead on my hands, and I have been thinking that it may have got amongst the food.' I found that brooding over this fancy had brought him to the verge of despair, and for weeks his life was a perpetual agony. He worries himself about his work of fixing advertisement-plates to walls, and can never persuade himself that they are securely fastened. He fancies the nails are bad, or the mortar loose, and makes himself ill over it. I have pointed out to him that if a plate fell it would almost invariably slide down the wall. This has not prevented him from painting a most elaborate mental picture of the decapitation of an unfortunate youngster, who happened to be playing marbles with his head against the wall. To enumerate all his troubles would take a small volume. I have a great pile of his letters before me now, and I suppose they constitute one of the most extraordinary analytical auto-biographies it would be possible to find. In reading them I cannot help marvelling at the strange unshapely wonder of such an imagination. He makes every incident in his life the foundation-stone of a castle of fancies; and of late years each castle has become a prison—a torture chamber in which he has dissected his motives and his actions, until he has ceased to believe in himself at all."

When I first saw the patient the *folie du doute* and *délire du toucher* were constant, and most varied in their manifestations. If he accidentally touched persons in the street, he began to fear that he might have injured them, and exaggerated the touch into a more or less violent push. If the person touched were a woman, he feared that she might have been pregnant, and that he might have injured the child. If he saw a piece of orange-peel on the pavement, he kicked it into the road, but soon afterwards began to think that this was a more dangerous place, as any one slipping on it might strike his head against the curb-stone; and so he was irresistibly impelled to return and put it in its former position. At one time he used to bind himself to perform certain acts by vowing he would give God his money if he did not do them. Then, sometimes, he was uncertain whether he had vowed or not: owing to this, he gave sums to religious objects which were quite disproportionate to his income. Apart from his peculiar fancies, I found the patient perfectly rational and intelligent; and, though his *délire du toucher* hindered him greatly in his work, he generally managed to execute it, but on some occasions he was compelled to abandon the attempt. At that time I tried to hypnotise him on twenty-four occasions, but apparently without success, and he was then compelled to leave town. He returned on April 2nd, 1895, for a week's further treatment: he told me that since his former visit his morbid ideas had neither been so frequent nor marked, and were accompanied by less mental agony. From that date, though the treatment was not again repeated, he rapidly recovered, and six months later wrote to say he could laugh at his former fears. His recovery was confirmed by a later report in 1902.

No. 84. Mr. ———, aged 33, tall, strong and athletic, was sent to me on March 7th, 1894, by Dr. Boulting, of Hampstead. The patient stated that he had always been of a sensitive disposition, and inclined to be morbidly self-conscious. Of late years this had greatly developed, and made his life a burden to him. He had the fixed idea that he was constantly making mistakes in business, and that all those with whom he was brought in contact considered him a fool. During a business interview he was embarrassed and spoke with difficulty, and felt that every one must notice this. He had the same feelings in reference to society, and shunned it as much as possible. He also had morbid and entirely unfounded fears about his physical condition. He was hypnotised ten times to July 11th, 1894, and his morbid ideas entirely disappeared. A year later he told me there had not been the slightest relapse, and that he was now fond of society and at his ease in it.

No. 85. Mr. ———, aged 35, was sent by me to Dr. de

Watteville, on October 29th, 1894. His illness had begun six months previously after the sudden death of his brother-in-law. From that time he slept badly, dreamt of his own death, and was haunted by constant fears about himself and his family. He developed agoraphobia, was unable to cross the road without assistance, dreaded losing his employment, and feared he would find his wife and children dead when he returned from work. One day, when sitting alone, he believed he saw two men bring his coffin into the room. He was utterly miserable and had strong suicidal impulses. He also had frequent attacks of giddiness, and felt he would fall unless he caught hold of something : on one occasion he lost consciousness. He was hypnotised five times up to November 12th : his morbid fears had then almost entirely disappeared ; but, as he still had attacks of giddiness, the treatment was repeated occasionally up to April, 1895. His recovery is confirmed by later reports. Case shown at Bethlem Hospital and elsewhere.

No. 86. Mr. ———, aged 32, April, 1895. Ten years previously this patient began to have peculiar doubts and fears. He felt that if he did anything opposed to popular superstition something dreadful would happen to the Almighty. He was capable of recognising the absurdity of this when it was pointed out to him ; but directly afterwards his morbid ideas returned and governed his actions. Every fresh superstition he heard of was added to his list ; and so many unlucky days and places were created by his doing, or failing to do, things against, or in conformity with, these superstitions, that his actions were seriously interfered with. Thus months often passed before he could find a propitious day for buying an article of clothing, and a still longer time would elapse before he found a suitable occasion to put it on. Sometimes there was nowhere for him to go, and nothing he could do. He was utterly wretched, but had succeeded in concealing his trouble from every one. After prolonged treatment he improved greatly, but his recovery could not be said to be complete.

I could cite many other and widely differing cases, but in all the essential conditions were the same—the patients were obsessed by ideas which interfered with their actions or happiness, and rendered their lives more or less miserable.

Braid reported two interesting cases of obsession. In one

the patient believed she was haunted by the spirit of a dead relative, and had visual hallucinations. In the other, the patient was unable to get rid of morbid ideas associated with death, which had arisen after seeing a dead body, and in addition had the fixed idea that she still smelt the corpse. Both patients recovered after hypnotic treatment.

Many equally successful cases are reported by more recent observers. Thus :—

No. 87 (Schrenck-Notzing). Mr. ——; fixed idea regarding catching cold kept this patient for six months in his room. Hypnotised. Recovered.

No. 88 (Schrenck-Notzing). Mr. ——, aged 24, had periods of terror and uncontrollable sensations and ideas, with the fixed idea that his *fiancée* did not love him. Hypnotised. Recovered.

No. 89 (Hecker). Mrs. —— was impelled to wash herself continuously and unnecessarily; had morbid ideas that the doors and windows were not properly fastened, and fancied that she dressed herself untidily. On one occasion, after having spent two hours trying to dress, she sent for Hecker, who found her in a state of great anxiety, putting on and off her clothes until exhausted. Hypnotised for a month. Recovered.

No. 90 (Wetterstrand). Mrs. ——, aged 42, for several years had a morbid dread of thunderstorms; did not dare go into the country in summer, and in winter dreaded what the summer might bring. Constantly watched the appearance of the sky. Hypnotised twenty times. Recovered.

No. 91 (de Jong). Mr. ——, agoraphobia of many years' standing. Hypnotised ten times. Recovered. No relapse after a year and a half.

No. 92 (de Jong). Mrs. ——, fear of storms and of travelling by rail. Hypnotised. Recovered.

No. 93 (van Eeden and van Renterghem). Mr. ——, aged 56. Psychical impotence for three years, with the fixed idea, which he recognised to be false, that his wife was unfaithful to him. Hypnotised eight times. Recovered. No relapse after twenty-two months.

This list might be largely extended, many other cases having been reported by Bernheim, Delbœuf, Gorodichze, Russell Sturgis, Voisin, Burot, Mavroukakis, Bourdon, etc.

Remarks.—Patients are generally ashamed to acknowledge

that they suffer from obsessions, and often conceal them from every one, including their medical attendant. Thus, few people have any idea how common the disease is, and it was only after I commenced to practise suggestive therapeutics that I constantly met with it. Fortunately hypnotic treatment frequently gives brilliant results in such cases: the majority of those I have seen recovered, and relapse has been rare. It is necessary to say something as to the mental conditions involved in obsessions, as these are very imperfectly understood, and English literature on the subject is particularly scanty.

One of the most important contributions to the subject is to be found in the late Dr. Hack Tuke's paper on "Imperative Ideas" (*Brain*, 1894). He stated that the mental phenomena he described had been more clearly defined by French and German than by English writers. This is undoubtedly correct; but, although the former have long recognised such conditions, it is only within comparatively recent times that they, like ourselves, have ceased to confound them with various forms of insanity. Ladame, of Geneva, for example, in referring to the different opinions expressed in reference to *folie du doute* and *délire du toucher* by Schüle, Magnan, Krafft-Ebing, Marcé, Jules Falret, Morel, Lesègue, Ball, Meynert, Kraepelin, and Scholz, says *folie du doute* is regarded by contemporary writers sometimes as a symptom of the most varied mental affections, sometimes as a psychopathic episode of hereditary degeneracy, sometimes as a special form of psychosis; and sometimes as a simple elementary psychic trouble, dependent on the general pathology of mental alienation. Thus "doubt," he says, does not only exist among the patients: it has passed into science, and could equally well be called *folie du doute* on account of its uncertain place in the chart of mental maladies, as well as for the strange symptoms which characterise it.

According to Ladame, Pinel, at the beginning of this century, first commenced to recognise *folie du doute*, while Esquirol, in 1838, published the first detailed clinical observation of *délire du toucher*, and laid stress on the patient's constant fight against obsessions and his recognition of their absurdity. Brierre de Boismont, in 1853, also stated that the irresistible idea keenly combated by the patient was characteristic of these cases. "The following distinction must be made," he said, "namely, that ideas may make one ill when they dominate the mind, but one is not really mad except when the will has become powerless to control the impulsions." That the patients fight against their obsessions, without succeeding in getting rid of them, was particularly insisted upon in the discussion upon monomanias at the Medico-Psychological Society of Paris on June 26th, 1854. Delasiauve, in 1859, made a first attempt to distinguish between pseudo-monomanias and recognised forms of insanity. After 1860, observations on *délire du toucher* became more numerous, and Baillarger appears to have been the first to notice that these conditions frequently commenced at puberty. Marcé, in 1862, though he failed to separate *délire du toucher* from insanity, clearly described the origin of imperative ideas. "In a predisposed person," he says, "feeble of character, endowed with keen sensibility, a word, an emotion, a fear, a desire leaves one day a profound impression. The thought, born in this manner, presents itself to the mind in an importunate way, takes possession of it, does not leave it, dominates all its conceptions; during this time the individual may have consciousness of all the absurdity, unreasonableness, or criminality of this idea; the acts themselves soon conform to these unhealthy preoccupations, and become absurd and extravagant."

The term, *folie du doute*, occurred for the first time in the celebrated discussion upon *la manie raisonnante*, at the Medico-Psychological Society of Paris, March 26th, 1866; but from what was said by Jules Falret on that occasion, it was evident that what he called *folie du doute* corresponded to *délire du toucher*, and not to the form of mental trouble described two years later by Griesinger as *Grübelsucht* and *Krankhafte Fragesucht*. In this discussion Baillarger stated that one of his patients never ceased to make suppositions and to lose herself in "if" and "perhaps." A clear distinction between these diseases and recognised forms of insanity was made for the first time in 1886 by Morel, and he stated that patients suffering from imperative ideas did not interpret their obsessions after the manner of the insane; that they neither experienced hallucinations nor illusions; nor did they undergo those transformations which change the personality of the insane, and make them radically different from what they were before. Heredity, including not only hereditary insanity, but also other nervous conditions, such as hysteria and hypochondria, he regarded as important exciting causes.

In 1868, Griesinger published cases which showed for the first time that the entire malady might consist in insoluble questions, which unceasingly pursued the patient, who could not escape from "why" and "how," and he considered the condition might be independent of emotional complications. In 1875, Legrand du Saulle showed that the same patients could present successively the symptoms of *folie du doute* and those of *délire du toucher*, and he attempted, by joining these two conditions, to form a special mental affection having a veritable morbid entity.

In 1877, Westphal published an important contribution to this subject. According to him, the obsession never becomes a true *idée fixe délirante*, but always remains a stranger to the patient's ego, while the insane conform logically to the deductions of their fixed ideas. This scientific distinction between the fixed ideas of the insane, and mere obsessions, has long been recognised by the Church, which has always made a difference between possession and obsession, saying for example: "This man is not possessed, he is only suffering from obsession." According to Westphal an obsession is not an emotion, nor is it ever produced by one, and if attacks of mental agony appear later, these are always secondary and simply concomitant phenomena. This opinion is opposed to the observations of Morel and the French *savants*. Wille holds that obsessions can have an emotional base, and thinks that they are sometimes followed by veritable mental alienation, while Westphal affirms that cases of obsession never become insane. Wille, as well as Legrand du Saulle, has noticed the frequent suicidal ideas and even attempts at suicide, sometimes followed by death, and considers *folie du doute* and its likes as an intermediate condition between the nevroses and the psychoses, and that obsession is always ready to pass into madness.

Westphal divides obsessions into three kinds :—(1) Those which remain purely theoretical, as the *folie du doute*, when it takes the form of questions. (2) Those which produce certain actions, as the *délire du toucher*. (3) Impulsive obsessions, which provoke immediate actions.

While other authors since Morel have emphasised heredity as an essential factor in obsessions, Magnan, in 1885, appears to have been the first to consider this mental trouble as a direct and immediate sign of morbid heredity.

In opposition to Legrand du Saulle, Ladame demands the separation of *folie du doute* and *délire du toucher* into two distinct clinical varieties. These, like pleuro-pneumonia, are certainly often associated, he says, but more often exist isolated. In illustration of this he cites the following cases :—

(a) A young man, aged 28, suffered from fear of contamination and frequently washed his hands as a method of purification. He never feared he would forget anything and never addressed questions to himself. This, according to Ladame, was a case of *délire du toucher* without *folie du doute.*

(b) Miss ——, aged 33, has had since childhood ideas which she cannot get rid of. She asks herself all sorts of questions and seeks in vain for their answers. These are particularly in reference to the other world and the Creation. Did everything make itself? Has God created all things? Did not the world make itself? Is there a God? How can one divide objects into infinitely little parts, when each little part can still be divided? How is it that an object infinitely divided can still be divided, notwithstanding that one cannot divide it any more? Is God able to divide it still further? God only can divide it and nevertheless this particle cannot be divided! How do you account for that? She has never suffered from *délire du toucher*.

Van Eeden says that in four cases treated by him the connection between *folie du doute* and *délire du toucher* could not be mistaken, and that in all these cases the *folie du doute* was evolved after the *délire du toucher* and was an evident consequence of it. One case commenced with the fear of catching syphilis. The patient avoided touching anything he suspected of being contaminated, and, if this happened, scrupulously washed his hands. His precautions became exaggerated, until he not only doubted their efficacy, but also the clearness of his judgment; and then, despite the excessive attention given to these washings, could not obtain a certainty of complete cleanliness. A similar progressive evolution was observed, says van Eeden, in another case, where the patient suffered from *crainte de souillure*, then doubt and finally mistrust of herself. The *délire du toucher* began with fear of soiling her food, she washed her hands incessantly, but afterwards the doubt returned. Another patient, who was nursing a case of cancer, became afraid of catching it. She washed her hands constantly, and avoided coming in contact with suspected persons.

In agoraphobia, claustrophobia, etc., van Eeden says the idea of fright arises suddenly from the impression of the surroundings, and it is only after having this that the patient avoids open or closed spaces. Here it is the fear which causes the obsession. He classifies these and similar conditions as follows :—(1) *Conceptions obsédantes ;* here the obsession springs from a precise and detailed conception of some act which acquires an impulsive force. (2) *Les émotions obsédantes ;* chiefly terror, in which a momentary emotion, an impression—which a normal man can equally well experience, but which he quickly represses—dominates the volition and the reason. The patients are not able to say what they fear, or if they give a reason it is evidently an invented one. (3) *Impulsions obsédantes ;* the irresistible tendency to commit strange or improper acts. (4) *Les idées obsédantes* properly so-called ; the intellectual obsessions of the French, the *Grübelsucht* of Griesinger and Berger. The patient is not able to escape from the obsession to think constantly about a certain subject or question. Here it is neither a question of a perception or emotion, nor of an impulse to commit an act; there is only one isolated idea—a word, a phrase, incessantly pursues the patient and continually occupies his thoughts.

Van Eeden regards what he calls "manias of superstition" as an interesting variety of obsessions. One of his patients, a man aged 40, of healthy constitution, has since childhood attached prophetic signification to puerile facts and events. To wear a certain necktie promises him happiness or unhappiness. If he does not touch a certain boundary-stone he thinks evil will happen to him. If he does not re-read a certain line, or make a certain letter thicker when writing, something horrible will befall him. At first his strange ideas were insignificant, or he was able to resist them; but, as he grew older they filled his life and rendered it intolerable. For twenty years he made a pilgrimage every Sunday to the railway station in order to kick a certain post three times with each foot. If he did not do this his father would die. In order to rid himself of these obsessions he made vows and associated threats with them. He said for example : " If I yield to one of my caprices in the course of an hour I shall have apoplexy before twenty-four hours have passed." At first this succeeded, but soon the effect of the vows diminished, and he was compelled to make them stronger. The unhappy man now stands sometimes for a quarter of an hour muttering the most fearful imprecations, in order to get the strength to go an errand. If he omits them he is forced to obey the most absurd impulses. He must stop before a certain house, retrace his steps, touch boundaries, stop passers-by or touch their clothes : in a word, he is obliged to act like a maniac. His intellect is perfectly normal, and he attends to his business as if nothing were the matter.

Bérillon thinks the professional character of these nervous troubles has not been sufficiently noticed, and he draws an analogy between them and the different functional spasms which show a tendency to professional localisation. In illustration of this he cites the following cases :—A young priest, not timid in the performance of his other religious duties, suffered agony on entering the pulpit. Another suffered in the same way when he received a confession. A medical student suffered extreme agony at the sight of a few drops of blood. A chemist made up a prescription which caused the death of a customer. He was able to prove that it was dispensed exactly as ordered by the doctor ; but, as his existence became a veritable torture from constant fear of making a mistake, he sold his business. A notary had morbid fears only when he had to give a professional opinion. A hairdresser noticed that his hand trembled one day, and then constantly dreaded that this would reappear when he shaved his best customers. The same anxiety did not exist when he had to shave a poor or unknown customer. Dr. Frémineau reports the case of an actor who abandoned his profession on account of extreme stage - fright. This condition only appeared after a successful career. Dr. Bérillon reports several similar cases. Riegler has noticed a morbid fear amongst railway mechanics, to which he has given the name of *sidérodromophobie ;* this is characterised by an extraordinary aversion to their habitual occupation, and the sight of a train or the whistle of an engine is sufficient to revive their anxiety. Grasset mentions that a distinguished Parisian surgeon commences to be anxious the moment a patient leaves his consulting-room with a prescription. He anxiously asks himself whether he could have written centigrammes instead of milligrammes ; and only recovers his mental calm when his servant, sent to seek the patient, brings back the prescription, and he can see that it is all right. Another doctor, he says, is rendered perfectly miserable by the fear of microbes. Brochin reports the case of a doctor who fears no contagious malady, except diphtheria, and who shows proof of veritable heroism every time he sees a diphtheritic patient. A case has recently been reported from abroad, where a medical man, dreading that his fees might be the means of contagion, invented elaborate methods of sterilising them; and I know of a similar case in this country.

These morbid fears are awkward enough when they occur in ordinary life, but, according to Bérillon, they acquire graver importance when the subjects of them are liable to enforced military service, especially in the ranks. In Legrand du Saulle's classic case of agoraphobia, a lieutenant of infantry experienced undefinable agony when obliged to cross an open space in civilian clothes, but this never happened when he was in uniform. When an officer suffers in this way he can escape from the intolerable situation by getting leave of absence, but it is not so with the soldier. Bérillon gives amongst others the following examples :—

Paul C., aged 25, illness dates from military service. When ordered to cross the horizontal bar at the gymnasium he was seized with extreme apprehension, and afterwards the idea of this exercise was always present. Again ordered to perform it he became terrified, and asked to be excused, but from that time his superiors insisted more and more upon the dreaded exercise. One day in attempting to cross the bar he became giddy and fell upon his head. A veritable agoraphobia developed; and since his return from military service he has been unable to cross a road by himself.

M., aged 37, commercial traveller, suffered from chronic diarrhœa, which caused him to dread leaving home; after this ceased he retained his nervous fears. Once, when a short distance from his house, the anxiety was so strong that he was obliged to return, and since then, seven years ago, he has lived in a circle having a diameter of about 200 metres, and nothing will induce him to leave it. When, as a member of the Reserve, he had to serve his first period of twenty-eight days, he was able to perform his duties; but at the second period the agoraphobia had developed, and by dint of diplomacy, ingenuity, and bribery, he managed to be kept constantly employed in the barracks.

According to Dr. Gélineau a crowd of sentiments of repugnance, etc., which the laity group as " aversions " closely resemble the conditions we are discussing. Henry the Third, for example, who showed his bravery at the Siege of La Rochelle and elsewhere, could not bear the sight of a cat. The Duke of Epernon fainted at the sight of a young donkey. Ladislas, King of Poland, got frightened and ran away when he saw apples; and Favoriti, a modern Italian poet, could not bear the smell of a rose. Dr. Pierre d'Apono was so frightened at the sight of milk and cheese that he fainted. Montaigne said: "I have seen more people driven to flight by the smell of apples than by arquebuses, others frightened at a mouse, made sick by the sight of cream, or by seeing a feather-bed shaken."

Ribot applies the term "fixed ideas" to the states we are discussing, and regards them as "chronic hypertrophy of the attention"; the "fixed ideas" being the *absolute*, "attention"[1] the *temporary* predominance of an intellectual state or group of states. The fixed idea is attention in its highest degree and marks the extreme limit of its power of inhibition. There exists, he says, both in normal attention and in fixed ideas, predominance and intensity of a state of consciousness: this is more marked, however, in the fixed idea, which is permanent and disposes of the important psychical factor—time. In attention, this exceptional state does not last long: consciousness reverts spontaneously to its normal condition, which is a struggle for existence between heterogeneous states. The fixed idea prevents all diffusion. There is no antagonistic state that is able to overthrow it. Effort is impossible or vain. Hence the agony of the patient who is conscious of his own impotency. The following is Ribot's conception of the probable physiological condition associated with fixed ideas:—In its normal state he says the entire brain works; diffused activity is the rule. Discharges take place from one group of cells into another, as the objective equivalent of the perpetual alterations of consciousness. In the morbid state only a few nervous elements are active; or, at least, their state of tension is not transmitted to other groups. Whatever may be their position in the cerebral organ, they are, as a matter of fact, isolated; all disposable energy has been accumulated in them, and they do not communicate it to other groups; whence their supreme dominance and exaggerated activity. There is a lack of physiological equilibrium, due probably to the state of nutrition

[1] *I.e.*, ordinary attention.

of the cerebral centres. Ribot refers to Westphal's recognition of the difference between fixed ideas and insanity, and his statement that "the fixed idea is a disturbance of the *form* of the process of ideation, but not of its contents." The "formal" perturbation consists, says Ribot, in the inexorable necessity that compels the association always to follow the same path. There is derangement, not in the nature, the quality of the idea, which is normal, but in its quantity, intensity, and degree. Thus it is perfectly rational to reflect upon the usefulness of bank-notes, or the origin of things, and this state differs widely from that of the beggar who thinks himself a millionaire, or the man who believes himself to be a woman.

As regards the connection between *folie du doute* and *délire du toucher*, it is interesting to note that the latter condition occurred in No. 83 (pp. 241-3) as soon as the patient's doubts took a material form, but was not associated with it when his obsessions were purely intellectual. Does not this show that the appearance of the *délire du toucher* simply depends upon the nature of the *folie du doute*, and that the incessant washings, etc., are the patient's natural physical efforts to rid himself of his material fears, while the character of the purely intellectual obsessions renders such relief impossible. Mr. —— (No. 83) sought and found its nearest equivalent in telling his religious troubles to an older friend, in whose opinions he tried to find consolation. From this point of view, the second of the cases quoted by Ladame shows *folie du doute* unassociated with *délire du toucher*. This separation is, I think, more artificial than real. In his first case, that of the young man who frequently washed his hands through fear of contamination, it is by no means clear that this was a case of *délire du toucher* without *folie du doute*. Surely the abnormal and incessant washing must have been the result of doubts which he thus tried to remove. The same objections might be raised to van Eeden's cases, where *folie du doute* is said to have resulted from *délire du toucher*.

Hack Tuke regarded imperative ideas, and the acts resulting from them, as essentially automatic, and considered this their fundamental characteristic. Are these acts automatic? An automatic act is simply an habitual voluntary one performed inattentively or unconsciously; while the so-called automatic acts of the sufferer from imperative ideas are carried out in opposition to his volition, and frequently associated with intense and painful consciousness. Possibly, with justice, they might be called *reflex*, seeing that they are the "fatal, unchosen, response to stimulation."

The fact that an imperative idea remains a stranger to the patient's ego distinguishes it, according to most authorities, from an insane delusion. This rule has its exceptions. One of my patients, as we have seen (No. 86, p. 244), commenced in 1885 to be "inhibited" by various superstitions. At first this rarely occurred; but later, owing to the number of his unlucky days, etc., the performance of many acts was often interfered with. Many people, by no means insane, actually believe in, and are influenced by, identical superstitions. This patient, however, did not believe in them, and keenly resented their interference with his actions. The non-assimilation of the imperative idea sometimes, then, constitutes the morbid element, and this apparently depends more upon the individual than upon the idea itself. The patient who made herself miserable about the Creation might, under other times and circumstances, have taken pleasure in discussing "the number of angels who could stand on the point of a needle; or whether, in passing from point to point, they had to traverse the intermediate space." Schliemann's imperative idea to discover the site of ancient Troy only differed from those we are discussing in the fact that it was assimilated by its possessor; but this did not constitute insanity.

In nearly all my cases the condition appears to have had an emotional origin. The shock of the sudden death of a relative caused one patient to fear his wife would die; another dreaded travelling after being frightened by a drunken man in a railway carriage. Although, in some instances, the emotional element changed its character, and in all became greatly intensified, it was certainly often associated with the commencement of the original trouble.

Imperative ideas are usually regarded as being typical of degeneracy, and especially of hereditary degeneracy. Some of my cases seem to confirm this: they were weak mentally and physically, and had unsatisfactory hereditary antecedents. In several instances their imperative ideas had become insane delusions; many of them had suicidal impulses; one attempted suicide, and another had halluoinations. On the other hand, the transition from the normal state to imperative ideas is almost insensible—the repetition of an insignificant saying being, according to Ribot, the slightest form, and preoccupation, such as anxiety about an examination, a degree higher. Most children, too, have suffered at one time or another from imperative ideas. This, as a popular writer has justly remarked,[1] appears to arise from an exaggerated sense of the importance of what they say and do, and also from an exaggerated fear regarding the notice taken of them by others. He says : " How miserable we sometimes make ourselves over some silly remark we have made. Some of us even keep a little store of foolish things we have said or done at various times—and take them out occasionally and blush over them. As a child I blushed for years at the thought of having piped out a response in church in the wrong place, before the clergyman's turn was over. I felt as if the whole congregation turned and gazed at me with scornful ridicule. As I walked away every one who glanced at me I felt sure was thinking, ' There goes the child who made that extraordinary squeak in church.' "

Every one cannot have fixed ideas, as for example idiots, who possess little spontaneous and no voluntary attention, while, as Ribot says: " In every sound human being there is always a dominant idea which regulates his conduct; such as pleasure, money, ambition, or the soul's salvation." Some of my patients were physically far above the average, and many of them possessed mental endowments of high quality, and their morbid ideas did not prevent them doing valuable work. Most of them, it is true, were of an emotional, nervous type, but is the sensitive, mobile brain necessarily degenerate ? May not the accidents to which it is liable be the result of its higher and more complex development ? The thoroughbred is more emotional and nervous than the cart-horse, but is this necessarily an evidence of its hereditary degeneracy ? The term " degenerate " is applied so freely and widely by some modern authors that one cannot help concluding that they rank as such all who do not conform to some primitive savage type, possessing an imperfectly developed nervous system.

[1] " To inculcate contempt of others." *Pall Mall Gazette*, April 4th, 1895.

(8) Epilepsy.

My results in the treatment of epilepsy have been encouraging but not conclusive. Out of ten cases, five were markedly improved, but none recovered completely. This, however, does not include two cases associated with dipsomania, which have remained without relapse, the one for four and a half, the other for five years. In the following examples the epilepsy was not complicated by other diseases.

No. 94. Miss ——, aged 19, January 5th, 1890. Good health up to 15, when menstruation and attacks of *petit mal* appeared simultaneously. A few months later *grand mal* commenced; first at night only, but soon in the daytime also. The convulsions were violent and generalised; and the patient bit her tongue and passed urine involuntarily. After a fit, she generally slept for several hours, and on awaking was either stupid and listless, or abnormally excited and violent. On several occasions she had been severely burnt and scalded; and her face, limbs, and body were scarred and disfigured. The memory and general mental condition began to deteriorate at an early stage of the illness, and she soon became almost idiotic. Despite treatment by bromides, etc., there had been a progressive increase in the number of seizures, which, when I first saw the patient, averaged about twenty a week.

She was hypnotised fifteen times from January 5th to the end of February, 1890; although no drugs were given, the fits ceased after the first induction of hypnosis. On March 7th, she had a fright followed by an attack of *grand mal*, and was hypnotised four times in the next fortnight; then, as there was no relapse, treatment was abandoned. The patient rapidly improved mentally and physically, and for the first time in her life was able to take a situation. She remained well until November, 1891, when attacks of *petit mal* reappeared. These were followed early in December by *grand mal*, there being ten fits up to January 19th, 1892. At that time hypnotic treatment, which had been delayed owing to my absence from home, was resumed and continued until the end of February. She had two attacks towards the end of January, after which the fits ceased. She returned to her situation in March, and up to November, 1892, when I left the neighbourhood, I was informed that she had only had

B

one or two very slight attacks of *petit mal.* During that time, as the patient lived some distance from me, I could not repeat the treatment, nor have I been able to get further news of the case. This patient was drawn from my general practice at Goole.

No. 95. Miss ——, aged 17, November 23rd, 1897. Began to have attacks of *petit mal* at the age of $2\frac{1}{2}$ years. These occurred frequently for several years, then disappeared under treatment.

In 1891, during convalescence from measles, she had her first attack of *grand mal,* followed by another attack the same year and one in 1892. No attacks in 1893. In 1894 she had five attacks; in 1895 thirteen; in 1896 five; while in 1897 she had twenty-one. During all this time she had careful medical treatment, and took bromides regularly in full doses.

The last of the attacks just referred to occurred on November 22nd, 1897, and hypnotic treatment was begun the following day. The sittings were repeated thirty times up to the end of 1898, and during that time there were no attacks.

The sittings were then reduced to one a month, and she had one attack in August, 1899. I saw her again in January, 1900, after which the treatment was discontinued until November, when she again had an attack. From that date, to April, 1901, the patient was hypnotised three times, and there were no further attacks. She then went abroad and treatment was discontinued. The attacks recommenced, and she had six between June 1st and October 19th, 1901. Hypnotic treatment was then recommenced, and she had twenty-nine sittings from October 21st, 1901, to February 24th, 1903. During that time, a period of seventeen months, there have been no attacks, and the patient has improved greatly both mentally and physically.[1]

In this case, on the advice of Dr. de Watteville, who saw the patient with me, medical treatment was also continued, and the patient took bromides more or less regularly, although not nearly to the same extent that she had done before hypnotic treatment was begun. It is to be noted that the attacks ceased when the patient was hypnotised regularly, and returned when hypnotic treatment was neglected.

Elliotson, Esdaile, and Braid, as well as more recent observers, have also reported cases, of which the following are examples :—

No. 96 (Elliotson). Mr. ——, aged 17, had suffered for four

---

[1] Up to the present date, May 28th, 1893, there has been no further relapse.

years from attacks of *grand* and *petit mal.* At first the convulsions were rare, but soon became frequent and severe: the tongue was often bitten, and the seizure always followed by profound coma. In addition to perfect fits, there were often fragmentary ones indicated by transitory deafness. There was neither hysteria nor any other nervous symptom. As the disease had resisted three years' medical treatment, drugs were abandoned and the patient mesmerised regularly. He recovered rapidly, and two years later there had been no relapse.

No. 97 (Esdaile). Mrs. Goodall, aged 33, epilepsy of nineteen years' duration. The attacks, preceded by an aura and accompanied by violent convulsions with loss of consciousness, occurred about twice a month. For six years she had also suffered from severe abdominal pain, and was unable to sleep without Cannabis Indica. She entered the Mesmeric Hospital on January 28th, 1847, and was under treatment for two months. Result: the fits ceased, she slept naturally without narcotics, and the abdominal pain disappeared. Later reports confirmed her recovery.

Braid also recorded a case of *grand mal* treated hypnotically, which had not relapsed eight years later.

No. 98 (Wetterstrand). Miss D. von B., aged 24, first seen September, 1891. Epilepsy of ten years' duration. The attacks became rarer under hypnotic treatment, and the last occurred on Christmas Day, 1891. The patient then got the fixed idea that the fits would return when she left Stockholm. Wetterstrand was unable to remove this by suggestion; he therefore put her to sleep on March 5th, 1892, and maintained the condition, with the exception of a few hours, until April 8th, 1892. When aroused she had lost her obsession, and there was no relapse.

From an early date in his hypnotic practice, Wetterstrand reported cases of epilepsy successfully treated by suggestion, but his results have been still more striking since he adopted the method of prolonged sleep. In 1893, ten cases treated in the latter way had already passed several years without relapse.

In 1897, Dr. Woods published fourteen cases, of which two —aged 13 and 8½ years respectively—are stated to have recovered, and ten to have been much improved. In the successful cases the duration of the disease had been two years in each instance, while in one two years, and in the other sixteen months, had passed without relapse.

Bérillon has published twenty cases with four recoveries, and Dr. Hilger, Magdeburg, seven, two of which were improved. Voisin, Spehl, Stadelmann, de Jong, and others have also reported successful cases.

Remarks.—No one has obtained results in epilepsy equal to those of Wetterstrand; and his success appears to be due to the employment of "prolonged sleep." His statistics are so startling that Forel only accepted them after personal investigation. It is possible that with the more general employment of "prolonged sleep" others may obtain results equal to those of Wetterstrand; but, to give hypnotism a fair trial, it should be commenced as soon as the disease shows itself, and not, as is usually done, put off until all other forms of treatment have failed.

It must be admitted, however, that some authorities cite cases which cannot be regarded as conclusive, as patients were stated to have been cured before sufficient time had elapsed to warrant this. Further, the description of the case sometimes casts doubt on the accuracy of the diagnosis, and it must not be forgotten that hystero-epilepsy, a disease frequently cured by hypnotic treatment, is common in France, and may be mistaken for genuine epilepsy.

(9) Chorea.

The following cases are from my own practice :—

No. 99. Master ——, aged 15, April 3rd, 1894, had good health up to two years previously, when he had influenza followed by chorea—the latter lasting four months. No history of fright or rheumatism. Heart normal. The present attack began at Christmas, 1893, and again after influenza. The right arm and leg were first affected, then the left. The condition had been growing steadily worse: the patient constantly dropped things, was unable to write, could not dress himself, and walked with difficulty. Treatment: iron, arsenic, cod-liver oil, change of air, etc. No improvement.

The patient was then sent to me by Dr. de Watteville, and hypnotised thirteen times from April 3rd to May 23rd, 1894. Before the termination of the treatment the spasms had entirely disappeared. Recovery confirmed by later reports.

In six other consecutive cases of chorea, recovery took place in each instance, while in none did the duration of the treatment exceed three weeks. One of these patients, a girl, aged 18, also suffered from headache, and frequent attacks of giddiness and drowsiness. These symptoms—suspiciously like those of the minor forms of epilepsy—also entirely disappeared after hypnotic treatment.

In another case, not included in the above list, the patient had had chorea three years previously, but twitching movements in the fingers had persisted after recovery. This patient was deeply hypnotised at the first attempt, and the abnormal movements entirely ceased after the second sitting.

Elliotson reported many successful cases, and asserted that mesmerism yielded better results than iron or arsenic; the latter being the remedies he had formerly recommended in place of purgatives, blisters, and the other debilitating measures with which chorea used to be treated in his day.

Numerous cases are also recorded by modern observers, and of these the following is an example:—

No. 100 (Dumontpallier). Miss ——, aged 12, October, 1892, had suffered from chorea since November, 1891. The spasms, which were frequent, practically affected all the voluntary muscles with the exception of the lower limbs. Heart normal. No improvement after nearly twelve months' careful medical treatment. Hypnosis was induced at the first attempt, and the choreic movements ceased for two hours: at the end of a week's treatment they had entirely disappeared.

(10) Stammering.

The following cases are from my own practice:—

No. 101. Dr. ——, aged 28, November, 1892, had always stammered, but was strong and healthy, and showed no other nervous symptoms. Hypnotised forty-six times up to July 7th, 1893; this was followed by marked improvement. Two years later the patient stated that he was practically well.

No. 102. Mr. ——, aged 17, December, 1893, had stammered badly since commencing to speak: at times he was quite inarticulate and, in addition, there were many words he could never pronounce at all. He was morbidly conscious of his infirmity, and led a solitary, miserable life. He suffered greatly from insomnia, and sometimes passed several consecutive nights without sleep.   Hypnotised seventy-two times from January to May, 1893.   He soon slept well, but it was only towards the end of the treatment that the stammering improved.

He again consulted me in September, 1898, and stated that there had been hardly any return of the stammering.   He confessed, however, that he had long been addicted to excessive masturbation, and that he had lost all power of mental work. He suffered from various neurasthenic symptoms; had recently failed in an important examination, and was in despair about himself.   He recovered under further treatment.   At the last report (1902) he was practising as a barrister, and could speak in public without difficulty.

Out of 48 cases of stammering treated by Wetterstrand 15 were cured, 19 improved, while in 14 there was no result. Successful cases are also reported by Ringier, von Corval, Hamilton Osgood, and others; but the results as a whole have not been so satisfactory as those obtained in other functional disorders. Most of the cases sent to me were severe and of long standing; while the patients and their friends, discouraged by the failure of other methods to which years had been devoted, seldom gave hypnotic treatment a fair trial.

(11) Sea-Sickness.

The following cases are from my own practice:—

No. 103. Mrs. ——, aged 41, March 20th, 1892. A full account of this case is given on pp. 191-4, but, in addition to her other symptoms, the patient invariably suffered from sea-sickness, even on the shortest voyage, or in the calmest weather.   This had been a great disadvantage to her, as her husband was captain of a merchant steamer, and often wished to take her with him. In April, 1892, I suggested during hypnosis that she should be free from sea-sickness.   Before the end of the summer she made eight voyages between the Humber and London: her husband reported that on the first outward voyage there was a strong north-east swell, while on returning the weather was rough and the steamer, which was in ballast, rolled heavily; rough weather was also encountered on some of the other trips. But the patient had not even the slightest feeling of nausea and ate hearty meals. Case shown at the International Congress of Psychology, London, 1892, and elsewhere.

No. 104. Miss ——, aged 19, September, 1891, had good health, but the shortest voyage produced violent and even dangerous sea-sickness. Profound hypnosis was easily induced at the first attempt, and curative suggestions given. During the following year, the patient crossed the Channel several times without being sick. The treatment was then repeated, as she wished to go to India. During the voyage a cyclone was encountered, and she alone amongst the passengers remained well. The return journey was equally successful, and further voyages to and from India were also free from sickness.[1]

The following cases were published by Gorodichze, in 1896 :—

No. 105. Mrs. ——, aged 36, was healthy, but of a nervous temperament. She lived by the sea and often went out boating, but was always sick, even when it was absolutely calm. After hypnotic treatment she remained at sea for seven hours in a small sailing boat in extremely rough weather, without feeling the least inconvenience.

No. 106. Mr. ——, aged 40, suffered from neurasthenia with obsessions. His business took him frequently to London, and every time he crossed the Channel he was sick. After hypnotic treatment sea-sickness ceased, and during a particularly rough voyage he was the only passenger who was not ill.

No. 107. Mr. ——, aged 46, nervous and a bad sailor, was cured by hypnotic treatment.

No. 108. Mrs. ——, aged 37, suffered from neuralgia and migraine. Formerly always sick at sea, but after treatment made many voyages without inconvenience, despite bad weather.

An extremely successful case is also published by Bérillon, while Farez cites instances of sickness caused by railway travelling which were cured by suggestion.

(12) Skin Diseases.

No. 109. *Pruritus vulvæ and Eczema.*—Mrs. ——, aged 49, August, 1889, had always been nervous and emotional. Three of her children had died of infantile convulsions; one suffered from epilepsy and two from hysteria. At an earlier date the patient

[1] See also Case No. 31, pp. 201-2.

had had several attacks of pelvic inflammation, associated with
endometritis and menorrhagia: the latter diseases, after lasting
five years, yielded to treatment in 1883. The menopause soon
followed, and the patient had good health for two years. In
1885, she began to suffer from pruritus vulvæ, and eczema of the
hips and thighs. Irritation was always present, but at night it
became intolerable and produced insomnia. She had long suffered
from constipation: the bowels never acted without medicine, and
rarely oftener than once a week. The uterus was retroflected,
and bound down by adhesions resulting from the former pelvic
inflammation.

For four years, I treated the patient by drugs and local
applications under the supervision of a skin specialist, but without improvement. I then sent her to Mr. Mayo Robson,
who thought the uterine displacement and chronic constipation
interfered with the rectal circulation, and played an important
part in the origin and maintenance of the disease. He stretched
the sphincter ani under ether, but this neither cured the constipation nor relieved the other symptoms.

In August, 1889, I tried to hypnotise the patient, other
treatment being abandoned. The attempt failed, and was repeated
unsuccessfully on sixty-six occasions during the next four months,
her condition meanwhile growing steadly worse. At the sixty-
eighth sitting somnambulism was induced. All irritation
vanished immediately, and she slept soundly on that and the
following nights. The bowels acted daily. In a fortnight all
trace of eczema disappeared, and treatment was abandoned. At
the last report, three years later, there had been no return of any
of the symptoms, and she had not required to take even a simple
aperient. Case seen after recovery by Dr. Churton, of Leeds,
and others.

No. 110. *Hyperhidrosis.*—Miss ——, aged 15, consulted me
in January, 1890, on account of frequent attacks of migraine,
accompanied by vomiting, from which she had suffered for three
years. Menstruation normal. I noticed that on the back of the
left forearm a patch of skin, about $2\frac{1}{2}$ inches long by $1\frac{1}{2}$ broad,
was the seat of constant perspiration. This condition, which
had existed from infancy, was always excessive, and invariably
rendered more so by emotion or exertion. The forearm was
always enveloped in bandages, but these rapidly became saturated,

and then the perspiration dripped upon the floor. The patient was frequently punished at school because she soiled her needle-work, and her condition distressed her greatly, as she wished to become a dressmaker.

On January 10th, the patient was hypnotised for the first time, somnambulism induced, and suggestions given as to the headaches and hyperhidrosis. The following day the perspiration had markedly diminished, and it ceased entirely after the re-induction of hypnosis. Treatment was then abandoned. The case was shown at the International Congress of Experimental Psychology, London, August, 1892, and neither up to that date, nor since, as far as I have been able to learn, has there been any return of either hyperhidrosis or migraine, and the patient now follows the occupation of her choice.

Elliotson reported various successful cases, notably one of *eczema impetiginoides*, of two years' duration and affecting the whole scalp, and another of long-standing psoriasis.

Other cases are reported by modern writers :—

➤ No. 111 (Hamilton Osgood[1]). *Eczema.*—Master ——, aged 11, had suffered from eczema since he was eighteen months old. In October, 1893, just before hypnotic treatment was begun, this extended from the umbilicus to the feet: the forearms were covered with crusts and sores, there were deep inflamed fissures on the wrists, and large sores in the armpits. The boy was irritable and nervous, and slept badly, owing to the constant irritation.

After the first sitting, the irritation ceased, and the child slept soundly the whole night. At the end of a month's treat-ment all trace of eczema had disappeared; and, although there was some return of it within the year, this again yielded to suggestion, and complete recovery took place.

No. 112 (Hamilton Osgood). *Eczema.*—Mrs. ——, aged 68, eczema of eight years' duration, which had resisted all treatment. Much irritation, insomnia and mental depression. Complete recovery after eighteen sittings, despite the fact that only slight hypnosis was induced, and the patient retained full memory of all that was said or done.

[1] Dr. Hamilton Osgood, of Boston, after studying Hypnotism on the Continent, has practised it with much success. He has also, by lecturing and writing, done much to call the attention of the profession in America to the subject.

No. 113 (Hamilton Osgood). *Eczema rubrum.*—Miss ——,
aged 28, suffered from eczema rubrum, affecting particularly the
scalp, face, hands, and feet: this had been unrelieved by
four years' careful treatment. The palms of the hands were
enormously thickened and intersected by deep fissures—the condition almost resembling elephantiasis; there was also insomnia
with much irritation. The patient commenced to sleep after the
first sitting, and at the end of the forty-seventh all trace of the
disease had disappeared.

No. 114 (Stadelmann). *Eczema.*—Miss ——, aged 46, seam-
stress, eczema of the hands and feet of eight years' duration; the
feet were swollen, and so hot and painful that the patient was
unable to keep them covered. Irregular menstruation, insomnia,
uric acid and rheumatism. Complete recovery, without relapse,
after a week's hypnotic treatment.

No. 115 (Charpentier). *Hyperhidrosis.*—Mr. ——, aged 22,
had suffered from hyperhidrosis of the palms of both hands for
seven years: this had come on suddenly after a fright, and had
been excessive ever since. If the patient wiped his hands drops
of sweat reappeared almost immediately, and dripped freely from
the fingers. The condition was neither affected by temperature
nor by the amount of liquid consumed, but was aggravated
by emotion and when the attention was drawn to it. Drugs,
external applications, and electricity had produced no effect; but
the patient recovered completely after four months' hypnotic
treatment.

Other successful cases, some as striking as those just quoted,
are reported by Farez, Bérillon, Grossmann, Backman, etc.

Remarks.—That suggestion should influence perspiration
seems reasonable, when one considers how much that secretion
is influenced by emotion. Farez has noticed that hospital
patients frequently perspire from the axilla when undergoing
medical examination. Bérillon and Magnin, who have vaccinated
a large number of adults, observed that a certain proportion of
them were frightened and perspired freely. Nervous and self-
conscious persons frequently suffer from a temporary hyperhidrosis,
when they are compelled to shake hands with strangers.

It is now generally recognised that eczema is sometimes of
nervous origin, and in this is probably to be found the explanation
of its occasional cure by hypnotism.

CHAPTER XI.

(I.) Surgical Cases.

As already pointed out, hypnotic anæsthesia is of more scientific than practical interest. It can, however, be evoked by suggestion in nearly all cases of profound hypnotic somnambulism. At first, on testing with the faradic brush, one may only find a slight amount of anæsthesia. If, however, appropriate suggestions are made, the anæsthesia may ultimately become deep enough to ensure absence of pain during surgical operation.

In cases of protracted operation it is sometimes necessary that the suggestions should be repeated, both as to the maintenance of the hypnosis and the presence of the anæsthesia. Before arousing the patient, the operator should suggest post-hypnotic anæsthesia, i.e. absence of pain on waking. Should the effect of this suggestion wear off and pain reappear, it can often be again arrested by rehypnotising the patient and repeating the suggestions. In good hypnotic subjects it may be advisable only to suggest analgesia, without loss of ordinary sensation, especially for the condition after operation.

(II.) Medical Cases.

Medical practice and experiment should be kept absolutely distinct; and no suggestions should ever be made to patients, except those necessary for the induction of hypnosis, and the relief or cure of disease. This rule does not apply after recovery, when the individual has ceased to be a patient: a certain proportion of my experimental work was conducted with former patients who placed themselves at my disposal.

The selection of patients for hypnotic treatment, and the hope of relief or cure held out to them, ought naturally to be regulated by the same principles as those governing ordinary medical practice. Thus, if the case is one of organic disease, it ought to be clearly explained to the patient that cure is absolutely out of the question. He should be told that at most there may be a thin overlying stratum of functional nervous disturbance; and that there is only a possibility, not a certainty, of this being removed by hypnotic treatment.

In cases alleged to be functional, the operator ought to satisfy himself that the symptoms, which he is about to attempt to relieve by suggestion, are not in any way associated with organic disease. Even then, he should never tell the patient that he is sure of curing him, but only hold out such reasonable hope as experience fully justifies.

Patients should always be given to understand that the operator neither claims nor possesses any mysterious or occult power, and that the phenomena of hypnosis are really dependent upon changes which take place in the subject's own brain. If the patient be intelligent, it may be advisable to tell him something about modern hypnotic theory, and to explain to him that possibly the phenomena of hypnosis may be due to the arousing of powers dormant in a secondary consciousness.

As a rule, the patients sent to me have exhausted all ordinary methods of treatment before consulting me. Under these circumstances, they come for hypnotic treatment solely, and receive that alone. If, however, other methods have not been exhausted, and any of them appear likely to help the patient, these are employed as well as hypnotism. Further, in certain cases—insomnia for example,—where the patients are more or less dependent upon narcotic drugs, these are not stopped until the curative effects of suggestion are able to replace them.

Patients treated by hypnotic methods may be divided into three classes: (1) Those in whom deep hypnosis has been induced. (2) Those slightly hypnotised. (3) Those in whom hypnosis has either been doubtful or entirely absent.

(1) *The first class*, which numbers—according to statistics already cited—about 13 per cent of those influenced, is the easiest to deal with. Such patients can be hypnotised or aroused at a word, and are generally markedly responsive

to curative suggestions. To take an illustrative case, let
us suppose that the patient is suffering from insomnia. He
is hypnotised and told that he is to sleep for half an hour.
During this time curative suggestions are given: *e.g.* that the
patient shall feel restful and drowsy at bedtime, fall asleep
as soon as he puts his head upon the pillow, sleep all night,
etc. These suggestions, if the case is one of deep hypnosis, are
likely to be responded to in whole or in part. If the success
has only been partial, the treatment is renewed on another day,
and the suggestions repeated. If this is not enough, the methods
may be varied with success. For example, if the patient suffers
from various symptoms, it is sometimes better only to suggest the
relief of one of these at a time: with other cases it is advantageous
to employ "prolonged sleep" in addition to suggestive treatment.
The latter method was largely used by Elliotson and Esdaile, and
possibly made up in a large measure for their ignorance of the
value of suggestion. According to Wetterstrand, too much
attention has been given to suggestion, while the curative value
of prolonged hypnotic sleep has been entirely forgotten. His
results, and those of Voisin, obtained in this way, are both striking
and valuable.

Patients treated by this method ought to be placed in charge
of a nurse who is put *en rapport* with them. At first, even in
cases where the patient has been deeply hypnotised, it is often
necessary that the suggestion to continue sleeping should be
repeated several times a day; for if this is not done, hypnosis
terminates spontaneously and the treatment is interrupted. The
action of the bladder and bowels should be regulated by suggestion,
and the patient fed at regular intervals without being aroused.

(2) *Cases of Slight Hypnosis.*—Here, with the exception that
prolonged sleep cannot be employed, the treatment is practically
the same as under Class 1. The patients rest in a more or less
lethargic condition while curative suggestions are given; and
these are varied, or repeated, to meet the requirements of each
individual case.

(3) *Cases in which Hypnosis is either doubtful or absent.*—In
this class suggestion frequently yields results as striking as those
found in the two others, but it is often extremely difficult to
determine whether the patient has been hypnotised or not. This
point, which is of distinct theoretical as well as practical interest,

will be again referred to when discussing hypnotic theory. The management of the cases in this group is more difficult than that in the two preceding ones, and the following points are important :—

Patients, who do not pass into a condition followed by amnesia on waking, generally believe that they have not been hypnotised, and thus conclude that they cannot be influenced by suggestion. The operator should, therefore, carefully explain that genuine hypnotic conditions are not necessarily followed by amnesia; and, further, that many patients, who present none of the usual phenomena of hypnosis, are still remarkably responsive to suggestion.

If possible, the patients belonging to this class should be trained to concentrate their attention on some soothing mental picture, while the operator makes his suggestions. In this way a dreamy condition is often obtained, which may be one of slight hypnosis or only the borderland of normal sleep. During this, the operator ought to suggest the deepening of this drowsy or quasi-hypnotic state, and also make appropriate curative suggestions. He should also explain beforehand the uncertainty which exists as to the fulfilment of the latter : they are made at this early stage because some patients respond to curative suggestions immediately, even when hypnosis is obviously absent, while with others it is the repetition of the suggestion which seems to bring about its fulfilment.

Another group, in this class, presents difficulties peculiarly its own. Thus, in cases of muscular tremor, spasms, convulsions, persistent hiccough, etc., it is often impossible for the patient to maintain physical, or mental, quietude even for a few moments. Despite this, many of them recover after a more or less prolonged suggestive treatment. In some instances improvement does not take place until hypnosis has been induced; in many others, however, the patients recover without having passed into any condition even remotely resembling the hypnotic. An example of the first variety is cited p. 185 : here the patient did not improve until hypnosis was evoked, and it was interesting to observe how at first the attacks of spasm appeared during that condition and invariably terminated it. An example of the second variety is cited pp. 178-80 : here the patient suffered continuously from either generalised convulsions or violent unilateral muscular spasms. Yet, under these unfavourable conditions, curative suggestions—repeated daily for half an hour at a time— were speedily responded to.

The nature of the curative suggestions made by the operator is of extreme importance, particularly in cases of slight or doubtful hypnosis. This statement requires further development. Certainly, if the patient has been deeply hypnotised, he will respond to any suggestion he understands, if this is neither opposed by his will nor beyond the range of his hypnotic powers. On the other hand, particularly where hypnosis is slight or doubtful, it is often essential to make a careful study of the patient and his surroundings; to gain his confidence, and to learn his hopes, fears, and difficulties. Here, suggestion should not only be employed in conditions obviously or possibly hypnotic, but carried on also in the patient's waking life, and extended to his friends and relatives. It is one thing to successfully suggest relief from some slight functional disturbance to a deeply hypnotised patient, and another, and much more difficult one, to induce the dipsomaniac to abstain from drinking. In the latter case, the suggestions must be varied to meet the carefully studied requirements of each individual, and everything done to incite him loyally to co-operate in the experiment. Friends and relatives, who possibly have given up in despair trying to help, must also be urged to renewed and more earnest efforts. The same rule applies to many forms of hysterical disease. In some cases, it is true, the illness has come on suddenly as the result of shock or over-strain, but in many others it is a culminating point in a life which has been characterised by lack of discipline and self-control. Convulsions or spasms, which the patients are incapable of influencing by their volition, have often had countless forerunners in tricks of gesture, bursts of passion, petulance, emotion, or the like. Such patients ought to be taught by friends, as well as physician, to try to control every unnecessary expression of emotion, and to make a voluntary effort in their waking life to check defects which have certainly preceded, and may possibly have provoked, their malady.

The central factor in all hypnotic treatment ought to be the development of the patient's control of his own organism. He should clearly understand that the operator exercises no mysterious power over him, but simply arouses forces which are latent in his—the patient's—own brain. It should be plainly pointed out to him that his disease frequently demonstrates the feebleness of his volition : he desires, for example, to resist drinking but cannot ; he wishes to escape from an obsession, but is unable to do so. The hypnotic training, which enables him to carry his wishes into effect, does so by increasing, not diminishing, his voluntary control of his own organism. He should be taught to apply this increased power for himself, not only in the immediate instance for which he seeks relief, but also on other occasions, for fresh troubles, should these arise.

CHAPTER XII.

BEFORE attempting to discuss hypnotic theories, it is necessary to clearly define the phenomena themselves. To facilitate this the latter may be divided into two groups: (1) Those observed in subjects who exhibit the widest range of hypnotic phenomena, and who are usually termed "somnambules." (2) Certain therapeutic results which sometimes follow suggestion, but are not associated with the usual phenomena of hypnosis.

Group 1.—Here in a typical case the following phenomena are to be observed. The subject, after undergoing one or other of the methods of hypnotisation, passes into a condition superficially resembling sleep. This state is characterised by "suggestibility," *i.e.* in it various phenomena can be excited by the suggestions of the operator.

Further, as the result of training, the subject can be taught to pass into the so-called hypnotic state in response to a given signal. Henceforth, hypnosis can be evoked immediately, without the subject closing his eyes or showing any symptoms resembling sleep.

Again, this condition, like the former, is characterised by "suggestibility," and in it the phenomena described in the chapter on "Hypnotic Phenomena" can be evoked.

The operator apparently has obtained a power of controlling the subject's organism, to an extent and in a manner which are without parallel in waking life. He can excite by suggestion physiological and psychological phenomena, which the subject had never previously been able to elicit by the action of his own volition.

Further, and the point is an all-important one in reference

T

to hypnotic theory, the subject can, and does, reject all suggestions which would be opposed to the feelings or prejudices of his normal state.

Finally, the subject can be trained to hypnotise himself, and can then evoke phenomena identical with those previously elicited by the operator.   In this condition, it is clearly to be seen that it is the subject himself who has gained this new and far-reaching power over his own organism.   Thus, every theory which fails to explain the phenomena of *self-hypnosis* must be rejected as unsatisfactory.

Group 2.—In typical examples of this group curative results are apparently obtained by suggestion, in cases where all the other characteristic phenomena of hypnosis are absent.   Thus, in the case of *grande hystérie* (No. 1, pp. 178-80), the patient's convulsive movements only ceased during normal sleep.   Here the only method employed was "suggestion"; and, if the patient's recovery resulted from it, the treatment was certainly carried out under conditions the opposite of those usually regarded as hypnotic.

Between the extreme examples of the two groups just referred to, many intermediate conditions are to be observed. Thus, amongst experimental cases, there are many in which the phenomena still demonstrate an increased control of the subject's organism, although not such a far-reaching one as in profound somnambulism.   Again, many patients treated by suggestion pass into a more or less marked lethargic condition, or show other symptoms which may be claimed, with more or less reason, to be hypnotic.

In discussing hypnotic theories in general it is impossible to keep these two groups distinct, as many authorities, notably Bernheim, regard increased suggestibility as the only distinction between the hypnotic and the normal state.   The existence, however, of two widely differing groups of phenomena ought not to be lost sight of, and I propose later to further contrast them; and to discuss the question whether the phenomena of the second group owe their origin to hypnotic influence, or to emotional states similar to those observed in normal life.

In attempting to present a picture of hypnotic theories the first difficulty encountered is due to their number and diversity. Max Dessoir, as we have seen, cited 1182 works by 774 authors in 1888-90; and it would be difficult to find two of them agreeing in every detail as to the theoretical explanation of all hypnotic phenomena.

Apparently, little of value has been discovered which can justly be considered as supplementary to Braid's later work, while much has been lost through ignorance of his researches. In the successful exposure of the errors of the Charcot school by Bernheim and his colleagues is to be found a reproduction of Braid's controversy with the mesmerists; while the Nancy theories themselves are but an imperfect reproduction of Braid's later ones.

THEORIES OF THE LATER MESMERISTS.

In order to understand the evolution of hypnotic theory it is necessary to know something of the views of the mesmerists.

According to Elliotson and Esdaile, the phenomena of mesmerism were entirely physical in origin. They were supposed to be due to the action of a vital curative fluid, or peculiar physical force, which, under certain circumstances, could be transmitted from one human being to another. This was usually termed the "od" or "odylic" force. Various inanimate objects, such as metals, crystals, and magnets, were also supposed to possess it; and to be capable of inducing and terminating the mesmeric state, and of exciting, arresting, and modifying its phenomena. One metal, for example, apparently produced catalepsy, another changed this into paralysis; and even a glass of water seemed to become charged with odylic force when breathed upon by the mesmeriser. Every one was not susceptible to these influences: those who were were termed "sensitives," and apparently developed many strange and new faculties. For instance, if they looked at a magnet in the dark they saw streams of light issuing from its poles, one colour from the negative another from the positive.

Esdaile thus summarised his theory of the therapeutic action of mesmerism :—"There is good reason to believe that the vital fluid of one person can be poured into the system of another. A merciful God has engrafted a communicable, life-giving, curative power in the human body, in order that when two individuals are found together, deprived of the aids of art, the one in health may often be able to relieve his sick companion, by imparting to him a portion of his vitality." The mesmeric influence, he said, was a physical power which one animal exerted over another, under certain circumstances and conditions of their respective systems: irregularity in the distribution of nervous energy being the cause of all mesmeric phenomena. He considered that there was a resemblance between the action of mesmerism and the effects of wine, opium, Indian hemp, etc. In the first stage there was stimulation; in the second, confusion of the mind, with exaltation of some organs and depression of others; while in the third stage, coma, with complete extinction of sensibility, occurred.

Esdaile held that a drug, or method of treatment, in order to be successful, should possess the power of producing such changes in the organism as were opposed to diseased action. In his opinion, no remedy rivalled mesmerism in its influence on the nervous system, and was at the same time equally devoid of danger. By its means, one could abolish pain and produce prolonged sleep, without the bad effects associated with narcotics; and this in itself was sufficient to cure a great variety of diseases.

Esdaile observed that local inflammation and sympathetic fever disappeared during mesmeric trance, and that the pulse and temperature became normal. Later, he successfully treated many different forms of inflammation by "prolonged sleep." His explanation of these results is particularly interesting, as it forestalled Delbœuf's ingenious theory as to the connection between pain and irritation. According to Esdaile, pain and irritation were the causes which maintained inflammation. If these were removed for a length of time the circulation recovered its equilibrium and the inflammation ceased, just as a fire expired for want of fuel.

It did not seem possible to Esdaile that suggestion, expectation, and imagination, alone, could explain what he had seen and done: he insisted that he had often operated on patients who had never heard of mesmerism, and to whom he had given no preliminary explanation. He could not, he said, have taught his patients the different phenomena they exhibited, as he himself was unacquainted with them when he commenced his experiments: he knew nothing of mesmerism, and concluded that the peasants and coolies of Bengal were equally ignorant.

Esdaile believed in clairvoyance, and held that the mesmeric influence could be exercised at a distance and conveyed by means of inanimate objects. He thought that a mesmerised subject acquired the power of understanding and prescribing for his own complaints: this he regarded as an exaltation of the natural medical instincts of animals. It was this secret monitor, he said, that prompted the dog to eat grass when sick, and the chick to peck gravel the moment it broke the shell. The same power enabled animals to choose wholesome plants and to reject poisonous ones. The medical instinct of somnambules was thus only a revival of ancient knowledge.

Esdaile asserted that mesmerism had long been known in India; but believed that its secrets, which had descended from remote antiquity, were confined to certain castes and families. Thus, when Dr. Davidson, late Resident of Jeypore, in Upper India, visited the Mesmeric Hospital in Calcutta, and saw the Native assistants stroking and breathing upon their patients, he said that he now understood what the *Jar-phoonk* of Upper India was: it was nothing but mesmerism. Many of his patients, after he had vainly tried to cure them of different complaints, used to ask leave of absence in order to be treated by the *Jadoowalla*, and to his great surprise, they often returned cured shortly afterwards. In reply to his inquiries, they all said they had gone through a process called *Jar-phoonk*, the meaning of which he could never make out. He now saw it before him in the continuous stroking and breathing of Esdaile's mesmerisers. *Jarna* meant in Hindoostanee to stroke, and *phoonka* to breathe, which very exactly described the mesmeric processes.

Dr. Thorburn wrote to Esdaile from Arracan, to tell him that mesmerism had been used from time immemorial amongst some of the rudest hill tribes in Assam, particularly the Mivis. Amongst the Assamese, the passes received different names, according to the sites over which they were made: thus, those used to relieve headache were called *Matapon*, while the long passes were known by the same name as in Upper India, namely *Jar-phoonk*.

Colonel Bagnold, of the Bombay Army, described the same practices as prevalent in Bombay; and related the case of a woman who was treated by a mendicant devotee, by means of what was evidently mesmerism, mixed up with incantations and religious ceremonies. The operator caused the patient to look at a string of sandal-wood beads, which he held before her eyes; then made passes with it from her head downwards, occasionally

stopping to breathe upon, or lay his hands on, her chest. Under
this treatment she soon became drowsy and went to sleep.

BRAID'S THEORIES.

As already mentioned, Braid first regarded mesmeric phenomena as the outcome of self-deception or trickery; later he
became convinced that a large proportion of them were genuine,
but all wrongly interpreted. Careful examination satisfied him
that such physical phenomena as cataleptic rigidity of the muscles,
and such psychic ones as inhibition of pain during operation,
were genuine. Further, other phenomena, which sceptics generally regarded as affording strong evidence of the falsity of
mesmerism, contained, according to Braid, a certain amount of
truth, although that was lamentably misrepresented. For example,
certain mesmeric subjects saw streams of light issuing from the
poles of magnets, others were supposed to possess the power of
clairvoyance. Braid was able to demonstrate that the first
phenomenon was a visual hallucination created by unconscious
suggestion; while the latter illustrated the hyperæsthesia of the
special senses that occurred during the mesmeric or hypnotic
state; and owing to this, the subjects received hints from the
operator and spectators, which they could not have obtained
in the normal state. These points, to which I will again refer,
are now mentioned to draw attention once more to the fact that
Braid's opposition to mesmerism was mainly from the theoretical
side. The cardinal point—on which all his theories were based
—was his discovery that the phenomena were *subjective* in origin,
and not due to any mysterious "force" or "fluid" possessed by
the operator. Braid's own theories differed widely: his earlier
ones were physical, his later more purely psychical; and I now
propose to give an outline of all of them.

At the *séance* of Lafontaine's, already referred to,[1] Braid had
observed that the mesmeric condition was induced by fixed
staring; and concluded that the inability to open the eyes arose
from paralysis of certain nerve-centres and exhaustion of the
levator muscles. He expressed his conviction that the phenomena
of mesmerism were due to functional changes in the nervous,
circulatory, respiratory, and muscular systems, induced by

[1] See p. 22, and also Appendix.

staring, physical repose, fixed attention, and suppressed respiration. He boldly asserted that all the phenomena depended on these physical and psychical conditions : they were neither due to the volition of the operator, nor to the power of his passes to throw out a magnetic fluid, or to excite the activity of some mystical universal fluid or medium. As we have already seen, he substituted the word "Hypnotism" for that of "Mesmerism," and invented the terminology we now use.

At first, Braid induced hypnosis by making the subject look at a bright object, held in such a position above the forehead as was calculated to produce the greatest possible strain upon the eyes and eyelids ; while at the same time he told him to rivet his mind on the idea of that one object. Braid not only maintained that the condition was a purely subjective one, produced in this mechanical way, but also claimed to have successfully demonstrated that it could be thus induced in persons who had never heard of mesmerism or hypnotism, and who were ignorant of what was expected of them. In illustration of this, he asserted that he had hypnotised one of his servants, who knew nothing of mesmerism, by giving him such directions as impressed him with the idea that his fixed attention was merely required for the purpose of watching a chemical experiment with which he was already familiar.[1]

The following is a summary of Braid's earlier conclusions :—

(1) Continued mental and visual concentration threw the nervous system into a new condition—that of hypnosis. In it phenomena could be excited, which differed from those observed in ordinary sleeping or waking life, and varied according to the methods employed.

(2) At first, during hypnosis, there was excited action of all the organs of special sense, sight excepted, together with a great increase of muscular power. Afterwards the senses became more torpid than during natural sleep.

(3) During hypnosis the operator could control the subject's nervous energy ; and was able to excite or depress it, either locally or generally.

(4) In the same way he could also alter the force and frequency of the subject's pulse, and modify his circulation.

(5) A similar influence could be exerted over the muscular system.

[1] Braid entirely abandoned this view at a later date. See p. 282.

(6) Rapid and important changes could be produced in the capillary circulation, and in all the secretions and excretions of the body.

(7) By means of hypnotism many diseases might be cured, even some that had resisted ordinary treatment.

(8) The same agency could sometimes prevent the pain of surgical operations.

(9) During hypnosis, by manipulating the cranium and face, the operator could excite certain mental and physical phenomena: these varied according to the parts touched.

At first, after inducing hypnosis, Braid resorted to various physical methods in order to produce changes in the muscular and circulatory systems; he believed this excited the different hypnotic phenomena, and played an important part in the cure of disease. He also held that cures could sometimes be effected by similar methods in the waking condition. From the description of his manner of inducing hypnosis it is evident that he employed verbal suggestion; but, at that time, this was certainly done unconsciously, and in ignorance of its value.

Amongst other interesting observations, Braid found that he could terminate the hypnotic condition by means of a current of cold air. He also noticed that he could make a rigid limb flexible by blowing on it; that he could restore the sight to one eye by the same means and leave the other insensible. Further, he could excite one-half of the body to action, while the other remained rigid and torpid; or make the subject pass from a general state of inactivity of the organs of special sense and tonic muscular rigidity, to the opposite condition of extreme mobility and excited sensibility. He acknowledged that he was unable to explain these extraordinary phenomena, but stated that he had no difficulty in reproducing them: that they were independent of any *rapport* between operator and subject; and invariably appeared, no matter whether the current of air came from the lips, the motion of the hand, a pair of bellows, or any other inanimate object.

The subjective explanation of the origin of hypnotic phenomena was not a new one, and had already been given both by the Abbé Faria and Bertrand. Their views, however, if not entirely forgotten, had exercised no practical influence on mesmeric theory; and Braid was evidently unacquainted with them when he commenced his mesmeric researches. Thus, his conclusions were arrived at independently, and successfully substituted for those universally held in his day. At a later date, when his opponents pointed out the similarity between the theories, Braid asserted that this was more apparent than real, as Faria had attributed everything to the effect of the imagination. On this point they certainly differed; although they were alike in asserting that neither contact nor magnetic fluid was necessary.

Braid did not believe that the phenomena of hypnotism were the result of the subject's attention to his own symptoms. Referring to some articles on Animal Magnetism which had appeared in the *Medical Gazette* in 1833, he said that in the writer's opinion the phenomena were the result of attention strongly directed to different parts of the body; whereas, by his method, the attention was riveted to something outside the body.

In opposition to the theory that hypnotism resembled reverie, Braid stated that reverie proceeded from an unusual quiescence of the brain, and the inability of the mind to direct itself strongly to any one point. There was a defect in the attention, which, instead of being fixed on one subject, wandered over a thousand, and was even feebly and ineffectually directed to these. That, he said, was the very reverse of what was induced by his method; because he riveted the attention to one idea and the eyes to one point, as the primary and imperative condition.

At first Braid was inclined to believe in phrenology; and considered it possible that the passions, emotions, and intellectual faculties could be excited during hypnosis, by touching or rubbing certain parts of the head and face. He cited twelve cases in which he thought he had observed these phenomena in subjects who were ignorant of phrenology, uninfluenced by previous training, or by leading questions and suggestions on the part of the operator. He admitted, however, that it was probable that errors might have arisen through the remarkable docility of hypnotic subjects, which made them anxious to comply with every suggestion or indication given by the operator. This, and other reasons, caused him to regard his results with distrust; and he stated that it was his intention to conduct a new series of experiments on fresh subjects, in order to ascertain to what extent it might be practicable, by arbitrary associations, to excite opposite phenomena by touching identical parts of the head. He hoped these would enable him to determine whether there was any necessary connection between the parts touched and the phenomena evoked; or whether they depended entirely upon associations, which had originated from some partial knowledge of phrenology, arbitrary arrangement, or accidental circumstances which had been overlooked or forgotten. In the latter case, the repetition of a definite sensation would be followed by a revival of the feelings with which it had been formerly associated.

Some experiments which Braid made in order to determine whether hypnosis could be induced by methods other than the stereotyped ones, appear to have first suggested alterations in his hypnotic theory, and shaken his faith in the purely physical explanation of hypnotic phenomena. At first, as already stated, he required his patients to look for a considerable time at some inanimate object, until the eyelids closed involuntarily. He frequently found, however, that this was followed by pain and slight conjunctivitis, and, in order to avoid this, he closed the patient's eyes at a much earlier stage. Despite this, he was able to hypnotise as easily as before, and without subsequent unpleasant symptoms. This led to further experiment, when he found he could induce hypnosis as readily in the dark as in the light, if the eyes were kept fixed, and the body and mind at absolute rest. Despite much perseverance, Braid never succeeded in hypnotising idiots: he always failed also with young children, and with persons of weak intellect, or of restless and excitable minds, who were unable to comply with his simple rules. As he succeeded with the blind, Braid concluded that the impression was made through the mind and not through the optic nerves. He observed also that the oftener subjects were hypnotised, the more susceptible they became; and thus, from association of ideas, the condition might ultimately be evoked entirely through the action of the imagination. If a subject believed something was being done which ought to hypnotise him, although he did not see what this was, hypnosis would probably be induced. On the other hand, the most expert operator in the world would exercise his influence in vain, if the patient were ignorant of his efforts.

Hypnotism; A Condition of Mental Concentration or Monoideism.

In opposition to his former physical theory, Braid attempted, in 1847, to explain all hypnotic phenomena by mental concentration or monoideism; whether the phenomena appeared in deep stages resembling sleep, or in "alert" ones, differing only in their suggestibility from the normal state.

After explaining what induced him to adopt the term "hypnotism," he now confessed that grave objections might be urged against it. Thus, under it had been grouped many conditions which varied widely, whereas only those subjects who passed into a state resembling sleep, and followed by amnesia on awaking, could be said to be really "hypnotised." Of those who were relieved or cured by hypnotic treatment not more than one in ten reached this stage. The word hypnotism, therefore, led them to think that they could not be benefited by methods that failed to produce the condition implied by the term. Braid, therefore, proposed that the term "hypnotic" should be restricted to cases of artificial sleep followed by amnesia on awaking, but in which the lost memory could be revived in subsequent hypnoses.

Further, Braid even proposed to abolish his old terminology altogether, and to substitute a fresh one, which he believed to be more in keeping with his advancing knowledge. He had become convinced that all the conditions which he had formerly grouped as hypnotic phenomena were really the result of mental concentration. Fixed gazing, concentration of the attention on a real or imaginary object—the usual hypnotic methods—all tended, he said, to produce monoideism. As the result of impressions received from without, either in the form of verbal suggestions or physical sensations, an individual in the normal state might have his attention fixed on one part or function of his body, and withdrawn from others. Such suggestions acted more powerfully during hypnosis; because, in that condition, the attention was more concentrated and the suggestions were aided by the subject's imagination, faith, and expectation. In this way dominant ideas were created—these reacted on the body and produced their physical equivalent.

To meet the requirements of his new theory, Braid invented the following terminology :—

Mono-ideology: the doctrine of the influence of dominant ideas upon mental and physical states.

Monoideism: the condition resulting from the mind being possessed by dominant ideas.

To *Monoideise*: to practise the method by which monoideism is induced.

Monoideiser: the person who monoideises.

Monoideised: the condition of the person who is in a state of monoideism.

Monoideo-Dynamics: the mental and physical changes which result from monoideism.

Psycho-Physiology: a generic term, comprising the whole of the phenomena which result from the reciprocal actions of mind and matter.

According to Braid, the fascination of birds by serpents, the phenomena of "electro-biology," of table-turning, the divining-rod, the gyrations of the odometer of Dr. Mayo, the movements of the magnetometer of Mr. Rutter, etc., were all examples of unconsciousness or involuntary muscular action resulting from dominant ideas. When the attention was absorbed by an idea associated with movement, a current of nervous force was sent into the muscles and a corresponding motion produced, not only without conscious effort, but even in many instances in opposition to volition. The subject lost the power of neutralising the dominant idea, and was irresistibly drawn or spellbound according to the nature of the impression produced; and might, in this way, be brought under the control of others, by means of audible, visible, and tangible suggestions.

The mental and physical phenomena, no matter what processes were employed to induce hypnosis, resulted entirely from dominant ideas: it mattered little whether these had existed in the subject's mind previously, or were afterwards verbally suggested by the operator. The latter acted like an engineer and called into action the forces in the subject's own organism, controlling and directing them in accordance with the laws which governed the action of the mind upon the body.

Braid thoroughly recognised that all the phenomena most characteristic of hypnosis could be induced without the subject having passed through any condition resembling sleep. He explained this by his "mental-concentration" theory. The condition, he said, was essentially a subjective one, due to the distribution of nervous energy within the subject's own body, which arose from the influence of his own mind upon his physical organism. While all was absolutely independent of the transmission of any occult influence from one person to another, both direct and indirect suggestions played an important part. Their influence depended, however, on the ideas aroused in the mind of the subject, and this involved no loss of "magnetic power" in the operator. If the mesmeric theory were true, a preacher or author would lose "vital fluid" in exact proportion to the numbers influenced by his spoken or printed ideas. This, of course, was absurd—a posthumous work might be quite as telling as one printed during the life of the author: the suggestion of new ideas to the mind of the reader, through the printed symbols of thought, being the only cause of whatever effect the book produced.

In *Neurypnology* Braid stated that he was unable to account for the fact that a current of air aroused hypnotised subjects from their trance; but, later, he thought he had found an explanation for this in monoideism. The particular function called into action, he said, occupied the whole attention of the person hypnotised, while others passed into a state of torpor: thus, only one function was active at any one time, and was hence intensely so. The arousing of any dormant function was equivalent to superseding the one in action. In this way, a state of muscular rigidity ceased when a current of cold air was directed to the skin, because this called the attention to the skin, and withdrew it from the muscular sense.

According to Braid, there was a difference between *spontaneous* and *induced* somnambulism; in the former the subjects were impelled to certain trains of action by internal impulses, while in the latter they tended to remain at absolute rest, and to pass into a state of profound sleep, unless excited by some impression from without.

Natural and artificial sleep were not regarded by Braid as identical: the principal difference between the two was to be found in their respective mental conditions. In passing into ordinary sleep the mind was diffusive and passive—flitting from one idea to another indifferently. Thus, the subject was unable to fix his attention on any regular train of thought, or to perform any act requiring much effort of will. This passiveness was

continued during sleep; and audible suggestions and sensible
impressions, if not intense enough to terminate it, only aroused
dreams, wherein ideas passed through the sleeper's mind without
exciting definite physical acts.   On the other hand, an active and
concentrated state of mind was produced by the methods for
inducing hypnosis.   This condition was favourable to suggestion;
the various impressions conveyed to the subject's mind, either
indirectly or by the verbal suggestions of the operator, were
quickly seized and responded to.   Finally, hypnosis had cured
many diseases, which had resisted natural sleep and every other
known remedial agency for years.   For instance, a few hypnotic
sittings of ten minutes each had cured a patient, who must have
had at least eight years' sleep during his long illness.

Magnets, etc.

In Braid's time the mesmerists held that magnets, certain
metals, crystals, etc., possessed a peculiar power over sensitive
subjects.   In their presence, some experienced an unpleasant
sensation like an aura, others got headache, or attacks of fainting
or catalepsy, with spasms so violent that they apparently
endangered life.   Frequently, there was hyperæsthesia of the
special senses; while many fancied they saw brilliant streams of
light flow from the poles of the magnet.   Braid investigated the
matter with the following results:—The phenomena appeared
either when the subjects knew beforehand what was expected of
them, or received the necessary information from the suggestions
or leading questions of the operator.   Apart from these conditions,
the phenomena never appeared; but imitation magnets produced
them when the subjects believed real ones were being used.

Reichenbach asserted that when a sensitive plate was placed
in a box with a magnet, it received an impression just as if it
had been exposed to the full influence of the light.   Braid
repeated the experiment, and also had similar ones performed for
him by an expert photographer; but, when all sources of fallacy
were eliminated, the results were invariably negative.

Braid constantly insisted that the effects attributed to magnetic or "odylic" force were entirely due to the action of suggested
ideas.   The following experiment, he said, illustrated this, and

also showed how, despite supposed *rapport*, a subject responded to suggestions, even when these were not given by the original operator.

One day Braid called on a London physician who used mesmerism in his practice. The latter told him that he had been obtaining wonderful results from the use of magnets, and offered to demonstrate this on a subject who was at that moment in a state of mesmeric trance. He asserted, for example, that when he touched the subject's limbs with the magnet, this produced catalepsy; and, certainly, what he had predicted happened. Braid, in his turn, stated that he had an instrument in his pocket which was quite as powerful, and offered to prove this by operating on the same subject. He then informed the doctor, in the subject's presence, that when he put the instrument into her hands it would produce catalepsy; and it at once did so, just as in the former instance. Having terminated the catalepsy by means of passes, Braid placed the instrument in another position, and stated that it would now have the very reverse effect—that the subject would not be able to hold it, owing to paralysis of her muscles: this, as well as many other experiments, was successful. Braid then privately explained to the doctor the real nature and powers of his apparently magical instrument. It was nothing more than his portmanteau-key and ring, and its varied powers were merely the result of the predictions which the subject had heard Braid make. The experiments, he said, simply illustrated the power of suggestion during hypnosis: neither magnet nor portmanteau-key played any real part in them.

In 1843, Braid referred to Elliotson's belief in the mesmeric powers of certain metals and to Wakley's test experiments. The latter, operating with a non-mesmerising metal, made the subject believe he was using a mesmerising one, whereupon she fell asleep: from this he concluded that all the subjects were impostors. Braid, on the contrary, asserted that the artificial sleep was genuine, but had been induced solely by suggestion: the metals were neither mesmeric nor non-mesmeric. In the same way, Braid explained the action of the "wooden tractors," which Dr. Haygarth, in 1799, substituted for the "metallic ones" of Mr. Perkins, with equally successful results. The latter consisted of two pieces of metal, one of iron and the other of brass, about

three inches long, blunt at one end and pointed at the other.
They were invented by Dr. Elisha Perkins, of Norwich, Connecti-
cut, who in 1796 took out a patent for them.   They were used
for the relief of headache, and other nervous pains, and were
applied by drawing them lightly over the part affected for about
twenty minutes.   This method of treatment, which was very
fashionable at one time, was termed Perkinism in honour of its
inventor.

According to Braid, it had long been recognised that various
anomalous sensations followed the prolonged direction of the
attention to any part of the body ; but, notwithstanding the fact
that remarkable cures had occasionally been caused by mental
excitement, and severe illness and even death had resulted from
fear, it was usually supposed that these sensations were unaccompanied by physical change.   With the exception of Dr. (afterwards
Sir Henry) Holland, who wrote on the influence of attention on
the bodily organs in his *Medical Notes and Reflections*, Braid said
no one believed that definite physical changes could be excited,
regulated, and controlled by the voluntary mental efforts of a
healthy individual ; or that the same results might be produced
involuntarily, by the direct or indirect suggestions of another
person.

Braid cited the following cases as illustrating the power of
suggestion to cause alterations in bodily functions :—

(1) *Increased secretion of milk* (case reported p. 88).

(2) *Cures of long-standing hysterical paralysis without organic
lesion.*   Here, if confident verbal suggestions were made to the
patient during hypnosis, the results were sometimes instantaneous ;
and the paralysis disappeared as if by the action of a magical
spell.

(3) *Activity of drugs in sealed tubes :* Braid had heard of the
discovery of certain drugs in America which were said to exercise
their influence through glass : *i.e.* if the patient held the bottle containing the medicine in his hand, it produced the same effect as
if he took the medicine by the mouth.   To those who laughed at
the idea Braid retorted that imagination, attention, and expectation
were capable of producing the effects attributed to the drug.   He
was soon able to prove this experimentally.   Having described
to a friend the wonderful properties of this American emetic,
which was capable of acting through glass, he placed a phial

containing coloured water in her hand. She immediately began to be sick, but this ceased when she was given another phial, which she was told was the antidote.

Braid believed that these and similar facts enabled us to understand how hypnotism cured or relieved disease. *Suggestion,* either verbal or indirect, aroused certain ideas in the mind of the patient. According to their nature, these acted as stimulants or sedatives, and either directed attention to, or withdrew it from, particular organs or functions. In ordinary practice, similar results were produced by prescribing medicines which acted as general or local stimulants or sedatives.

If blushing, a phenomenon due to altered capillary circulation, appeared immediately as the result of a mental impression, dominant ideas might equally well produce powerful effects on other parts of the body. According to Braid, homœopathy, as well as hypnotism, illustrated the action of suggestion. Sir J. Y. Simpson had proved that one homœopathic dilution was so weak that a patient would have to take a dose every second of time, night and day, for thirty thousand years, before he consumed one grain of the original drug; while another was so attenuated that it would require a mass of the dilution, equal to sixty-one times the bulk of the earth, to contain a single grain of medicine!

Further, Braid held that the mental element associated with the administration of drugs in general had been far too much ignored. It was worth finding out, he said, how much of the benefit derived from ordinary treatment was due to the effects of medicine, and how much to suggestion. A mental impression was produced whenever a drug was consciously taken; and this might account for the remarkable changes of opinion as to the value of particular medicines. At one time a universal favourite appeared to possess every valuable quality, then was discarded as worthless, while later it regained its former position. All this arose naturally: a sanguine doctor prescribed the remedy with confidence, and his patients caught the inspiration. Every successful result increased the faith of both physician and patient. Thus the medicine acquired curative powers in excess of its physical properties. Later, when the same remedy was prescribed doubtfully by others, the mental influence on the patients was unfavourable; and so the drug was robbed of some of the value that naturally belonged to it.

Braid's views as to clairvoyance, telepathy, etc., have already been referred to, as also his rules for the avoidance of experimental error.

Phrenology.

Braid's increased knowledge of the power of mental influences over hypnotic phenomena soon led him to discard even the slightest belief in phrenology. He complained, however, that the author of an article in the *North British Review*, for November 1854, confounded him with the "Phreno - Mesmerists," and attributed to him the belief that touching particular parts of the head would make a hypnotised subject laugh, pray, sing, steal, fight, etc. In reply, Braid stated that his earlier experiments had neither proved nor disproved the doctrine of phrenology; but left that precisely where they found it. The phenomena might arise in various ways: (1) From a previous knowledge of phrenology. (2) From training during hypnosis, so that when points were touched, with which particular ideas had been associated by verbal suggestion, the phenomena appeared. This arbitrary association, however, could be equally readily established by touching parts of the body other than the head. The touch simply called into action the "muscles of expression," and thus excited in the mind of the subject the ideas with which these were usually associated in the waking condition. This latter method was the natural one, and was simply an inversion of the usual sequence subsisting between mental and muscular excitation. Thus, first, the touch called into play the muscles constituting the "anatomy of expression" of any given passion or emotion; and, secondly, this physical expression suggested to the mind of the subject the corresponding passion or emotion, with which it had been associated in the waking condition. Under ordinary circumstances, the mental impression would have come first and excited its corresponding physical manifestation; but here the physical condition preceded the mental one and acted as its exciting cause.

This theory was published by Braid in 1843; and, in 1844, he practically demonstrated that he could induce all the so-called phrenological phenomena by verbal suggestion, no matter what part of the body was touched.

Suggestion, Passes, etc.

At first Braid employed mechanical methods for the induction of hypnosis and its phenomena. Later, he stated that these acted mainly as indirect suggestions, and that direct verbal suggestion was best for all hypnotic purposes. After hypnotising his subjects, he stated in a confident manner the results he wished to obtain, and often found that these could be varied by simple change of voice. Thus, if he made a subject see an imaginary sheep, and then asked him in a cheerful manner what colour it was, this tone usually elicited the reply "White," or some light colour. If he then asked : " What colour is it *now* ? " giving a sad intonation to the word *now*, the reply would usually be, " Black."

Braid explained the action of passes and other physical methods in the following manner :—Every fresh impression modified existing functions, whether the new impression was a mental or a physical one. The brain received many impressions which subsequently influenced the mind, although they were not all perceived when conveyed to it by the organs of sense ; while others, too slight ever to become conscious, might nevertheless be sufficient to produce a local influence on the nerves and capillaries. Thus, a person might be so absorbed in a book as not to notice he was sitting in a draught, and yet this might cause rheumatism. In like manner, passes, which the subject was hardly conscious of, might produce a physical effect either through pressure, agitation of the air, changes in temperature, or electrical states. They were most powerful, however, when they directly excited mental action, either by fixing the attention on one part or function of the body and withdrawing it from others ; or by arousing ideas previously associated with the physical impression. All these effects, however, could be neutralised by direct suggestion ; and thus by training it was quite possible to make passes produce results opposite to those formerly evoked by them. If, on making the passes, the operator verbally stated what would happen, this did happen instead of the usual result. From that time, "through the double conscious memory,"—to use Braid's own words—a like impression would recall the idea that had been arbitrarily associated with it.

Dangers.

Some of the opponents of hypnotism asserted that it could be used to excite the animal passions : thus, they said, virtuous women might become the victims of unprincipled men, and afterwards retain no consciousness of what had taken place. This charge, Braid stated, was not in keeping with observed facts. In replying to it he cited many reasons for his belief that the practice of hypnotism was devoid of danger, and amongst these the following are the more important :—

(1) He had successfully demonstrated that hypnosis could never be induced without the subject's knowledge and consent.

(2) Perception and judgment were not abolished in hypnosis; this was not only true of the "alert" condition, but extended also to the "deep." Even when the subjects were in the latter state, if anything were done which was opposed to their moral sense, they at once passed into the "alert" stage, and were then as capable of defending themselves as when in the waking condition.

(3) Hypnosis undoubtedly increased the moral sense, and rendered subjects more fastidious as to conduct than when awake.

(4) Even supposing, for the sake of argument, that it were possible for an unprincipled person to commit an immoral act upon a deeply hypnotised subject, the latter's loss of memory on awaking would not protect the criminal. Consciousness was never abolished during hypnosis; and everything which had taken place during it could be recalled by the subject in subsequent hypnoses.

Further, Braid objected that, while hypnotism had been credited with dangers which it did not possess, those who attacked it raised no objections to the use of chloroform or ether. Although in no way an opponent of the latter, he drew attention to the following facts :—

(a) On several occasions he had witnessed the most intense manifestations of erotism arise spontaneously during the earlier stages of etherisation.

(b) Ether, chloroform, and other narcotic drugs had frequently been administered for criminal purposes. Sometimes this had been done without the subject's knowledge, and various crimes had been perpetrated during the unconsciousness of the victim.

Analogous States.

Braid thought that the voluntarily suspended animation of Colonel Townsend, and the prolonged trance of the fakirs, might be explained by hypnotism. Some instances of the latter were remarkably well authenticated by the evidence of English officers of position. On one occasion, a fakir was buried at a depth of four feet; it was arranged that the experiment should last nine days; and an English officer had the grave constantly watched by sentinels. At the end of the third day, the officer, fearing the fakir might be dead, and that this might be the cause of trouble to himself, insisted on the termination of the experiment. When the man was dug up, he was as cold and stiff as a mummy and apparently lifeless; he revived, however, after being manipulated for about a quarter of an hour.

Braid also found a resemblance between the condition produced by hashish and certain hypnotic states; and, in support of this, quoted the experiments made by Dr. O'Shaughnessy at Calcutta, and already cited, p. 45.

In discussing other theories, Braid's will be again referred to; meanwhile I wish to draw attention shortly to the following points. Braid's theories changed as his knowledge increased, and he held in all three distinct and widely differing ones. In the first, he explained hypnosis from an almost purely physical standpoint; in his second, he considered it to be a condition of involuntary monoideism and concentration of the attention. His third theory differed from both of these. In it he recognised that reason and volition were unimpaired, and that the attention could be simultaneously directed to more points than one. The condition, therefore, was not one of involuntary monoideism. Further, he recognised more and more clearly that the state was essentially a conscious one, and that the losses of memory which followed on awaking could always be restored in subsequent hypnoses. Finally, he described as "double consciousness" the condition which he had first termed "hypnotic," then "monoideistic." As already noted, few students of hypnotism are acquainted with any of Braid's theories except the

earliest ; and his third and latest one, which he promised to put
before the public in a more complete form, never saw the light
in the manner he intended.   My account is drawn from little-
known pamphlets, unpublished MS., etc.

The following is a summary of Braid's latest theories :—
(1) Hypnosis could not be induced by physical means alone.
(2) Hypnotic and so-called mesmeric phenomena were subjective
in origin, and both were excited by direct or by indirect suggestion.   (3) Hypnosis was characterised by physical as well as by
psychical changes.   (4) The simultaneous appearance of several
phenomena was recognised, and much importance was attached
to the intelligent action of a secondary consciousness.   (5) Volition was unimpaired, moral sense increased, and suggested crime
impossible.   (6) *Rapport* was a purely artificial condition created
by suggestion.   (7) The importance of direct verbal suggestion
was fully recognised, as also the mental influence of physical
methods.   (8) Suggestion was regarded as the device used for
exciting the phenomena, and not considered as sufficient to
explain them.   (9) Important differences existed between
hypnosis and normal sleep.   (10) Hypnotic phenomena might
be induced without the subject having passed through any condition resembling sleep.   (11) The mentally healthy were the
easiest, the hysterical the most difficult, to influence.

In this country, during Braid's lifetime, his earlier views
were largely adopted by certain well-known men of science,
particularly Professors W. B. Carpenter and J. Hughes Bennett,
but they appear to have known little or nothing of his latest
theories.   Bennett's description of the probable mental and
physical conditions, involved in the state Braid described as
"monoideism," is specially worthy of note.   Not only is it interesting in itself, but it serves also as a standard of comparison
with which to measure the theories of later observers, who have
attempted to explain hypnosis by cerebral inhibition, psychical
automatism, or both these conditions combined.

BENNETT'S THEORIES.

(A) Physiological.

According to Bennett, hypnosis was characterised by alterations in the functional activity of the nerve tubes of the white

matter of the cerebral lobes. He suggested that a certain proportion of these became paralysed through continued monotonous
stimulation; while the action of others was consequently exalted.
As these tubes connected the cerebral ganglion-cells, suspension
of their functions was assumed to bring with it interruption of
the connection between the ganglion-cells.

(B) Psychical

From the psychical side, he explained the phenomena of
hypnosis by the action of predominant and unchecked ideas.
These were able to obtain prominence from the fact that other
ideas, which, under ordinary circumstances, would have controlled
their development, did not arise; because the portion of the brain
with which the latter were associated had its action temporarily
suspended, *i.e.* the connection between the ganglion-cells was
broken, owing to the interrupted connection between the "fibres of
association." Thus, he said, the remembrance of a sensation
could always be called up by the brain; but, under ordinary
circumstances, from the exercise of judgment, comparison, and
other mental faculties, we knew it was only a remembrance.
When these faculties were exhausted, the suggested idea pre-
dominated, and the individual believed in its reality. Thus, he
attributed to the faculties of the mind, as a whole, a certain
power of correcting the fallacies which each one of them was likely
to fall into; just as the illusions of one sense were capable of
being detected by the healthy use of the other senses. There
were illusions mental and sensorial: the former caused by predominant ideas, and corrected by proper reasoning; the latter
caused by perversion of one sense, and corrected by the right
application of the others.

In hypnosis, then, according to this theory, a suggested idea
obtained prominence and caused mental and sensorial illusions,
because the check action — the inhibitory power — of certain
higher centres had been temporarily suspended. These theories
were first published by Professor Bennett in 1851.

Remarks.—In many respects the theories of modern observers
resemble those we have been discussing. The Salpêtrière school
has revived many of the errors of the mesmerists. Heidenhain
reproduced the physical side of Braid's theories as to monoideism,

while Bernheim did the same thing for the psychical side. Other observers, instead of regarding the phenomena of hypnosis entirely from a physical, or entirely from a psychical, point of view, have recognised, like Braid and Bennett, that the mental changes were of necessity associated with physical ones, and *vice versâ*.

In the latest of modern theories is to be found a reproduction and development of Braid's views as to double consciousness. This theory stands apart. In all others, the phenomena of hypnosis are supposed to depend on some inhibitory action, in some limitation or arrest of the functions that subserve normal life. In the "double" or "secondary consciousness" theory, on the other hand, the subject is credited with an augmented power of controlling his own organism; his volition is supposed to be increased, and his consciousness unimpaired.

MODERN HYPNOTIC THEORIES.

CHARCOT'S THEORY, OR THAT OF THE SALPÊTRIÈRE SCHOOL.

The theories of this school are now almost universally discredited by those practically engaged in hypnotic work. Even as far back as the Second International Congress of Psychology (London, 1892) they had almost ceased to attract attention; and it was obvious that the views of the Nancy school had almost entirely supplanted them.

On the other hand, they cannot be passed by without examination, for many in this country, who have not studied hypnotism practically, still regard them as affording a satisfactory explanation of hypnotic phenomena. The following is a summary of the principal points in the theories of this school:—

(1) It was asserted that hypnosis was an artificially induced morbid condition; a neurosis only to be found in the hysterical. Women were more easily influenced than men, children and old people were almost entirely insusceptible.

(2) Hypnosis could be produced by purely physical means; and a person could be hypnotised, as it were, unknown to himself.

(3) Hypnotic phenomena were divided into three stages, lethargy, catalepsy, and somnambulism, which were induced and terminated by definite physical stimuli.

(4) Hypnotism, so far, had not proved of much therapeutic value.

(5) While there did not exist a single case in which a hypnotic somnambule had acted criminally under the influence of suggestion, hypnotism was not without its dangers. Hysteria might be evoked in trying to induce hypnosis.

(6) Certain hypnotic phenomena could be induced, transferred, or terminated, by means of magnets, metals, etc.

(7) There was a difference between suggestion in normal life and in hypnosis. The former was a physiological phenomenon, the latter a pathological one. Suggestibility did not constitute hypnosis, it was only one of its symptoms.

The above theory has been strongly attacked, chiefly by the so-called Nancy school. Before referring in detail to the objections they raised to it, I wish to draw attention to the fact that they pointed out the insufficiency of the data upon which it had been founded, and cited the confession of one of its own supporters that only a dozen cases of true hypnosis had occurred in the Salpêtrière in ten years, and that a very large proportion of the experiments had been made upon one subject, who had long been an inmate of that hospital. On the other hand, the Nancy school called attention to the extended nature of their own observations, and to the fact that their conclusions had been drawn from the study of many thousands of cases.

(1a) Is Hypnosis a Morbid Condition which can only be induced in the Hysterical?

This question must, I think, be answered in the negative. Charcot argued that hypnotism and hysteria were identical, because in both the urine presented similar characteristics. In reply to this, Moll pointed out that all Charcot's subjects suffered from hysteria; and, as the phenomena which characterise waking life are readily induced in hypnosis, Charcot easily created a complete type of hysteria by suggestion.

If the hysterical alone can be hypnotised, we must conclude from the statistics already cited (pp. 57-67) that at least 80 per cent of mankind suffer from hysteria.

Further, the highest percentage of successes was obtained amongst those classes most likely to be free from hysteria. Thus, the majority of the 152 undergraduates hypnotised by Wingfield at Cambridge would be drawn from our public schools; and, if these do not always turn out good scholars, they cannot at all events be accused of producing hysterical invalids. Liébeault found soldiers and sailors particularly easy to influence, while Grossmann, of Berlin, recently asserted that hard-headed North-Germans were very susceptible. Professor Forel, of Zurich, told me that he had hypnotised nearly all his asylum warders; that he selected these himself, and certainly did not choose them from the ranks of the hysterical. Most of Esdaile's patient's were males, and he drew particular attention to the fact that they were free from hysteria.

These and similar facts apparently justify the statements of Forel and Moll, that it is not the healthy, but the hysterical, who are the most difficult to influence. Forel, as we have seen, considers that every mentally healthy man is naturally hypnotisable; while Moll says, if we take a pathological condition of the organism as necessary for hypnosis, we shall be obliged to conclude that nearly everybody is not quite right in the head. The mentally unsound, particularly idiots, are much more difficult to hypnotise than the healthy. Intelligent people and those with strong wills are more easily hypnotisable than the dull, the stupid, or the weak-willed. Forel says that the most difficult to influence are without doubt the insane; while the number of mentally healthy persons hypnotised by Liébeault and Bernheim alone amounts to many thousands. My personal experience accords with these views. I formerly found no difficulty, for example, in hypnotising healthy Yorkshire peasants for operative purposes, and amongst that class obtained 100 per cent of successes. Now, when my patients are usually chronic nervous invalids, I find the difficulty of inducing hypnosis greatly increased. This experience is not alone a personal one; for, on visiting hypnotic cliniques in France, Switzerland, Holland, and Sweden, I invariably found that others encountered similar difficulties.

(1b) Are Women more Susceptible than Men?

All observers, with the exception of the Salpêtrière school, agree in stating that sex has little or no influence upon suscepti-bility. According to Liébeault, the difference between the two sexes is rather less than 1 per cent. All Wingfield's, and the majority of Esdaile's, subjects were men.

(1c) Are Children and Old People Insusceptible?

As we have already seen, Wetterstrand found that children from 3 or 4 to 15 years of age could be influenced without exception. Bérillon, out of 250 cases in children, hypnotised 80 per cent at the first attempt. Liébeault also found children peculiarly susceptible; and one of his statistical tables records 100 per cent of successes up to the age of 14. In adult life age apparently makes little difference. In the same table we find that from the ages of 14 to 21 the failures were about 10 per cent, and from 63 years and upwards about 13 per cent.

(2) Can Hypnosis be induced by Mechanical Means alone?

This question is answered by the Nancy school in the negative, and my own experience agrees with this. I know of no single instance where hypnosis has followed the employment of mechanical means, when mental influences have been carefully excluded, and the subjects have been absolutely ignorant of what was expected of them. No one was ever hypnotised by looking at a lark-mirror, until Luys borrowed that lure from the birdcatchers, and invested it with hypnotic power. On the other hand, any physical method will succeed with a susceptible subject who knows what is expected of him.

(3) Are Hypnotic Phenomena divided into Three Distinct Stages?

The production of the definite stages described by the Salpêtrière school as arising from their respective physical stimuli, has never been noticed by other observers. Amongst the many hundreds of hypnotised subjects I have seen, none have responded to the manipulations which produced such striking phenomena at the Salpêtrière. On the other hand, I and many others have found that we could easily evoke these stages by verbal suggestion, and train the subjects to manifest them at a given signal. The condition, however, was always an artificial one.

Further, the Salpêtrière stages cannot be accepted until it is proved that suggestion was rigorously excluded. Instead of this, we know that in many instances the experiments were discussed before the subjects themselves. It is specially worthy of note that Charcot's stages, as described by his followers, have lost much of their original clearness and precision. Other phenomena, in addition to the characteristic ones, have appeared; and the latter have not been confined to their proper places, *i.e.* the stages have become mixed. Again, the phenomena, instead of only appearing in response to definite physical stimuli, have become more capricious in their origin; and one method, instead of only exciting its appropriate stage, sometimes produces all three. This tends to show that the phenomena really result from varying mental states, the outcome of direct or indirect suggestion, and not from definite and unvarying physical stimuli—a view further strengthened by the fact that it is admitted that the physical stimulus only acts when given by the person who is *en rapport* with the subject.

(4) Is Hypnotism of little Therapeutic Value?

On the one hand, we have the negative evidence of a few cases observed at the Salpêtrière, where experiment, not cure, seemed the main end. On the other, we have the positive evidence drawn from many thousands of cases, where hypnotism has been successfully employed for the cure or relief of disease.

(6)[1] Can various Physical and Mental Phenomena be excited by the Application, or near Presence, of certain Metals, Magnets, and other Inanimate Objects?

Here, in the assertions of the Salpêtrière school, and their refutation by that of Nancy, we have an exact counterpart of the controversy between Braid and the mesmerists. All the old errors, the result of ignoring mental influences, are once more revived. Medicines are again alleged to exercise an influence from within sealed tubes. The physical and mental conditions of one subject are stated to be transferable to another, or even to

---

[1] No. (5) will be discussed later.

an inanimate object. It is useless to enter into any arguments to refute these statements; for this would be needlessly repeating the work of Braid. Indeed, in many instances, their absurdity renders argument unnecessary: for example, when a sealed tube containing laurel-flower water was brought near a Jewish prostitute, she adored the Virgin Mary! From this it might be inferred that different religious beliefs were represented by different nerve centres, and that these could be called into action by appropriate physical stimuli. The chief apostle of these doctrines was Luys; and considerable attention was drawn to them in this country in 1893, by popular articles in the daily papers and elsewhere. Indeed, the editor of a well-known medical journal thought them of sufficient importance to demand his writing a book in order to disprove them. He apparently was ignorant of the fact that M. Dujardin-Beaumetz had, in 1888, reported to the *Académie de Médecine* that Luys' experiments were conducted so carelessly as to rob them of all value, and that among students of hypnotism they were entirely disregarded.

The Salpêtrière theory not only resembles that of the later mesmerists, in attributing to magnets, metals, etc. the power of exciting varied and wonderful phenomena, but also differs little, if at all, from it in other respects. Thus, the mesmerists stated that all were not susceptible to the influences just referred to, and called those who were "sensitives." The Salpêtrière school say the same thing, but call their sensitives "hysterical." Again both schools regarded the influence as a purely physical one, which could be exerted without the knowledge and against the will of the subject. There was one important difference, however, between the later mesmerists and the Charcot school. When Elliotson commenced to investigate the subject, nothing was known about its mental side or about the influence of suggestion. Thus, his errors were excusable, and almost unavoidable. When Charcot started his researches, not only had Braid already demonstrated as fallacious all the errors Charcot and his followers adopted later, but Liébeault also had pointed out the influence of suggestion, and how, through ignorance of its powers, false conclusions were sure to be drawn. Despite all this, Elliotson's pioneer work brought upon him bitter attacks and threatened ruin, while Charcot's fallacies did not injure the reputation he had established in other departments of science.

The remaining points (Nos. 5 and 7), namely, the alleged
dangers of hypnotism and the nature of suggestion, will be
referred to in discussing the theories of the Nancy school, and in
the chapter on the " So-called Dangers of Hypnotism."

HEIDENHAIN'S THEORY.

The Salpêtrière theory, which assumed that hypnosis could
only be induced in the hysterical, gave us an explanation of
hypnotic phenomena, which was at the same time both entirely
physical and pathological. Heidenhain's theory, on the other
hand, may be taken as a type of the purely physiological one.
According to him, the phenomena of hypnotism owed their origin
to arrested activity of the ganglion-cells of the cerebral cortex.
He held that these higher centres were inhibited by the monotonous stimulation of other nerves, *i.e.* by fixed gazing, passes,
etc., and that sensory impressions, which usually produced movements after passing to the higher centres and evoking consciousness, now did so by passing directly to the motor centres.   This
was essentially a " short-circuiting of nervous currents" theory.
Heidenhain regarded the hypnotised subject as a pure automaton,
who imitated movements made before him, but who was entirely
unconscious of what he did.   To have caused him to move his arm,
he said, the image of a moving arm must have passed before his
retina, or an unconscious sensation of motion must have been
induced through passive movement of his arm.   The subject had
no idea corresponding to the movements he made : the sensory
impression led to no conscious perception and to no voluntary movement, but sufficed to set up unconscious imitation.   In reference
to the playing of different parts by hypnotised subjects, Heidenhain
said that it was a mistake to suppose that the subjects realised
what they did : this was quite out of the question ; the hypnotised
individual neither thought nor knew anything about himself.
Heidenhain held that the fact of the subject's forgetfulness of the
sensations he had experienced during hypnosis afforded satisfactory
evidence that these sensations had been unconscious ones.   This
theory was first published in 1880, and attracted considerable
attention.   It was accepted, for example, by Professor M°Kendrick,
of Glasgow, and restated by him in the ninth edition of the

Encyclopædia Britannica, as giving a true and scientific explanation of the phenomena of so-called animal magnetism.

To this explanation many objections may be urged, thus :—

(1) It is a mistake to call the hypnotic action on the cortical functions *inhibition*, without stating explicitly that the normal action of these functions in respect to motion is always to a large extent inhibitory; and that the complete description of the method by which the so-called automatic reflex responses are brought about is thus " inhibition of the inhibitory functions."

(2) While giving an elaborate exposition of the theory of cerebral *inhibition* produced by peripheral stimulation, Heidenhain omitted to take into consideration the result of central *stimulation* by means of an idea or emotion. As hypnosis can be equally well induced in that way, Heidenhain's theory cannot be accepted, as he wished it should, in substitution for that of " dominant ideas." It cannot justly be considered as an alternative to it, as it is simply the physiological statement of psychical facts.

(3) The theory itself is not a new one; with the exception of a few details, it is essentially an imperfect reproduction of that of the late Professor John Hughes Bennett, of Edinburgh, published in 1851. But Bennett, as we have seen, possessed a clearer view of the whole problem, and did not fall into the mistake of attempting to substitute the physiological statement of psychical facts for the facts themselves.

(4) Hypnosis can be induced, not only in the absence of *monotonous* peripheral stimulation, but even without any peripheral stimulation at all. At the present day, it is usually evoked by central stimulation, which, in those who have been previously hypnotised, need not be persistently monotonous; the single word " Sleep " being then sufficient to excite the condition. In such cases, the factor which Heidenhain regarded as essential to the production of hypnotic phenomena, *i.e.* monotonous peripheral stimulation, is absent.

(5) Instead of a hypnotised subject imitating a movement which he sees, and failing to perform one which is verbally suggested to him, the reverse is actually the case. As a rule the slightest verbal suggestion is sufficient to induce the movements described by Heidenhain; on the other hand, hypnotised subjects never copy movements made before them unless they have been trained to do so. The imitative movements only take place,

according to Moll, when the hypnotic subject is conscious of them, and knows that he is intended to make them. If they were unconscious reflexes, the subjects would imitate any person's movements; but they only imitate the one person who exists for them, *i.e.* the operator, and him only when they know he wishes them to do so. When such experiments are often repeated the imitation may become automatic in later hypnoses, as is the case in waking life. At first, however, a clear idea of the movements to be made is necessary; and since we regard the cerebral cortex as the seat of ideas, and as there is no reason for shifting them to another part of the brain in hypnosis, there can be no doubt of the activity of the cortex.

(6) Heidenhain's only argument is based upon the subject's subsequent defect of memory; he thus assumes, as his sole test for present consciousness, the subsequent remembrance of its content. Yet, if the reality of that test be granted, the question whether a man was conscious when he read an article in the *Times*, may depend on whether or not he received a blow on the head when he had finished it. Further, there is a more radical objection to all these arguments founded on subsequent loss of memory, the very fact, indeed, that memory is frequently present. Braid, for example, found that only some 10 per cent of his subjects were unable to recall the events of hypnosis, while Schrenck-Notzing's International Statistics give 15 per cent. Again, if on awaking the act performed during hypnosis is forgotten, the lost memory can be revived in subsequent hypnoses; and, finally, the amnesia which would otherwise follow deep hypnosis can be entirely prevented by suggestion.

THEORIES OF VINCENT AND SIDIS.

Various other modern theories are based more or less entirely on a supposed cerebral inhibition. Thus, Bennett's theory crops up again in Vincent's *Hypnotism*. Thirty-two pages are devoted to "neurons" and "dendrons," "inaptic" and "aptic" acts, and reasons for rejecting the term "reflex." Finally, we arrive at Vincent's hypnotic theory, which is founded simply on an inhibition of one set of functions—with an increased capacity of action in the others—the inhibition and dynamogenia of

Brown-Séquard. "The stimulus," Vincent says, "instead of being dissipated amongst an indefinite number of neuronic groups, is confined to those whose function is the pure appreciation of the stimulus; the other groups, whose function is the consideration of the reasonableness of the suggestion and the development of the stimulus in other conscious directions, are inhibited."

Sidis, in the *Psychology of Suggestion*, explains the phenomena of hypnosis in exactly the same way. "There is," he says, "a functional dissociation between the nerve-cells. The association-fibres, that connect groups into systems, communitiés, clusters, and constellations, contract. The fine processes of the nerve-cells, the dendrons, or the terminal arborisation, or the collaterals that touch these dendrons, thus forming the elementary group, retract and cease to come into contact." He further discusses which association-fibres give way first, and whether the neuraxon is contracted as a whole, or whether the fibrillæ alone contract, and so withdraw the terminal arborisations for minute distances. All this might be of interest if it were related in any way to the subject in dispute. The phenomena to be explained, however—increased volition, memory, intelligence, etc.—are just the exact opposite of those which have been assumed; and theories, no matter how elaborate, nor how learned in terminology, are valueless when founded upon imaginary mental states, the existence of which is simply assumed by the operator. What does it matter whether lack of consciousness or loss of memory be produced by interruption of association-fibres, arrested action of ganglionic cells of the cerebral cortex, retracted dendrons or disconnected neurons, or even by *an inhibition of the amœboid movements in the pseudopodic, protoplasmic prolongations of the neurospongium*,[1] if the problems we are dealing with actually involve an increase of intelligence, consciousness, volition, and memory?

MR. ERNEST HART'S THEORY.

Another physical theory was published by the late Mr. Ernest Hart ("Hypnotism and Humbug," *Nineteenth Century*, January 1902) in the following complicated and somewhat

---

[1] Rückardt's theory, afterwards elaborated by Lépine, Golgi, Ramon y Cajal, Duval, and Lugaro.

obscure sentence :—" Ideas arising in the mind of the *subject* [1]
are sufficient to influence the circulation in the brain of the
person operated on, and in such variations are adequate to produce
sleep in the natural state, or artificially by total deprivation, or
by excessive increase, or local aberration in the quantity or
quality of the blood to produce coma and prolonged insensibility
by pressure of the thumbs upon the carotid ; or hallucinations,
dreams, and visions by drugs, or by external stimulation of the
nerves, or to leave the consciousness partially affected, and the
person in whom sleep, coma, or hallucinations is produced,
subject to the will of others and incapable of exercising his
own."

The existence, however, of cerebral anæmia in hypnosis is by
no means established.   The belief in its existence is an old one,
which recent investigations have done much to discredit.   Many
years ago Carpenter suggested it as a possible explanation of at
least some hypnotic phenomena, and Hack Tuke also considered
there was a partial spasm of the cerebral blood-vessels in
hypnosis.   Heidenhain, too, at first supposed that anæmia of the
brain was the cause of hypnosis.   He soon gave up this opinion
for several reasons.   (*a*) He saw hypnosis appear in spite of the
inhalation of nitrite of amyl, which causes hyperæmia of the
brain.   (*b*) The investigations of Förster discovered no change
in the vessels at the back of the eye during hypnosis.   (*c*)
Salvioli and Bouchut stated that they found cerebral hyperæmia
during hypnosis.

Mental activity varies in hypnosis just as it does in normal
life, and in both is doubtless associated with changes in the
blood supply; but, even granting that cerebral anæmia exists
in hypnosis, to assume that it explains its phenomena is un-
scientific.   For, as Professor William James points out, the
change in the circulation is the result, not the cause, of the
altered activity of the nervous matter.   Many popular writers,
he says, talk as if it were the other way about, and as if mental
activity were due to the afflux of blood : this belief has no
physiological foundation whatever ; it is even directly opposed
to all that we know of cell life.   The stomach does not digest

---

[1] Here "subject" is an obvious misprint for "operator" ; while the description
of the wonderful feats performed by "ideas" might lead one to suppose that the
writer believed in spiritualistic materialisations and the like.

because more blood flows into it, nor do the muscles of the arm contract for a similar reason: on the contrary, their increased blood supply follows their increased functional activity. If one desired to be hypercritical, one might still further object that when a correlation had been established between a physical condition and a psychical state, the one did not in any true sense explain the other. As Tyndall said: "There is no fusion possible between the two classes of facts. The passage from the physics of the brain to the corresponding facts of consciousness is unthinkable."

THE THEORIES OF THE NANCY SCHOOL.

It is difficult to condense the views of the so-called Nancy school, for not only do marked differences of opinion exist between its various members, but the views held by some of the more prominent among them have changed greatly of late years. It must be noted too, in justice to them, that Liébeault and his followers do not claim to have founded a school. As Professor Beaunis said: "We hear frequently nowadays of the school of Nancy, but there is something in this term which has been applied to us which does not correspond with the reality. The term 'school' implies a community of which all the members hold the same ideas. This we are not; but the public quickly accept ready-made labels without troubling themselves much about the ideas underneath them. In our researches, undertaken with mistrust and doubt, we have arrived at similar results upon a certain number of points. Each observer, however, retains his own ideas and individuality, and it is easy to note the profound and even radical differences that separate us. These diversities of opinion are easily explained, and their non-existence would be impossible in a science still in its infancy. What is common to all of us is the conviction of the importance of these questions, 'and the belief in their future—the profound conviction that this method so ridiculed constitutes one of the greatest advances of the human mind, and one of its most precious possessions."

Taking Bernheim as the leading representative of the so-called Nancy school, we find the essential part of his theory to be a reproduction of the psychical half of Bennett's. In hypnosis Bernheim recognises certain mental changes, not of a pathological character; but to these he denies any physical equivalent. Thus, if we join Heidenhain's purely physiological theory and Bernheim's purely psychical one, we obtain an accurate reproduction of Bennett's two theories.

BERNHEIM'S THEORIES.

In hypnosis, according to Bernheim, the whole nervous force of the subject is concentrated upon a single idea. This nervous concentration may be changed from one point to another in response to the suggestions of the operator; but, though the focus shifts its place, the same concentration continues to exist.

In the normal state, he says, we are subject to errors illusions, and hallucinations. Sometimes these are spontaneous, or follow imperfect sensorial impressions; sometimes they are suggested to us, and accepted without being challenged. In the normal state there is a tendency to accept ideas suggested by others, and to act upon them; but every formulated idea is questioned, and, as the result of this, either accepted or rejected. In the hypnotised subject, on the other hand, there exists a peculiar aptitude for transforming the suggested idea into an act. This is so quickly accomplished that the intellectual inhibition has not time to prevent it; and, when it comes into play, it does so too late, as the idea has been translated into its physical equivalent. If consciousness follows the suggested act, it at all events follows it too late to interfere with its fulfilment.

Bennett, as we have seen, regarded the phenomena of hypnosis as the result of a definite physical change in the subject; Bernheim, on the other hand, attempts to explain them (a) by finding an analogy between them and the phenomena of the normal state, and (b) by means of suggestion.

According to Bernheim, hypnotic phenomena are analogous to many normal acts of an automatic, involuntary, and unconscious nature; and nothing, absolutely nothing, differentiates natural and artificial sleep. If any distinction at all exists between the normal and the hypnotic state, this can be explained by means of suggestion. Both the normal and the hypnotised subject can be influenced by it; but, as it has been suggested to the latter that he should become more responsive, a peculiar aptitude for transforming the idea into an act has in this way been artificially developed. *In other words, every one is suggestible, and if you take some one and suggest to him to become more suggestible, that is hypnotism!* Thus, suggestion not only excites the phenomena of hypnosis, but also explains them. Suggestion, *i.e.* the mental impression, including the preliminary suggestion to become more suggestible, conveyed from the operator to the subject, is the only essential factor in the equation; all else is practically unimportant.

This theory contains five distinct propositions, none of which can be accepted without discussion :—

(1) Nothing differentiates natural and artificial sleep.

(2) Hypnotic phenomena are analogous to many normal acts of an automatic, involuntary, and unconscious nature.

(3) An idea has a tendency to generate its actuality.

(4) In hypnosis the tendency to accept suggestions is somewhat increased by the action of suggestion itself. Such increased suggestibility, one of degree, not of kind, alone marks any difference between the hypnotic and the normal state.

(5) The result of suggestion in hypnosis is analogous to the result of suggestion in the normal state.

It is also asserted that in the five preceding propositions is to be found a complete explanation of hypnosis and its phenomena.

(1 and 2) Explanation of Hypnosis by Means of a Supposed General Analogy between it and the Normal Sleeping and Waking States.

My chief objections to this are :—

(1st) That an analogy, no matter how successfully established between two sets of phenomena, by no means explains either of them.

(2ndly) That many important points of difference exist between hypnosis and ordinary sleep.

(3rdly) That the automatic, involuntary, and unconscious acts, in which Bernheim seeks to find his analogy, rarely, if ever, occur in hypnosis, and are certainly by no means characteristic of it.

(1) The Supposed Identity of Hypnosis and Ordinary Sleep.

Braid considered that marked differences existed between hypnosis on the one hand, and natural somnambulism and the normal sleeping state on the other. These, he thought, consisted mainly in the increased mental and physical powers of the hypnotised subject. Many other authorities agree with Braid. Thus, Moll says, the memory is not at all affected in slight hypnosis; we always presuppose, however, a great decrease of self-consciousness in sleep, and it is just this self-consciousness which remains intact in slight hypnosis.

According to Max Hirsch and Spitta—whose views are shared by Lehmann, the distinguished Danish psychologist— hypnosis and sleep are far from being identical. In reply to Liébeault's assertion that the latter condition results from the concentration of the subject's attention upon the idea of sleep, Hirsch points out that little children fall asleep easily, simply because they do not concentrate their attention; and they, at the same time, are quite unacquainted with the idea of sleep.

Sully finds the following differences between sleep and hypnosis: (a) The greater part of our dream material in nightly sleep comes from within the organism, and not from without, as in hypnosis. (b) The natural dream is more complex and varied than the hypnotic. (c) The hypnotised subject tries to translate his hallucinations into actions in a manner that finds no parallel in ordinary sleep.

Delbœuf said: " I put the subjects to sleep; or more correctly speaking, they believe that they have been asleep." This conception of the condition is, I think, the true one. In deep hypnosis the subjects believe that they have been asleep, because on awaking they are unable to recall what has happened. The condition, however, may have been characterised by great mental and physical activity, presenting in subsequent amnesia its solitary point of resemblance to normal sleep. Finally, this amnesia itself is not a necessary concomitant of the state, and can be easily prevented by suggestion.

(2) The supposed Analogy between Hypnotic Phenomena, and the Automatic, Involuntary, and Unconscious Acts of Normal Life.

According to Braid's conception of hypnosis, the state was characterised by mental and physical phenomena, which were not to be found in other conditions. The hypnotised subject had acquired new and varied powers, but had not at the same time lost his volition or moral sense. He asserted that he had proved that no one could be affected by hypnotism at any stage of the process, unless by voluntary compliance. The subjects were docile and obliging; but, despite this, they refused all criminal suggestions, and even developed a higher sense of propriety than characterised their normal condition.

Totally different views were formerly held by Bernheim and certain other members of the Nancy school. They believed that the subject's volition was weakened or destroyed, and considered this condition to be one of automatism. To both these points I wish to draw attention.

The hypnotic state was described as one of cerebral automatism; and, according to Bernheim, its phenomena found their analogy in various automatic movements of normal life, such as walking. Suggested crimes, which would really seem to differ essentially from acts like these, were, however, described as illustrating "automatism" in its highest form. It is with this illustration that I desire to deal at present. Let us take a typical case. It is suggested to a high-principled girl in the somnambulistic state that she shall take a piece of sugar from the basin and put it into her mother's tea-cup, after having been informed that this is really a lump of arsenic, certain to cause death. Let us now attempt to understand the supposed mental condition with regard to consciousness and volition, and then compare it with the usual scientific conception of automatism. It is, I think, generally conceded by the Nancy school that hypnotic acts are conscious ones; and that, if amnesia follows on awaking, the lost memory can be restored in subsequent hypnoses. Indeed, Professor Bernheim, when discussing the Salpêtrière experiments, insists upon the fact that the hypnotised subject is conscious in all stages. Therefore, the alleged criminal act was a conscious act.

Again, we are told that somnambules, before accepting criminal
suggestions, frequently struggle against them. This would
indicate that, in some instances at all events, they are carried
out in opposition to volition as it exists in hypnosis. Further, it
must be conceded that a criminal act would not be performed
voluntarily by a virtuous person in the normal state. The suggested act, then, is one which would have been opposed by volition
in the waking state.

Now let us turn to "automatism," as defined by Professor
Waller, the well-known physiologist. "The word," he says, "has
received two diametrically opposed meanings, viz. (1) self-
moving, self-rising, spontaneous; (2) automaton-like, that is to
say, like a mechanism, that appears to be self-moving, but that
we know to be moved by secret springs and hidden keys." The
second sense is the one in which he employs it, and is also, I
think, the one now generally adopted by science. As the supposed
essential characteristic of the suggested crime is the fact that it
arose not spontaneously, but in response to the desires of the
operator, it is obvious that if it is automatic at all, it must accord
with the second conception of automatism. Now let us follow
Dr. Waller in his further definition of the second condition, and
then see how this agrees with the so-called "hypnotic automatism."
According to him, the automatic action is essentially a reflex
action, and differs from it only in that it is, as a rule, the habitual
or serial effect of habitual or serial stimuli. An automatic act is
the repeated or rhythmic motor response to a repeated or continuous excitation. Usually it is carried on unconsciously.
Automatic actions may be divided into two sub-groups : (1)
primary or inherited, of which the act of sucking is an example;
(2) secondary or acquired, as, for example, walking. In this
discussion I think we may disregard primary or inherited automatic
acts. Obviously, to kill one's mother cannot be regarded as an
inherited automatism; and if such a crime be automatic at all,
it must fall under the group of secondary ones. Of this form of
automatic act the winding of one's watch may be taken as a
typical example. This is first performed consciously and voluntarily. After a time consciousness sometimes ceases to participate
in the action. On attempting to wind our watch many of us
must have occasionally found that we had already done so,
although quite incapable of recalling the fact. Now, this

automatic act is simply a voluntary one, performed inattentively or unconsciously—one that has previously been frequently performed, and follows well-worn nerve-channels. It has commenced as a conscious, voluntary act. It has become unconscious by repetition, but still remains voluntary, in the sense that it is an act which the consciousness would generally approve of, did it happen to participate in it.

Let us consider the so-called automatic crime of the hypnotised subject, and see how it agrees with this conception of automatism. (*a*) The crime has not been a habitual one. In the present instance the very nature of the act renders this impossible. Obviously, the subject could not have habitually killed her mother. The alleged automatic act must, then, in this instance, have been performed for the first time. Now the essential character of the secondary or acquired automatic act is that it has been frequently, consciously, and voluntarily performed previously to becoming automatic, and follows in consequence well-worn nerve tracts which offer no obstacle to its fulfilment. (*b*) The hypnotic act, on the contrary, is performed consciously; and the attention, instead of being directed in other channels, as in genuine automatism, is supposed to be intensely concentrated on the operator, or on the signal given by him—a signal sometimes so faint that the subject is only enabled to recognise it by means of the hyperæsthesia of his special senses. (*c*) The hypnotic crime is sometimes supposed to be performed in opposition to volition as it exists in hypnosis, and is always supposed to be in opposition to the normal volition. The genuine automatic act, on the other hand, has only been enabled to become automatic owing to the fact that it has previously been frequently performed as a voluntary one; and now, when performed unconsciously, it still remains such an act as the volition, as a general rule, would approve of. The so-called " automatic crime " of the hypnotised subject not only *differs*, then, from the general scientific conception of automatism, but is its exact *opposite* in every detail.

While holding, and holding strongly, that the hypnotic crimes we are discussing cannot in any sense be termed automatic, I do not deny that the hypnotic subject can be trained to perform automatic acts. If I suggest some simple movement to a subject, which his volition does not disapprove of, doubtless after a time it may be performed automatically, *i.e.* after having been fre-

quently, voluntarily, and consciously performed, it may at length
be executed unconsciously as a genuine automatic act, in response
to the habitual stimulus which has excited it.

Putting aside the question whether the so-called hypnotic
crimes are executed automatically, there remains another and
very important one, whether hypnotic subjects are more or less
under the control of the operator, and thus can be compelled to
perform criminal or other acts, which would be opposed by their
normal volition.   Formerly the writings of the Nancy school
indicated a belief that the hypnotic state was essentially characterised by the obedience of the subject to the operator.   Some
years ago most stress was laid upon complete obedience, and
Liébeault said : " We may postulate, as a first principle, that a
subject, during the state of hypnotic sleep, is at the mercy of the
operator, and carries out suggestions with the fatality of a falling
stone."   Bernheim says : " In profound somnambulism, or the
sixth degree, the subject remains asleep, becoming a perfect
automaton, obeying all the commands of the operator " (*Suggestive
Therapeutics*, p. 8). . . . Again, " the subjects more deeply
influenced by hypnotism pass into a condition known as
somnambulism.   Then new phenomena appear.   The automatism
is complete.   The human organism has become almost a machine,
obedient to the operator's will " (p. 29). . . . " The most striking
feature in a hypnotised subject is his automatism " (p. 125). Now,
possibly as the result of the influence of the late Professor Delbœuf,
a greater power of resistance is conceded.   In a more recent
article Liébeault admits that he has only encountered 4 to 5
per cent of hypnotised subjects to whom one could with absolute
certainty successfully suggest crime.   This admission is an
important one ; but despite it, the so-called automatism is still
regarded as the essential characteristic of the hypnotic state.   At
the Moscow Congress in 1897, Bernheim veered round from his
previous automatic theory, and admitted that many subjects
resisted suggestions.   They also retained, he said, sufficient
volition for some things, and only carried out suggestions which
were agreeable or indifferent to them.   Certain subjects also
realised the experimental nature of the crimes it was suggested
they should commit.   He still believed, however, that a certain
small proportion could be induced to commit real crimes.

If only four or five out of a hundred subjects evince the so-called automatism, surely one is not justified in describing this phenomenon as the essential characteristic of the whole group. If five out of a hundred unhypnotised individuals presented certain phenomena which were absent in the remainder, one would surely not choose these rarely occurring phenomena as the descriptive characteristics of the class, and those upon which the belief in other, and more frequently observed phenomena, should depend. Yet, strange as it may seem, this was the position assumed by Durand de Gros, who assured Delbœuf that if he succeeded in proving that the suggested crimes of the Nancy school were recognised by the subject as experimental ones, he would destroy hypnotism entirely. The existence, then, of many undisputed phenomena, which are common to all hypnotic subjects, is to depend upon the acceptance of others, which it is alleged occur in 4 or 5 per cent alone out of the same number.

Putting aside the question of the average number of subjects in whom it is alleged crime can be successfully suggested, I desire first to refer to some of my own observations, and afterwards to consider them in conjunction with the so-called suggested crimes of Bernheim and others, in order to gain, or at all events to strive after, a clearer conception of the mental states involved.

When I commenced hypnotic work some twelve years ago, I, as Delbœuf at first did, believed that the hypnotic subject was entirely at the mercy of the operator. I was soon awakened from this dream, however, not by the result of experiments made to test the condition, but from constantly recurring facts which spontaneously arose in opposition to my preconceived theories. Of these facts the following cases are illustrations :—

Miss C., aged 19, an uneducated girl, had been frequently hypnotised, and was a good somnambule. She had had sixteen teeth extracted at Leeds during hypnotic anæsthesia (p. 165). At a later date, having examined her mouth and found that a fragment of one of the stumps remained, I asked her to come to my house to have it removed. She mentioned this to one of her neighbours, an old woman, who advised her to have no more teeth extracted, as this would cause her mouth to fall in. The following day she presented herself, and was at once hypnotised ; but refused to open her mouth, or to permit me to extract the tooth. Emphatic suggestion continued for half an hour produced no result. This was the first occasion on which she had rejected a suggestion. I then awoke her, and asked why she refused to have the tooth extracted. She told me what her neighbour had said, and expressed her determination to have nothing more done. I explained the absurdity of this, and pointed out that, as she had only the fragment of one tooth remaining, its removal could not affect the appearance of her face. As she was still obstinate I said: "Unless this fragment is removed you cannot have your artificial teeth fitted." This argument was sufficient. She gave her consent in the waking state, was at once hypnotised, and operated on without pain.

Sarah L., aged 20, was a good somnambule, who had been the subject of two painless operations (Case No. 6, pp. 161-2). At a later date I wished to satisfy myself of the depth of the hypnotic anæsthesia, as another and more serious operation was contemplated. Having obtained her consent to test the condition, I hypnotised her and pricked the pulp of her thumb deeply with a needle, and also pinched her arm severely. She showed no sign of pain, and afterwards remembered nothing of what had occurred. A few days later, I wished to repeat the process. She again permitted me to prick her thumb, but when I attempted to pinch her arm she drew it away, and refused to let me touch it. Her mother, who was present, gave the following explanation. After the first experiment, her daughter noticed that her arm was blackened in several places, and asked the cause. When told what I had done, the girl said: "I don't object to being pricked with a needle; but I won't allow Dr. Bramwell to pinch my arm again, because the neighbours might notice the marks." On both occasions her arm was covered, and I did not know it had been marked. I awoke the patient. She had no recollection of what she had said or done. I told her she had refused to let me pinch her arm, and asked the reason. She laughed, and gave the same explanation as her mother. One day, when I had hypnotised the patient, her mother said to me: "Ask her what she did on a certain occasion." I questioned her, but could obtain no response. I afterwards learnt what she had done. It was something which her mother regarded as a joke, but which was slightly indelicate. Many persons, even fairly refined ones, would have told this without blushing; and I have little doubt the patient would have done so when awake.

Miss P. had been frequently hypnotised and was a good

somnambule, in whom anæsthesia could be easily induced. She was maid to one of my patients, a chronic invalid, whose house was managed by a sister of uncertain temper. On one occasion, when I had hypnotised P., her mistress requested that I would ask her what had been said to her by this sister. A quarrel had taken place, of a somewhat amusing nature, and her mistress wished to hear P.'s account of it in hypnosis; but, despite energetic suggestion, she absolutely refused to say a word on the subject.

Miss S., aged 19, in good health, intelligent and well-educated. This subject was a good somnambule, in whom anæsthesia and other phenomena of deepest hypnosis could be easily induced. She had a bad memory for words, and was extremely shy in reading, singing, or playing before others. I suggested to her that she should, on awaking, recite some verses with which she was previously unacquainted, and which I had read twice to her when asleep. Shortly after awaking, she repeated them with very few mistakes, and without apparent embarrassment. Her mother assured me that, under ordinary circumstances, this feat of memory would have been entirely beyond her power, and that nothing would have induced her to read or recite before me. On another occasion, her mother asked me to suggest during hypnosis, that on awaking, she should go to the sideboard in my room, pour out a glass of water, and drink it. This suggestion was not carried out, and was the first which had not been fulfilled. In a later hypnosis she explained the reason for her refusal—she did not know me well enough to help herself to a glass of water in my house without being asked.

Mr. E., aged 25, a shopkeeper, had been frequently hypnotised for medical and surgical purposes, and was a good somnambule On one occasion I showed him at the York Medical Society. At the close of my lecture I was requested to give an example of changed personality, by making this subject believe he was a dissenting minister preaching a sermon. He refused to do this, and I was then asked to make him believe he was a hawker selling fish. This was also rejected; but he accepted the suggestion that he was Barnum, and that the medical men were wild beasts, and proceeded to describe them in a highly amusing manner. I afterwards tried to make him accept the first two

suggestions, but invariably failed.   On one occasion, however, he
accepted the suggestion that he should poison a personal friend.
The subject, at that time, was in the "alert" stage of hypnosis,
with his eyes open.   I took a lump of sugar from the basin, and
assured him that it was a piece of arsenic sufficient to kill a
dozen persons.   I then put it in a cup of tea, and told him to
give it to his friend to drink.   He did so at once.   I asked him
why he had poisoned his friend, and he replied laughingly, but
in an unnaturally gruff voice, "Oh, he has lived long enough."
Another young man who was present, also a good somnambule,
would carry out suggestions like those rejected by E., but refused
to execute the fictitious murder.

The last two subjects, S. and E., accepted suggestions which
were apparently in opposition to their normal character.   I made
no attempt to ascertain E.'s mental condition in reference to the
supposed crime, but I think one can without much difficulty
imagine it.   E. was a respectable tradesman, and a somewhat
devout Dissenter ; and it was not unnatural to suppose that he
refused the part of fish-hawker as this was not in keeping with
his social position, and that of minister as it offended his religious
susceptibilities, but accepted that of showman because it contained nothing objectionable to him.   Would it be reasonable to
suppose that he should at the same time be capable of weighing
fine distinctions between suggested alterations in personality,
and be unable to understand the experimental nature of the
crime ?   He, by the way, affords the only instance in which an
imaginary crime has been carried out by one of my own
subjects.   All others, without exception, have absolutely refused
such suggestions.

Why should S. have recited the poem and refused to take a
glass of water from my sideboard ?   The answer to the first
question is obvious.   She was extremely anxious to get rid of the
nervous embarrassment from which she suffered, and thus the
suggestion contained nothing opposed to her volition.   She
herself explained the second.

In the cases above recorded, although a certain amount of
evidence was obtained from the patients themselves in reference
to their mental condition, no systematic attempt was made to
investigate this.   I am well aware that this admission is a
startling one, and can only say in self-excuse that this all-

important point has been equally neglected by others. I have since attempted to repair the mistake, and with interesting results. For example, Miss D., who was the subject of the most striking series of "time appreciation" experiments I have recorded, also refused certain suggestions. These I will now relate, as well as her own description of her mental and physical condition during hypnosis. On one occasion during hypnosis, I asked her to put her fingers to her nose at Mr. Barkworth, a member of the Society for Psychical Research, who assisted at the experiments. She laughed, and, despite repeated suggestions, absolutely refused to do so. At a later date, in hypnosis, I asked her for an explanation. She told me she did not want to, and would give no other reason. On another occasion, during hypnosis, I suggested that she should steal Mr. Barkworth's watch. The watch was placed upon the table, and Mr. Barkworth hid behind a screen. I told the subject that Mr. Barkworth had gone and had left his watch, that he was very absent-minded, would never remember where he had left it, would never miss it, etc.; suggested that she should take it, that no one would ever know, etc. I awoke Miss D.: she took no notice of the watch. I asked her, "Where is Mr. Barkworth?" "Gone away." "He has left his watch; would you not like to take it?" She laughed and said, "No, of course not." I rehypnotised her and asked, "What did I suggest to you a little while ago when you were asleep?" "That I should steal Mr. Barkworth's watch, that he was absent-minded, would never miss it, etc." "Then why did you not do so?" "Because I did not want to." "Was it because you were afraid of being found out?" "No, not at all, but because I knew it would be wrong."

On another occasion I again questioned her in hypnosis in reference to this suggested theft. I said, "Did you recognise that it was an experiment?" "Yes, perfectly." "How did you know it was?" "I can't tell you; I only felt sure it was." On being questioned further, she said, "Well, I knew you would not ask me to do anything really wrong." "Well, then, if you were quite certain in your own mind that it was only an experiment, why did you not carry it out?" "Because I did not wish to do what was wrong, even in jest." She admitted, however, that she would put a lump of sugar into her mother's tea-cup, even if I said it were arsenic. When asked why she would do this, and yet would not take the watch, she replied as follows : " I would not take a watch, even if I knew the suggestion were made as an experiment, because this would be pretending to commit a crime. I would, however, put a piece of sugar into my mother's tea-cup if I were sure it was sugar, even though some one said it was arsenic, because then I should not be the one who was pretending to commit the crime. I should only have put sugar into the tea." So subtle a distinction would not, I think, have occurred to the subject in the waking condition.

In reply to further questions in hypnosis, she said she felt sure she could refuse any suggestion; that she felt she was herself; that she knew where she was and what she was doing. " Are you the same person asleep as awake ? " I asked. " Yes," she replied, with a laugh. She described the condition as a sort of losing herself and yet not losing herself. She knew and heard all that was going on, and yet seemed to take no notice of it. When Mr. Barkworth was put *en rapport* with her, she remembered his voice, and recalled the fact that she had heard it on a previous occasion, when not *en rapport* with him. She said she was resting all the time, and that nothing she did or thought tired her. I asked her what it felt like to have her arm made cataleptic by suggestion. She replied, " I did not feel frightened, but I felt startled. I think it would surprise any one." " When you awake and find your arm still rigid, what do you feel then ? " " I feel amused." " When you are sleeping here, and no one is talking to you, do you ever think of anything ? ". " Yes. One day I was troubled about my dressmaking. My employer was ill, and I had more responsibility than usual. I had a difficult piece of work to do, and could not understand how it was to be done. When asleep here I planned how I would do it, and carried this out successfully when I returned home. When I awoke I did not know that I had done this. The way out of the difficulty suddenly came into my head on my way home, and I thought I had found it out at that moment. I now remember planning while asleep what I afterwards carried out."

On one occasion after being hypnotised, and when she was apparently in the lethargic condition, she suddenly volunteered the statement that her mother wished to speak to me. Shortly afterwards the latter entered the room. The subject was still asleep, and no suggestions of *rapport* were made. Mrs. D. commenced to tell me about a friend in whom she was interested, with a view to finding out whether I thought hypnotic treatment would be of benefit in his case. The subject suddenly joined in the conversation, and added some important details which Mrs. D. had forgotten. On awaking she remembered nothing in reference to this.

On another occasion, under similar circumstances, Mrs. D. questioned me in reference to a trivial indisposition from which her daughter was suffering, and asked me whether I thought she might give her a certain simple remedy. Upon this the subject commenced to laugh, and recounted in a highly amused manner an experiment of her mother's in domestic medicine, of which she had been the unfortunate victim.

One day, I successfully suggested a visual hallucination of her own-photograph to Miss D., when she described her appearance, dress, etc. A further suggestion that she should see a *décolleté* photograph of herself was not realised. Questioned regarding this in a subsequent hypnosis, she replied as follows : "I never should have had my photograph taken in such a low-necked dress; and did not wish to see it or describe it to you, as the idea offended me."

I obtained the following account of the hypnotic condition from another subject, an educated, intelligent woman. She said : "When asleep I still feel that I am myself, and can think and reason just as well as when I am awake. I could resist any suggestion if I wanted to do so. The sensation is a pleasant one, as if I were getting rested all over. I am conscious of no other sounds, except your voice. When you are not talking to me, the condition is generally a blank. At such times I occasionally, but rarely, think, or spontaneously recall the events of past hypnoses."

Another educated subject, a very good somnambule, described her state in similar terms. She said : "I feel a kind of restfulness which I do not get in any other condition in life. I feel no fatigue. External sounds, other than your voice, I hear vaguely as if in a dream, but pay no attention to them. I still feel that I am myself and can reason just as well as if I were awake." She also said that she felt certain that she could refuse any suggestion which she disapproved of, and would not carry out an imaginary crime, even if she knew it was only an experiment.

Y

This subject readily accepted suggestions of anæsthesia and analgesia, and was unable to remember in the waking state either painful sensations or tactile impressions. On being re-hypnotised, however, though she could not recall any sensation of pain, she was able, in response to suggestion, to state where she had been pinched or pricked, and to describe the tactile impressions associated with these operations.

Further experiments with Miss D. were made in conjunction with Dr. Hyslop, of Bethlem, and of some of these he gives the following account in his work entitled *Mental Physiology*, pp. 423-424. "In the state of artificially induced hypnosis, the will power is sometimes retained intact. Bramwell has demonstrated that although there is an extreme readiness to react to suggestion from without, yet there still remains a higher controlling influence or auto-suggestion, which enables the hypnotised person to deliberate, choose, and inhibit at will.

" During the waking state of one of Dr. Bramwell's subjects we made the suggestion to her that she ought to resist a certain movement during her hypnotised state. Dr. Bramwell was not present at the time the suggestion was made, and was quite unaware of the restriction imposed upon the subject. On testing the movements suggested during the hypnotic state, he found that the subject absolutely refused to carry out his suggestion with regard to this particular movement. The auto-suggestion proved as efficacious during the artificial state as during the normal state. How we are to explain this retention of the individuality of the subject we do not know. The facts alone would appear to warrant the conclusion that the memory image of the special act to be restrained was present during the artificial state, and that there existed a certain degree of continuity between the primary mental conception and the secondary inhibition. On again awaking this subject remembered our suggestion, but had not the faintest recollection as to what had happened during hypnosis.

" This question becomes one of extreme importance from a medico-legal point of view. Dr. Bramwell believes that subjects in the hypnotic state invariably refuse to perform acts which would be criminal or even indecent. Whether the refusal is only a manifestation of an *acquired* tendency to resist or to act in certain directions, or whether there is some mentalisation possible apart from true consciousness, we cannot attempt to decide. In the present instance the refusal to perform the movement (to make her arm stiff) was evidently the result of the ante-hypnotic suggestion. We have yet to learn how far an individual is truly responsible for his actions during certain mental states; and, as the student may gather from such instances, the mere absence of memory of the events which have taken place during those states need not entirely negative the possibility of there having been some freedom of choice and the power of restraining certain actions."

In most of the cases referred to the subjects refused to carry out suggestions in hypnosis, which they would have rejected in the waking state. Sometimes, however, in hypnosis they refused things they would readily have done or submitted to when awake. For instance, Dr. Allden, when Resident Physician at the Brompton Hospital, hypnotised a girl, suffering from chronic pulmonary disease, to relieve insomnia. She rapidly became a good somnambule. On one occasion, after he had hypnotised her, the nurse reminded him that it was his day for examining the patient's chest; but, to his astonishment, she, although naturally docile and obliging, refused to allow it to be bared. She had previously been examined dozens of times by himself and others, and had never made the slightest objection. He insisted upon her submitting, but was unable to overcome her resistance. He asked her why she objected now, when she had never done so previously. She replied: "You never tried before to examine my chest when I was asleep." On awaking she remembered nothing of what had occurred, and he said nothing to her about it, but examined her chest as usual. Afterwards the nurse told her what she had said, whereupon she was greatly distressed, and wondered how she could possibly have been so rude to her doctor.

These, and many similar facts, have forced me to abandon all belief in the so-called "automatism," or better termed "helpless obedience," of the subject: still I must refer to some of the arguments in support of it, before attempting to analyse further the mental condition in hypnosis. Of these arguments the following are examples :—

(a) When subjects successfully resist suggestion, it is usual to explain this by assuming that they have not been so deeply hypnotised as those in whom no resistance has manifested itself.

I cannot admit the correctness of this in my cases. During the last twelve years, I have had frequent opportunities of examining hypnotic subjects at home and abroad, and have nowhere observed more profound somnambules than amongst my own subjects—rarely, in fact, seeing cases to equal some of them. Not only did all the subjects to whom I have referred exhibit the phenomena of profoundest somnambulism, but nearly all had undergone painless hypnotic operations.

(b) The personality of the operator, and his method of training his subjects, have been supposed to play an important part in the acceptance or rejection of suggestions. Granting that this be true, it does not explain the resistance which I encountered. I commenced by believing that the subjects were entirely under my control, and did my best to develop their supposed obedience.

(c) The existence of one class of phenomena is considered as necessarily implying the existence of another, and a totally differing class. Durand de Gros asked: " Is it possible that suggestion should have the power of producing extraordinary physical changes, and yet be without this particular effect upon the moral state ? " The facts I have already cited answer this question in the affirmative. Putting these aside, the assumption that the physical phenomena necessarily imply certain moral ones is unreasonable. What inevitable connection exists, for example, between an alteration in the pulse-rate and the murder of one's mother ? Should I not be equally logically justified in assuming that the subject in the normal state who, in response to suggestion, would play the violin or paint a picture, would be equally willing to rob a church ?

(d) Evidence in favour of obedience afforded by cases in which the subjects are alleged to have accepted criminal and analogous suggestions. This is important. The fact that the phenomenon of helpless obedience was invariably absent in my subjects, does not justify me in concluding that it did not sometimes occur in those of others. These cases of so-called automatism fall into two classes: (1st) Where an imaginary crime has been suggested ; (2ndly) where a real act has been performed, which it is assumed the subject would not have submitted to in the normal state.

(1st) First, as regards imaginary crime: here, as Professor Delbœuf has pointed out, it is supposed that the subject passes through a mental state similar to that of the operator. Assumption, without experimental proof, is a frail and unsatisfactory basis on which to erect a theory. Let us first examine the facts. A somnambule puts a piece of sugar into her mother's tea-cup, while her medical attendant makes various absurd and untruthful assertions as to its composition. Bernheim and Liégeois believe that the subject accepted these absurd statements as true, because, being hypnotised, she was unable to distinguish between truth and falsehood. Delbœuf claimed that she had sufficient sense left to know exactly what she was doing. *To neither did it occur to ask the subject during hypnosis what she thought about the matter herself.* If they had done so, she would have promptly solved the difficulty, and told them that, while they were discussing probabilities, she was quietly laughing in her sleeve at the grotesque absurdity of the whole performance. It may be noticed in passing that while Bernheim considered the Salpêtrière subjects so abnormally acute that they could catch the slightest indication of the thoughts of the operator, and so destroy the supposed value of the phenomena alleged to be induced by metals, magnets, drugs in sealed tubes, etc.; he, on the other hand, supposes the Nancy subjects to be so abnormally devoid of all intelligence as to be unable to understand when a palpable farce is played before them.

(2ndly) When a real act has been performed which it is assumed the subject would not have submitted to in the normal state. Of this Bernheim cites an example. He states that he uncovered a young woman, presumably a hospital patient, in the presence of his assistants, and that she appeared perfectly calm and indifferent. Bernheim also quotes a case in which he entirely failed in persuading another young woman, also a good somnambule, to allow him to uncover her or to accept the suggestion that she should commit an imaginary crime, despite the fact that he varied his suggestions in every conceivable way. To another subject he suggested profound sleep and insensibility to all sensations coming from him. She remained insensible when he plunged a pin deeply into her nose and touched the mucous membrane of her eyes. When, however, he attempted to disarrange her clothes, she immediately blushed, resisted, and spontaneously passed into the waking state. Let us take the case of supposed helpless obedience. The mere fact that a

woman permitted herself to be uncovered does not necessarily
imply that she was incapable of resisting. Before this can be
used as an argument in favour of the helpless obedience of the
hypnotised subject, one is justified in demanding that it should
be clearly proved that, under similar circumstances, the subject
would have objected to being uncovered in the waking condition.
Medical men are frequently obliged to uncover their female
patients for examination, and rarely encounter resistance. The
first time I visited Professor Bernheim's wards I was struck by
the fact that, in order to show some hysterical muscular movements in the abdomen of a non-hypnotised subject, he threw off
the bed-clothes, drew the patient's nightgown up to her neck,
and left her in that condition while we examined other cases.
Though such treatment is opposed to the practice of English
hospitals, I do not propose to criticise it. I only desire to draw
attention to the fact that a patient was stripped in the waking
state, from my point of view unnecessarily so ; and that she and
every one else apparently regarded this as devoid of importance.
The particular hypnotised subject referred to above did not
object to be stripped : why should she ? She must have been
accustomed to see other hospital patients examined ; and, apparently, there was no special reason why she should have objected
to the ordinary routine. Cases such as these appear to me
absolutely valueless, since the subject's supposed obedience
remains so easily accounted for in other ways. To render such
a case worthy of serious consideration, it would be absolutely
necessary to eliminate many important factors, such as (a) the
fact that the subject was ill; (b) that she was in a hospital
where patients were stripped as part of the ordinary routine ;
(c) that the examination was made by a medical man.

Strangely enough, the most marked case of resistance to
suggestion that I have observed was shown by Liébeault's
celebrated somnambule, Camille. When I first visited Nancy
in 1889, Liébeault showed me this subject, who had been
frequently hypnotised, and whom he regarded as a typical
specimen of profound somnambulism illustrating hypnotic
automatism in its highest degree. He assured me that the
suggestions he made to her were carried out with the fatality of
a falling stone. He hypnotised her, and suggested that on
awaking she should find, on opening the outer door, that there

was a violent snow-storm; that she should at once return, complain of this, and proceed to the stove to warm herself. While doing so one of her hands would touch the stove, and she would believe that she had burnt it. It was a warm summer's day, and, of course, the stove had not been lighted. The subject refused to accept the suggestion. Liébeault insisted for some time, and then gave up the attempt, saying that she sometimes refused suggestions. He then asked her: " Will you do this another time if you will not do it to-day ? " She replied: " Yes, to-morrow." On the following day the suggestion was repeated and carried out in all its details. In this instance, then, the " classic " hypnotic automaton, the one who was supposed to carry out a suggestion with the fatality of a falling stone, refused one, not on moral grounds, but apparently from pure caprice.

The difference between the hypnotised and the normal subject is to be found not so much in conduct, as in the increased mental and physical powers of the former. Any changes in the moral sense that I have noticed have invariably been in favour of the hypnotised subject. As regards obedience to suggestion, there is apparently little to choose between the two. A hypnotised subject, who has acquired the power of manifesting various physical and mental phenomena, will do so in response to suggestion for much the same reasons as one in the normal condition. In the normal state we are usually pleased to show off our various gifts and attainments, more especially if we think they are superior to those of others; and in this respect the hypnotised subject does not differ from the normal. Both will refuse what is disagreeable: in both this refusal may be modified or overcome by appeals to the reason, or to the usual motives which influence conduct. When the act demanded is contrary to the moral sense, it is usually refused by the normal subject, and invariably by the hypnotised one. I have never observed any decrease of intelligence in hypnosis. In the alert stage it is often conspicuously increased, while in the lethargic it is only apparently, not really, suspended. Forel's warders, who could sleep by the bedside of suicidal maniacs, and awake immediately at a given signal, or who could inhibit their own hearing of the purposeless noises of the insane, and acutely hear everything which demanded their attention, did not in so doing show any loss of intelligence. The power of concentration in the normal state, with its accompanying inhibition of undesirable impressions, is a well-known and somewhat analogous condition, but one which is not usually regarded as indicative of mental degeneration.

When one turns to the later works of Braid, and sees how clear was his experimental proof that the hypnotised subject not only had the power of choosing between suggestions, but invariably refused those repugnant to his moral nature, one cannot help feeling surprised at the revival of theories in reference to so-called automatism or obedience, which are identical with the views of the mesmerists. This is the more astonishing when one considers that Bernheim, who holds these views, also boldly asserts that there is nothing in hypnotism but the name; that it does not create a new condition, and that hypnotic acts are only exaggerated normal ones. According to Bernheim, however, the moral state in hypnosis differs widely from the normal : which is in obvious contradiction with his own conception of hypnotism. One can understand, for example, how a prolonged muscular rigidity may be a hypnotic exaggeration of a somewhat shorter normal one ; but it is difficult to comprehend how a hypnotic willingness to murder one's mother can be an exaggeration of the *refusal* to hurt a fly when awake. Bernheim's view of the moral state does not follow logically from the supposed resemblance between the hypnotic and normal condition, but apparently has its origin in an erroneous estimate of the nature and the power of suggestion. On the one hand, he tells us that the hypnotic and normal conditions are practically identical, and their only distinction a slight difference in suggestibility. On the other hand, we are informed that a virtuous individual will sometimes commit crime in response to hypnotic suggestion. If this were correct, we should be justified in describing the origin of hypnotic crime thus :—

(*a*) A virtuous girl in the normal state has a natural tendency to accept the suggestion that she should murder her mother.

(*b*) In hypnosis suggestibility is slightly increased, and thus, when it is suggested to her to murder her mother, she does so.

The views which I have long held regarding the hypnotised subject's power of rejecting disagreeable or criminal suggestions are now shared, more or less completely, by a good many other observers. These, however, as far as I have been able to learn, have based their statements solely on cases where suggestions have been rejected, and have not attempted to ascertain the subjects' mental state by questioning them in hypnosis.

Thus, Professor Beaunis says hypnotised subjects usually reason very logically and evince striking powers of deduction; they are certainly not unconscious machines incapable of judgment. He frequently observed that subjects refused suggestions which were disagreeable to them.

Dr. Crocq, of Brussels, also admits that subjects frequently reject distasteful suggestions.

Richter believes that a somnambule may entirely refuse to perform certain acts, and oppose no resistance to others.

According to Gilles de la Tourette, the hypnotic somnambule is not a pure automaton, a simple machine that one can turn at will. He possesses a personality, sometimes, it is true, subdued or weakened, but which in certain cases persists in its entirety, and shows itself clearly by the resistance it opposes to suggested ideas. The hypnotised subject always retains his individuality, and can manifest his will by resisting suggestions.

Brouardel says that, if agreeable or indifferent suggestions are made to a somnambule by a person whom he likes and trusts, he will accept them; but, if they are contrary to his personal affections or his natural instincts, he opposes an almost invincible resistance to them. He cites the case of a Jewess supposed to be the absolute machine ("*chose*") of the operator, but who refused to empty the ink-bottle on her best dress.

Pitres mentions a case of a somnambule who refused to awake whenever a disagreeable post-hypnotic suggestion was made to him.

According to Dr. Charpignon, it is much easier to restore moral rectitude, by means of hypnotic suggestion, to a somnambule who has lost it, than to pervert, by the same means, a person of high moral character.

Dr. de Jong cites many cases of resistance to suggestion. One of his subjects, a profound somnambule, apparently accepted criminal suggestions as readily as she did innocent ones. She refused, however, to undress before another person, and would not tell an insignificant secret she had promised not to reveal. Another subject refused to tell Dr. de Jong something of an indelicate nature which she had seen, and which she had already confided to a friend of her own sex. These subjects, according to de Jong, refused certain suggestions, because they involved real facts which were disagreeable to them; while they executed others alleged to be criminal, because they recognised that these were laboratory experiments devoid of danger either to themselves or others.

Delbœuf relates an experiment with J., the somnambule already referred to (p. 84). She was a courageous young woman, and sometimes took care of Delbœuf's country-house in his absence. She was armed with a revolver, owing to the serious strikes and riots existing at that time. One night a man tried to force the door. The barking of the dogs awakened J.; she opened the window, saw the man, took out her revolver, went into the hall and watched for his entry in order to fire at him. The man, possibly frightened by the noise, disappeared. On a subsequent occasion, Delbœuf secretly discharged the revolver; then hypnotised J., and suggested that two persons in another room were robbers, and insisted that she should fire at them. In obedience to his suggestions she fetched the revolver, but, despite his reiterated and emphatic commands, absolutely refused to fire; on the contrary, she stepped backwards and placed the revolver cautiously on the floor.

SUGGESTED CRIMES.—SUMMARY.

(*a*) I have never seen a suggestion accepted in hypnosis which would have been refused in the normal state.

(*b*) I have observed that suggestions could be resisted as easily in the lethargic as in the alert stage.

(*c*) I have frequently noticed increased refinement in hypnosis: subjects have refused suggestions which they would have accepted in the normal condition.

(*d*) I saw Camille refuse a suggestion from mere caprice.

(*e*) Examination of the mental condition in hypnosis revealed the fact that it was unimpaired.

(*f*) The arguments of Bernheim are devoid of value, as they are founded exclusively on cases where (1) a simple and harmless act has been assumed to be thought criminal by the subject, because the operator has stated it to be so; and (2) where the subject has permitted something in hypnosis, which he would probably have submitted to in the normal state.

(3) An Idea has a Tendency to generate its Actuality.

According to Bernheim, the suggestive phenomena of hypnosis depend upon the fact that, in the normal subject, an idea has a tendency to generate its actuality : and this power is supposed to be artificially increased by suggestion. But it is not the hypnotised subject alone who receives suggestions, as these are often made even more forcibly in normal life.

Now, if we confined our attention to the hypnotic state, and considered how frequently a suggested idea, unassociated with violent emotional conditions, produced a rapid and definite response, we should be inclined to admit that in hypnosis an idea not only had a tendency to generate its actuality, but almost invariably did so.

A similar statement, however, in reference to normal life, cannot be accepted without question. If an extended statistical inquiry were made as to the results of suggestion without hypnosis, we should find that these would fall under three classes :—

(A) Where the suggested idea had produced no result.

(B) Where the result was different, or even opposite, from that intended.

(C) Where the suggestion had been responded to with more or less exactitude.

(A) Where the Suggested Idea had produced no Result.

A very casual glance at the events of everyday life would compel us to conclude that this class is the commonest of the three. This is evident, if we think of the numberless things ineffectually suggested in the family circle to domestics, workmen, tradespeople, friends, acquaintances, etc.

(B) Where the Result produced was opposite to, or, at all events, different from that intended.

Numerous examples of this class could easily be cited. Thus, if a thief snatches my watch and runs away, and I suggest to him to stop, he, on the contrary, runs the faster. If a street arab is making a noise under my window, and I tell him to cease and go away, he not only persists, but incites others to join him. If I hold up a good boy as a pattern to a naughty one, the latter, instead of imitating the former, kicks him !

(C) Where the Suggestion has been responded to with more or less Exactitude.

When we compare the results of this class, with those obtained in the others, they must, I am afraid, sink into insignificance. For one suggestion which has generated its actuality, we must count at least a hundred which have produced nothing, and possibly ten where the result has been an unexpected or disagreeable one. I would, therefore, re-state the proposition as follows :—

(1) A suggested idea has generally a tendency to generate nothing.

(2) A suggested idea has frequently a tendency to generate its opposite.

(3) A suggested idea rarely tends to generate its actuality.

When the theory first crept into psychology that a suggested idea had a greater tendency to evoke its actuality than to produce other or negative results, I do not know, but certainly it is now frequently quoted as an accepted truth. The production of the flow of saliva by the sight of food is the stock illustration of the alleged phenomenon. The most important factor in the equation—hunger in the subject of the experiment—is apt to be lost sight of. It is quite possible that the sight of a couple of pounds of raw beefsteak might produce a flow of saliva in a very hungry man. But, after these had been cooked and eaten, if he were shown a similar piece of raw steak, its sight, instead of inducing a flow of saliva, would in all probability simply evoke feelings of disgust.

To this point, namely, that the result of an idea does not depend so much upon the fact that it has been suggested, as upon the nature of the idea itself, and its relationship to the character of its recipient, I will again refer when discussing " Suggestion." Meanwhile, I wish to emphasise the fact that " tendency " implies numerical proportion. For example, if I fire a dozen times at a target, and if on five occasions the bullet strikes it, and on seven misses and passes to the right, the *tendency* must be in favour of the results which are numerically the greater of the two. In the same way, before concluding that an idea has a tendency to generate its actuality, one must be able to prove that out of a given number of cases this result follows more frequently than others.

(4) In Hypnosis the Tendency to accept Suggestions is somewhat increased by the Action of Suggestion itself: this alone distinguishes the Hypnotic from the Normal State.

Granting for the moment that the normal and hypnotic states are practically identical; that both are characterised by susceptibility to suggestion; how far are we justified in concluding that the increased suggestibility of the hypnotic subject is due to "Suggestion" alone—without the previous production of mental or physical change? Let us consider the means by which the alteration has been stated—by Bernheim and others—to have been brought about. The phrase, "You are to become more suggestible," or the like, is supposed to have artificially created it. Now, if we admit that this or a similar formula is sufficient to change a normal into a hypnotic subject, and to account for his increased suggestibility, we must be prepared to show, in order to maintain the distinction between the two, that the individual who is still regarded as normal, *i.e.* less suggestible, has escaped similar influences. Suggestions in normal life, however, are frequently associated with those of increased suggestibility. A beggar, in appealing for alms, not only asks that they should be given him, but also suggests in various ways, directly or indirectly, according to his skill and ingenuity, that the object of his petition should become more responsive to his prayer, *i.e. more suggestible.* There is an important difference between the two. In hypnosis, to gain increased suggestibility it is often only necessary to repeat quietly some recognised formula once or twice; while in normal life we frequently attempt to obtain a like result in a much more forcible and varied manner. We must conclude, then, that if, as assumed by Bernheim, the hypnotic and normal states are practically identical, and suggestion a factor

common to both, suggestibility, as the result of the methods
employed to develop it, ought to be more markedly characteristic
of the normal than of the hypnotic condition.

(5) The Result of Suggestion in Hypnosis is Analogous to the Result of Suggestion in the Normal State.

If we confine ourselves to cases in which suggestion in the
normal subject has been employed in the same manner as it is
used in hypnosis, the analogy is at once seen to be an extremely
imperfect one. The results of the workings of the mind acting.
so to say, in cold blood upon the body, are extremely rare and
generally unimportant. On the other hand, if we turn to the
effects of strong emotional states, we find many phenomena
which more or less closely resemble those of hypnosis. Similarity
of result, however, does not necessarily imply identity of cause;
and an attempted analogy which is based solely on the former
and ignores the latter must ever be an imperfect one. Fear,
hope, faith, religious excitement, and the like, are almost invariably
present in cases which are cited as analogous to hypnotic ones.
Not only are these conditions unnecessary for the induction of
hypnosis, but some of them, such as fear, absolutely preclude its
production: thus, hypnotic phenomena can be evoked in the
absence of all those conditions that are essential for the production
of similar phenomena in the normal state; and, further, the
presence of some of these conditions, instead of favouring
hypnosis, prevents or hinders it. Putting aside this important
objection—the difference between the conditions associated with
the development of the phenomena—there still remain certain
points of contrast between the phenomena themselves. These I
now enumerate:—

(A) SUGGESTION IN HYPNOSIS.

(1) Once deep hypnosis has been induced, a wide range of
phenomena, both mental and physical, can be evoked at any
time, and, with the consent of the subject, by any one. Further,
a considerable number of phenomena can be simultaneously
produced in the same subject.

(2) One phenomenon can be immediately changed into its

opposite, *i.e.* muscular rigidity into paralysis, anæsthesia into hyperæsthesia, etc.

(3) Hypnotic phenomena can be terminated at will.

(4) The date of the appearance of the phenomenon can be delayed, *e.g.* it can be suggested during hypnosis that it shall not appear till twelve months afterwards.

(5) With two important limitations, the suggestion will invariably be responded to, *i.e.* it must contain nothing in opposition to the subject's moral sense : it must not be beyond the range of his hypnotic powers.

(6) Under the conditions just mentioned, the exact nature of the response can be predicted, *i.e.* similar stimuli will produce identical results.

(7) Subjects who readily respond to suggestions when hypnotised, are frequently the very ones who have for years resisted suggestion in the waking condition, even when this has been associated with emotional states. For example, a patient who had long suffered from dipsomania had received many and varied suggestions in the waking state. The grief of his friends and relatives, and their repeated remonstrances, were powerful suggestions. So, too, were the loss of fortune and self-respect ; and the physical sufferings, associated with keen remorse, which followed his drinking-bouts. Twelve months passed in a home for inebriates must also have been full of suggestions of many kinds. All these, however, produced no result ; and yet, after a few weeks' hypnotic treatment, the patient abandoned the alcoholic habit, and still, after a lapse of eight years, remained an abstainer.

(8) Hypnotic suggestion tends to gain strength by repetition.

(B) Suggestion by Means of Emotional States.

(1) The resultant phenomena are usually isolated ones, or, at all events, much more limited in number than those which can be simultaneously evoked in the hypnotised subject. Further, they cannot be produced by any one. Thus, the subject who had been influenced by the "touch" of a king, would probably be unresponsive to that of a peasant.

(2) One phenomenon cannot be immediately changed into

its opposite without an alteration in the emotional state which had produced it.

(3) Emotional phenomena cannot be terminated at will.

(4) The date of the appearance of the phenomena can rarely be delayed or fixed.

(5) The phenomena are evoked with less certainty than in hypnosis: an emotional state which will produce a physical effect in one subject may produce nothing in another.

(6) Identical emotional states do not always produce similar physical phenomena. On the contrary, opposite conditions are frequently evoked in different subjects by identical emotions, *e.g.* fear will paralyse one, and excite violent muscular movements in another.

(7) Subjects who are unable to respond to certain suggestions in the normal state often readily carry out similar ones when hypnotised.

(8) An emotional suggestion frequently loses strength by repetition, *i.e.* a subject may quickly come to disregard former fears.

So far we have been occupied in discussing the facts upon which Bernheim's theoretical explanation of hypnosis is founded. To these exception has been taken on every point, viz. :—

(I.) To the supposed identity of normal and hypnotic sleep.

(II.) To the supposed analogy between the phenomena of hypnosis, and the automatic, involuntary and unconscious acts of normal life.

(III.) To the general principle that, in normal life, an idea has a tendency to generate its actuality.

(IV.) To the statement that suggestion—regarding this as a thing apart, unassociated by mental or physical change—increases suggestibility in the hypnotised subject; and that this alone forms the sole distinction between hypnosis and normal life.

(V.) To the supposed general analogy between the result of suggestion in the normal state and in hypnosis.

In all these statements there is only one I am prepared to accept, namely, that suggestion plays an important part in evoking hypnotic phenomena. There remains for our consideration the question how far suggestion *explains* the phenomena of hypnosis.

Does Suggestion explain Hypnosis and its Phenomena ?

The answer to this question must, I think, be a distinctly negative one. The success of suggestion depends not so much on the suggestion itself as on the conditions inherent in the subject. These are: (1) willingness to accept and carry out the suggestion, and (2) the power to do so. In the hypnotised subject, except in reference to criminal or improper suggestions, the first condition is generally present. The second varies according to the depth of the hypnosis, and the personality of the subject. For instance, I might suggest analgesia, in precisely similar terms, to three subjects, and yet obtain quite different results. One might become profoundly analgesic, the second slightly so, and the third not at all. Just in the same way, if three jockeys attempt to make their horses gallop a certain distance in a given time, the suggestions conveyed by voice, spur, and whip may be similar, and yet the results quite different. One horse, in response to suggestion, may easily cover the required distance in the allotted time; it was both able and willing to perform the feat. The second, in response to somewhat increased suggestion, may nearly do so; it was willing, but had not sufficient staying power. The third, able, but unwilling, not only refuses to begin the race, but bolts off in the opposite direction. With this horse we have the exact opposite of the result obtained in the first instance; and yet possibly the amount of suggestion it received largely exceeded that administered to the others. As Myers has pointed out, the operator directs the condition upon which hypnotic phenomena depend, but does not create it. " Bernheim's command, ' Feel pain no more,' is no more a scientific instruction *how* not to feel pain, than the prophet's ' Wash in Jordan and be clean' was a pharmacopœial prescription for leprosy." In hypnosis, the essential condition is not the means used to excite the phenomena, but the peculiar state which enables them to be evoked. Suggestion no more explains the phenomena of hypnotism than the crack of a pistol explains a boat-race. Both are simply signals—mere points of departure, and nothing more. In Bernheim's hands the word " suggestion " has acquired an entirely new signification, and differs only in name from the " odylic " force of the mesmerists. It has become

z

mysterious and all-powerful, and is supposed to be capable, not only of evoking and explaining all the phenomena of hypnotism, but also of originating—nay, even of being—the condition itself. According to this view, suggestion not only starts the race, but also creates the rowers and builds the boat !

Braid's later Views regarding Suggestion, etc.

(1) ORIGIN OF THE SUGGESTED IDEA.

While Braid held that hypnotic phenomena resulted from dominant ideas in the mind of the subject, he, at the same time, stated that it was a matter of indifference whether these had existed previously, or were afterwards audibly suggested by the operator, or indirectly created by the sensory impressions resulting from his manipulations.

(2) SELF-SUGGESTION.

Braid cited many instances in which hypnosis and its phenomena were entirely the result of self-suggestion, although they were supposed to be due to other causes.

(3) PASSES AND OTHER MANIPULATIONS.

Braid's views, as to the influence of passes and other manipulations being mainly mental, has already been given (see p. 291).

Points of Difference between Braid and the Nancy School as to Suggestion.

The difference between Braid and the Nancy school, with regard to suggestion, is entirely one of theory, not of practice. Braid employed verbal suggestion in hypnosis just as intelligently as any member of the Nancy school. This fact is denied by Bernheim, who says : " It is strange that Braid did not think of applying suggestion in its most natural form—suggestion by speech—to bring about hypnosis and its therapeutic effects. He did not dream of explaining the curative effects of hypnotism by means of the psychical influence of suggestion, but made use of suggestion without knowing it." This statement has its sole origin in ignorance of Braid's later works. In these his references to the use of verbal suggestion in therapeutics are both clear and numerous, and various examples have already been given. Braid, however, while anticipating Bernheim as to the practical use of suggestion, differed entirely from him in his theoretical conception of it. He did not regard suggestion as explanatory of hypnotic phenomena; but, like Myers at a later date, looked upon it simply as an artifice used in order to excite them. He considered that the mental phenomena were only rendered possible by previous physical changes; and, as the result of these, the operator was enabled to act like an engineer, and to direct the forces which existed in the subject's own person.

The Views of Braid and of Forel as regards Passes.

While Braid believed that the mental effect resulting from the indirect physical action of mechanical means could be checked or reversed by stronger and more direct verbal suggestion, he still held, and I think justly, that physical impressions were capable of producing both physical and mental results. Forel, on the other hand, denies the physical influence of mechanical processes, on the ground that suggestion is capable of altering their supposed action. He says: "Blowing on the face no longer awakens my subjects, because I have suggested that this would remove pain instead of arousing them." From this he concludes that the act of blowing produces no result, and considers this a powerful argument against the Somatic school. Would it not be equally logical to contend that the prick of a pin produced no physical effect because the subject, when rendered insensible to pain by suggestion, had been taught to regard the pin-prick as a signal to evoke some other condition?

Attention in Hypnosis.

While Braid and Bernheim differ as to the physical changes which precede or accompany hypnosis, they both attach much importance to the question of attention in reference to the induction of hypnosis and its phenomena.

Attention in the Induction of Hypnosis.

According to Braid, the induction of hypnosis is facilitated either by : (1) the concentration of the attention on some external object, or (2) concentration of the attention on some idea connected with hypnotism.

Liébeault and Bernheim consider that ordinary and hypnotic sleep are both due to the fixation of the attention and the nervous force upon the idea of sleep. The individual, they say, who desires to go to sleep chooses a quiet spot, meditates, and keeps still. His nervous force is concentrated upon a single idea, and deserts the nerves of sensation, emotion, and special sense. The conditions that induce the hypnotic state are identical : the subject is told to concentrate his mind upon the idea of sleep ; and, to aid himself in doing so, is directed to look fixedly at some object. Bodily repose results from this ; the senses become less acute and more and more isolated from the external world, and finally thought is arrested.

A connection undoubtedly exists between the subject's power of attention, and the facility with which hypnosis can be induced. For example, idiots, who possess little spontaneous and no voluntary attention, cannot be hypnotised at all ; and others, such as those suffering from mania, hysteria, etc., whose attention is actively turned into other channels, are extremely difficult to influence.

In reference to the connection between the attention and the induction of hypnosis, the following points seem worthy of notice :—

(a) It is not necessary that the attention should be concentrated on the idea of sleep. Braid, as we have seen, easily induced hypnosis when the patient gazed steadily at an external object, and concentrated his attention on the idea of that object. Moreover, primary hypnosis need not resemble sleep, and the subject may at once pass into the alert stage, without having even closed his eyes.

(b) Primary hypnosis has sometimes been induced in cases where it would be difficult to prove that any concentration of attention had existed, either upon any external object or upon the idea of sleep. In these cases, the subject, after having given his consent to the experiment, has rested quietly, and voluntarily reduced his mental activity. He has, as nearly as possible, emptied his mind of all thought, and produced, not a condition of concentration, but its opposite—abstraction.

(c) The phenomena of natural somnambulism, which, as Gurney pointed out, in respect to the absorption of the mind in one direction, present the closest analogy to those of hypnotism, demand no previous concentration of attention at all.

(d) Once hypnosis has been induced, the condition can be evoked at any time, and practically instantaneously, in response to a previously arranged signal. Here, then, although the attention of the subject has been momentarily directed to the signal, prolonged concentration of attention has been absent.

Does Concentration of Attention cause Hypnosis?

As Gurney said, even if we confine ourselves to cases where attention is actually present during the production of hypnosis, what ground is there for describing it as the cause of that state? The general effects of a one-sided strain of mind or body are pretty well known, and " tonic cramp of the attention " may be a very satisfactory description of the one-sided absorption in a particular direction which characterises many isolated stages of hypnotic trance. But what tendency should the cramp of an attention, which is directed to a button held in the hand, have to produce, or to facilitate, a fresh cramp or series of cramps, when the attention is diverted to quite fresh objects. He had, he said, again and again found the complete change to a new genus of ideas to be absolutely effortless and instantaneous— found, that is, that the attention, which had as usual been fixed during the process of hypnotisation, became quite abnormally mobile afterwards. This great mobility of attention seems an odd result of previous rigid attention to a button. If I am told, he said, that a particular mental attitude—that of fixed or one-sided attention—is the cause of certain mental phenomena which are new to me, I am surely justified in demanding that the order of events shall present some perceptible coherence—shall at least not run directly counter to what my general experience has led me to expect.

Again, taking the case where the attention is concentrated

during the production of the state, how does this explain the fact that, when a subject is left to himself in hypnosis, his condition is usually one of abstraction ?   Here, then, as a supposed result of a previous concentration of attention, we have the spontaneous development of its opposite.

Thus, preliminary fixation of attention cannot be accepted as an explanation of subsequent mobility.   All that we can concede so far is : (1) That fixation of the attention frequently precedes, and usually facilitates, the induction of hypnosis.   (2) That the attention in hypnosis can easily be rendered excessively mobile.

Rapport and Attention.

The following is Liébeault's view :—" It is observed," he says, " that nearly all artificial somnambules are in relation by their senses with those who put them to sleep, but only with them. The subject hears everything the operator says to him, but hears him alone, provided the sleep is sufficiently deep.   He only hears the operator when he is addressed directly by him, and not when a third person is spoken to.   This *rapport* extends to the other senses."   According to Liébeault, the subject remains *en rapport* with the hypnotiser because he goes to sleep while thinking of him, and this does not differ from what sometimes happens in ordinary sleep.   A mother who goes to sleep close to the cradle of her child does not cease to watch over him during her sleep, but, while she hears his slightest cry, is insensible to other louder sounds.   The concentration of the subject's attention upon the operator, and his mental retention of the idea of the one who put him to sleep, is the cause of the *rapport.*

In *rapport,* Bernheim, on the contrary, finds his solitary point of difference between normal and hypnotic sleep.   He says : " In ordinary sleep, as soon as consciousness is lost, the subject is only in relationship with himself.   In induced sleep his mind retains the memory of the person who put him to sleep, hence the hypnotiser's power of playing upon his imagination, of suggesting dreams, and of directing the acts which are no longer controlled by the weakened or absent will."

The following was Braid's view of the condition of the attention in hypnosis :—

The principal difference between hypnotic and normal sleep

is to be found in the mental condition. When falling into ordinary sleep the mind passes from one idea to another indifferently, and the subject is unable to fix his attention on any regular train of thought, or to perform any act requiring much voluntary effort. As the result of this, audible suggestions and sensory impressions received by the sleeper, if not intense enough to entirely awaken him, seldom do more than arouse dreams, in which ideas pass through his mind without exciting definite physical acts. On the other hand, the concentration of attention, which is the result of the means employed for inducing hypnosis, is continued into the state itself; and verbal suggestions or sensory impressions excite definite trains of thought or physical movements, instead of dreams.

Certain points of difference and resemblance are to be noticed between these views.

According to Braid, the condition of the attention in hypnosis favoured response to external suggestion, but not to suggestion conveyed by any particular person, such as the hypnotiser. It was possible by suggestion to create an artificial state in which the subject seemed only to be *en rapport* with the operator, but this condition was only an apparent, not a real one. The subjects really heard the suggestions of others, though special artifices might be necessary in order to make them respond to them. In illustration of this, Braid cited a case in which he made a somnambule respond to his indirect suggestions, conveyed in the form of confident predictions of what was going to happen, though the subject was asleep when he entered the room, and apparently only *en rapport* with the original operator (see p. 287). Carpenter drew attention to the fact that *rapport* was unknown to Mesmer and his immediate disciples, and was not discovered until long after the practice of mesmerism had come into vogue. The phenomena of *rapport* only acquired constancy and fixity in proportion as its laws were announced and received. Mesmerists ignorant of *rapport* produced a great variety of remarkable phenomena, but did not discover this one until the idea had been put into their minds, and thence transferred to their subjects.

Bernheim and Liébeault believe that a real *rapport* exists between the subject and the operator, and that this follows as a natural consequence from the methods employed in inducing hypnosis. Not only does it exist, but, according to Bernheim, the operator's power of evoking hypnotic phenomena depends on it. While Bernheim and Liébeault agree on this point, they differ, as we have seen, on another. For Bernheim finds in *rapport* the sole difference between hypnotic and ordinary sleep ; while Liébeault, on the contrary, tries by means of it to establish an analogy between them.

My own observations in reference to *rapport* have led me to conclusions similar to those of Braid, viz.: (1) That *rapport* does not appear unless it has been directly or indirectly suggested. (2) That the condition is always an apparent—never a real— one. Thus, it could always be experimentally proved that the subjects actually had been cognisant of what had been said and done by others who had not been placed *en rapport* with them. In those who did not know what was expected of them, and to whom neither direct nor indirect suggestions of *rapport* were made, this condition did not appear. On the contrary, they heard and obeyed any one who might address them.

Moll, in *Der Rapport in der Hypnose*, published in 1892, comes practically to the same conclusion as Braid in regard to *rapport*, viz., that it is caused by direct or indirect suggestions of the operator, or by self-suggestions which result from the subject's conception of the nature of the hypnotic state.

It is true, as Liébeault has pointed out, that *rapport* frequently exists between the sleeping mother and her child, and that she will hear its slightest cry and yet be unconscious of louder sounds. This, however, has no analogy in the hypnotic state. The *untrained* somnambule responds with equal readiness to the voice of any one, and, if he has been taught only to respond to one voice, he still hears others. Again, the difference between hypnotic and normal sleep is not, as Bernheim says, that *rapport* exists only in the former. On the contrary, we might with justice establish a distinction between hypnotic and normal sleep, on the ground that *rapport* is absent from the former and is a frequently recurring phenomenon in the latter.

Bernheim's Explanation of Hypnotic Amnesia.

According to Bernheim, every one possesses a certain definite amount of nervous force or cerebral activity. During the waking state this is concentrated in the higher nervous centres—the reasoning part of the brain—while in hypnosis it is concentrated in the lower centres—the imaginative or automatic part. All the impressions received during hypnosis, all the phenomena induced—conceptions, movements, sensations, images—owe their origin to this concentrated and accumulated nervous force. When the subject awakes and resumes his self-control, however, the nervous activity is again diffused through the higher centres of the brain and to the periphery. The impressions received during hypnotic sleep fade, because, having been perceived, as it were, if the simile may be permitted, by a quantity of nervous light, they are no longer bright enough to be conscious when this light ceases to be concentrated upon them. When hypnosis is again induced, the former state of concentration reappears, and, at the same time, the lost memories are revived.

This explanation is ingenious, but unfortunately not in accordance with observed facts. If I suggest to a subject that on awaking he will remember the events of hypnosis, he invariably does so. Yet, in accordance with this theory, the redistribution of nervous force to the higher centres should have inevitably prevented this. Again, suggestion may rob the hypnotised subject of the power of recalling the events of previous hypnoses. But, if Bernheim's explanation were correct, the lost memories could not escape revival, seeing that they must have reappeared when the nervous force was again concentrated in the lower centres.

The Influence of the Operator in inducing the so-called Automatism.

In the estimation of the part played by the operator, Braid differed from certain members of the Nancy school. According to the former, the operator merely acted as an engineer who directed the forces in the subject's own body ; and the phenomena of hypnosis could also be evoked by ideas previously existing in the subject's mind. The latter regard the operator's rôle as a much more important one : not only are his suggestions a mighty force in themselves, but their power is increased by a constant undermining of the volition.

For the successful manifestation of hypnotic phenomena,

Forel considers it essential that the subject should be under the dominion of the operator, and have lost his own power of concentration and attention. He regards the condition as a battle between operator and subject, in which the former, after capturing outpost upon outpost, at last reigns supreme in the central citadel itself. " The mind of a man, *A.*, imposes itself," he says, " upon the mind of another man, *B.*, takes possession of it by entering through some crevice in its armour, and finishes by reigning there more or less as master, and by employing the brain of *B.* as its docile instrument."

According to Bernheim, the natural tendency that exists in every one to accept suggestions is gradually and skilfully developed by the operator.

In opposition to the views of Bernheim, etc., I would insist on two classes of cases :—

(1) *Instances where the operator has deliberately tried to minimise his own importance in reference to the induction of hypnotic phenomena.*

Although I soon ceased to believe that the subject's volition was dominated by that of the operator, I still found, as the result of sensational writings on the question, that a considerable number of my patients objected to be hypnotised, on the ground that it would interfere with their volition. To obviate this difficulty, I changed my method of inducing and managing the hypnotic state. I commenced by informing every new patient that I did not believe it possible for the operator to dominate the volition of the subject, and that, even if such a thing were possible, it could certainly be prevented by suggestion. I explained to my patients that nothing would be suggested without their consent having been previously obtained in the normal state. Under these circumstances, if the suggestions were successful, this would not imply any interference with volition, seeing that their consent had already been obtained. I pointed out that the fulfilment of a hypnotic suggestion frequently demonstrated an increased, not diminished, power of volition. For example, a patient who desired to resist a morbid impulse, but was unable to do so by the exercise of his normal volition, might gain this power by hypnotic suggestion. Thus, the suggestion did not suspend the volition of the subject, but removed the obstacle which prevented the wish from being carried into action. Further, as resistance was manifested despite suggested obedience, it was reasonable to expect that this might be enormously increased by training. I suggested, therefore, to all patients during hypnosis, that they should invariably possess this power of resistance, and also, that neither I nor any one else should ever be able to reinduce hypnosis without their express consent. This change of method did not affect the results. Notwithstanding the fact that the patients were convinced, and justly so, that they possessed complete control of the whole condition, hypnosis was evoked as easily as formerly, and as wide a range of phenomena was induced.

(2a) *Cases where an attempt has been made to teach the subject to evoke hypnosis and its phenomena without the intervention of the operator.*

As already stated (pp. 52 and 53), I have frequently instructed patients to hypnotise themselves, and to evoke the phenomena of hypnosis by self-suggestion.

(2b) *Cases where, after very slight hypnosis, the patient has taught himself to evoke hypnosis and its phenomena.*

An account of a case of this kind is given pp. 201-2.

In such cases it would be difficult, I think, to explain hypnotic phenomena as the result of arrested or weakened volition, and of outside interference by the operator. It might be objected, perhaps, that the influence of the operator had not been entirely eliminated, o:. the ground that he had been associated with the induction of the primary hypnosis. The conditions, however, that are more or less frequently associated with the origin of a particular state are by no means essential for its after-manifestation. For instance, the art of swimming is usually taught either by means of a life-belt, or by attaching the pupil to a cord which the teacher holds and guides by means of a rod. These artificial aids, however, are not essential to the art of swimming : they are only useful in its acquirement. It would be illogical to ascribe a champion's power of winning a race to the life-belt he discarded years before. In the same way, it would be unjustifiable to attribute a subject's power of influencing forces within his own body by suggestions arising in his own mind, to the influence of

the operator who had formerly instructed him how to evoke and
direct this power. And the objection applies with additional
force where the subject, having been hypnotised (slightly, if at
all), without any instruction in self-suggestion by the operator
has taught himself the practice from books.

Monoideism.

Bernheim, as we have already seen, still holds the theory of
monoideism, which Braid originated, but afterwards discarded.
In hypnosis, according to the former, the mind of the subject is
concentrated on a single idea. Impressions which under ordinary
circumstances would reach consciousness now cease to do so, not
only because they do not happen to be attended to, but also
because the subject has no faculty left wherewith to attend to
them. Thus, this is not only a " *concentration of attention* " theory,
but a " *concentration and limited quantity of attention* " theory.

Beaunis, while admitting the influence of attention in the
production of the phenomena of hypnotism, does not believe that
all the facts can be explained by the " concentration of attention "
theory. " If," he says, " a hallucination is suggested to a subject
and realised on awaking immediately afterwards, it may be
possible to explain this on the assumption that the attention was
still concentrated upon the suggested idea." He does not believe,
however, that, when the appearance of the phenomenon has been
delayed for a lengthened period, it can be explained in the same
way; for he does not consider it possible that the subject's
attention can have been concentrated on the suggested idea all
the time.

Gurney, who also rejected the " concentration of attention "
theory, said the energy of attention was not a fixed quantity,
bound to be always in operation in one direction or another;
nor did the human mind, any more than Nature, abhor a vacuum.
What did we gain, then, by employing a general term to describe
such special effects ? When once the (gas) chandelier metaphor
was abandoned—when once it was recognised that in a multitude
of cases the quantity of attention turned on in one direction was
in no way connected with its withdrawal from any other—the
idea of a common psychic factor seemed out of place and misleading.

This theoretical objection is in accordance with observed facts. Doubtless certain hypnotic states exist in which all the attention, so far as it is called into action, is concentrated upon one idea. In order to prove, however, that directing the attention upon a new point necessarily withdraws it entirely from the old one, it must be shown that the phenomenon which resulted from the former concentration inevitably ceased when the latter one arose. A cutaneous analgesia of the arm might, with some show of reason, be said to result from attention directed to the muscles during suggested catalepsy : on the ground that no attention was left wherewith to attend to painful sensations. But while the catalepsy still exists, how, by this theory, can one explain, for example, a cutaneous tactile hyperæsthesia of the same limb, by means of which the subject can distinguish the two points of the compass at half the normal distance? If the subject is unconscious of painful sensations because his attention is entirely concentrated on his muscular condition, this same lack of attention to the skin ought not only to have prevented abnormal distinctness of tactile impressions, but even to have inhibited the usual ones. The experiment can be still further complicated ; for, while still permitting the catalepsy to persist, the cutaneous tactile hyperæsthesia can be associated by suggestion with a cutaneous analgesia over the same area. Now the subject's whole attention cannot be directed to maintaining a condition of muscular rigidity, if he still has enough of it left to suffice, not only for the increased perception of certain tactile sensations, but also for the selection[1] and inhibition of other painful ones. Further, the opposite of these phenomena can be simultaneously evoked on the other side of the body ; the subject's muscles can be paralysed by suggestion, his tactile sensibility abolished, and his sensibility to pain increased. The attention is now directed upon six different points, and could, with equal ease, be simultaneously directed on many others. A psychic blindness, for example, could be suggested on one side, a psychic deafness on the other ; hyperæsthesia of the sense of smell and taste on the one side, and diminished or abolished sensibility on the other, etc., etc. But this is not all ; for while the attention is presumably turned in all these different directions, the subject may be engaged in the

---

[1] Before the painful sensations can be inhibited they must be sorted out, as it were, from the other sensations the subject is experiencing.

successful solution of some intellectual problem. A still further complication is possible. Let us suppose, as in the case of one of my own subjects, that at an earlier date, in a previous hypnosis, a suggestion to record the time at the expiration of 40,845 minutes, or some such complicated number, had been made; this may be carried out, despite the existence of the various muscular and sensorial conditions already referred to, and the fact that, at the moment of its fulfilment, the subject is engaged in some other mental effort.

This picture of the hypnotic state is neither fanciful, nor dependent solely on my own personal observation. The fact that numerous and varied hypnotic phenomena can be simultaneously evoked in the same subject has been repeatedly observed and recorded by others, and, strange to say, even by those who attempt to explain hypnosis by the concentration of the attention upon a single point. It is solely the important bearing of these facts upon this particular theory which has hitherto been so largely overlooked.

Granting that hypnotic phenomena are the result of .changes in the attention, one is forced to conclude that these are the exact reverse of those stated by Bernheim as explanatory of the hypnotic state : the simultaneous presence of many phenomena clearly shows that hypnosis cannot be explained by the concentration of the attention on any one given point. Again, the fact that the multiple phenomena are sometimes similar in character to the isolated ones, indicates that the explanation of hypnotic phenomena by means of the *amount* of the attention concentrated is also fallacious. If *all* the attention is requisite for the production of one phenomenon, and, while this one still lasts, many other hypnotic phenomena are simultaneously induced, whence do the secondary ones derive that excessive amount of attention which is said to be necessary for the induction of the primary one ? The hypnotic condition differs, then, from the normal, not because only one phenomenon can be manifested in it at once, but because it may present simultaneously many and more varied phenomena than can be induced in the normal state at any one time. In a word, hypnosis is frequently a state of *poly-ideism*, not one of *mono-ideism*.

MOLL'S THEORY.

Dr. Albert Moll, of Berlin, attempts to explain the phenomena of hypnosis by seeking, like Bernheim, an analogy between them and those of normal life. There are, he says, two cardinal facts that we ought to keep in mind: (1) We are liable to be influenced by the ideas of others, and to accept as true statements which we ourselves have not investigated. (2) When a physiological or psychological effect is expected it has a tendency to appear.

The two facts just cited are sufficient, Moll thinks, to explain many of the phenomena of slight hypnosis. The increased susceptibility to suggestion evinced in this state, as the result of the subject's weakened volition, alone separates it from the ordinary waking condition. Moll does not believe that any analogy exists between slight hypnosis and sleep, for in the former there is neither loss of memory nor alteration in consciousness.

In order to explain the phenomena of deep hypnosis, in addition to the factors just referred to, Moll introduces a third, *i.e.* a *dream consciousness* similar to that which exists in natural sleep. He thinks the *positive* hallucinations of deep hypnosis are similar to those that occur in dreams, and that they are caused in the same manner by peripheral or central stimuli. The character of the dream aroused, the nature of the mental picture excited, by the *peripheral* stimulus, depends, in sleep as well as in hypnosis, upon the personality of the subject. The dividing line between sleep and hypnosis is merely a quantitative difference in the movements occurring in both : in hypnosis these are easily induced ; in sleep they are duller, slower, and rarer.

For the production of *negative* hallucinations, Moll considers that the three following factors are necessary :—

(a) The subject's conviction of the absence of an object or sensory impression.

According to Moll, if, in the waking state, we are convinced of the absence of something actually present, this belief tends to prevent our perceiving it. Thus, he says, if a man is working in some place which is generally quiet, and where he does not expect to hear a noise, he would not notice if one were made !!

In Moll's opinion, the hypnotised subject's conviction of the non-existence of an object or sensory impression arises in the following manner. The suggested idea cannot be supplanted by a voluntary one, for, owing to the alterations in the attention which result from the methods of the operator, the subject is unable to control the ideas conveyed to him or to put forward his own. External ideas dominate his consciousness. The conviction of the non-existence of an object arises from the subject's weakened will, and his dependence on the operator. The fact that many motor suggestions have already been made, which the subject has been unable to resist, renders further suggestions easy.

(*b*) Diversion of attention.

The diversion of the subject's attention follows the conviction of the non-existence of the object : he believes that no object is present, and, therefore, ceases to direct his attention to it.

(*c*) Dream consciousness.

Moll considers that the existence of a " dream consciousness " is also necessary for the explanation of negative hallucinations. In it not only do former memory-pictures reappear as hallucinations, but sensory impressions no longer, as in normal life, induce feelings or perceptions.

Moll explains the sudden and often nearly systematic forgetfulness, in reference to hypnotic states, by means of Max Dessoir's theory of the " *Doppel-Ich.*" He also considers that the punctual execution of post-hypnotic commands is only comprehensible if, in addition to the primary consciousness, *a secondary one works intelligently in us.*

To this theory the following objections might, I think, with justice be raised :—

(1) According to Moll, in light hypnosis there is a slight inhibition of the will, which becomes more profound in deep hypnosis. This point has already been referred to in discussing the so-called automatism and the influence of the operator ; and I have endeavoured to show that this inhibition of the will was not present in cases which I have personally observed. Further, in self-hypnosis, where the influence of the operator has been entirely eliminated, hypnotic phenomena can be readily induced.

(2) The objections which have already been raised to the supposed identity of normal and hypnotic sleep are equally

applicable to Moll's "dream-consciousness" theory. Sully's views as to the difference between the movements occurring in these conditions have already been referred to (p. 310).

(3) I know of no instance in which a dream has spontaneously arisen in the hypnotised subject as the result of a peripheral stimulus. It is true that subjects can be taught to exhibit various hypnotic phenomena in response to peripheral stimuli; but, as Moll himself has pointed out regarding the movements occurring in Heidenhain's cases, the subjects must first have a clear idea of what is expected of them.

(4) Moll assumes a loss of consciousness in deep hypnosis, on which he largely bases the supposed resemblance between that condition and normal sleep. Various objections to this view have been raised in discussing Heidenhain's theory: the hypnotic state is almost invariably a conscious one; and, though amnesia usually follows on awaking, it can be prevented by suggestion.

(5) The supposed analogy drawn from normal life, which Moll selects as an illustration of the way in which negative hallucinations arise—from the conviction of the absence of an object or sensory impression—is a peculiarly unfortunate one. A noise is not the less likely to be heard because of previous quietness: on the contrary, a particular noise would be less likely to be detected if it followed numerous others. Again, the cessation of a habitual noise, which we expect to be continued, does not on that account escape notice. When the screw of a steam-boat stops, this almost invariably arouses the attention of the passengers; and, even if they are asleep, it usually awakes them immediately.

(6) Moll's analogies drawn from normal life to explain hypnotic memory are somewhat strained. For example, in reference to the recollection in hypnosis of the events of previous hypnoses, he cites Max Dessoir's statement that he had heard of one person who once during sleep took up a dream at the point where he had left it off on the former night. Surely this is attempting to explain the little-known in terms of the less-known.

(7) To Moll's explanation of certain hypnotic phenomena by means of the "intelligent action of a secondary consciousness" I shall again refer. Meanwhile, I would point out that this does not agree with the "involuntary dream-consciousness theory"; the two explanations contradict each other.

2 A

Before describing this latest hypnotic theory—that which attempts to explain hypnotic phenomena by *the intelligent action of a secondary consciousness*—I wish to draw attention to the analogy which is supposed to exist between hypnosis and certain, and often widely differing, pathological conditions.

The Supposed Analogy between Hypnosis and certain, and often widely differing, Pathological Conditions.

As we shall presently see, Moll drew attention to the contradictory nature of these supposed analogies; but, nevertheless, a further illustration of them is to be found in "Hypnotism in Court," and "Hypnotism," two articles which appeared in the July and October numbers of the *Journal of Mental Science* for 1898. Both are apparently from the same pen, and as they are unsigned, I will, for convenience' sake, call the writer X.

According to X, hypnotism is related to hysteria, stupor, "látah," etc.

(I.) **Hysteria.**—As we have seen, the supposed connection between hypnotism and hysteria, disputed by Esdaile and Braid more than fifty years ago, was restated by the Salpêtrière school, and successfully disproved by that of Nancy. X's attempt to revive an ancient fallacy is not likely to be successful, especially as he does not support it by a single observed fact.

At the International Congress of Experimental Psychology, London, 1892, it was generally recognised that susceptibility to hypnosis did not indicate the existence of hysteria or any other morbid condition. Hypnotism was found to increase the patient's volition: thus hypnotic cure was due to the intensification of an entirely normal moral process, and was not essentially dependent upon assistance from without.

According to X, self-control is weakened in hypnosis. This view is an old mesmeric fallacy which was successfully exploded by Braid over fifty years ago. My subjects, no matter how deeply hypnotised, could always choose between suggestions, and invariably rejected what was distasteful.

X asserts that therapeusis admits the principle that a lower tissue may be sacrificed to save a higher, but that it is distinctly bad practice "to harm the higher organ to release the lower, as hypnotism does." This, however, concerns ordinary rather than hypnotic practice. Most of the diseases which are treated hypnotic-ally are central in their origin, as, for example, dipsomania, hysteria, obsessions, etc. In such cases it is the cure or relief of the higher organ which is at stake, and no sacrifice of any kind, either higher or lower, is involved. Lost or weakened self-control is at the root of the diseases just referred to; and, when hypnotism cures them, it does so by developing the patient's own volition.

If, however, we judge ordinary practice by X's standards, the administration of narcotics and anæsthetics must be condemned, and their employment for the relief of pain considered bad practice. His opinion, I think, is not now generally held by the profession, although, as we have seen, in 1842, Dr. Copland asserted, at the Royal Medical and Chirurgical Society, that "pain was a wise provision of nature, and patients ought to suffer pain while their surgeons were operating; they were all the better for it, and recovered better."

(II.) **Stupor.**—Stupor has been divided into two forms—(1) Anergic: (2) Delusional.

(1) *Anergic.*—In typical cases there is blueness and swelling of the hands and feet, slow and feeble circulation, vacant expression, retention (or in some cases incontinence) of urine and fæces; complete absence of mental function in the region of will, per-ception, memory, and often even of consciousness.

(2) *Delusional.* — This form is the outcome of profound melancholia, in which the mental activity is terminated by a melancholic delusion.

Stupor is supposed to be due to pathological changes in the brain and its blood-vessels: it is generally associated with grave disease, and frequently has a fatal termination (*Dictionary of Psychological Medicine*, Hack Tuke).

Here, again, X contents himself with simple assertion, and omits to adduce a single fact in support of the supposed connection between stupor and hypnosis. Hypnotised persons do not turn blue, nor do their hands and feet swell; they do not lose control over the bladder or bowels. Their volition is unimpaired, their perception and memory are often abnormally acute, and conscious-ness is rarely, if ever, lost. Hypnosis is not associated with profound melancholia, nor does it end in a cessation of mental activity. On the contrary, the hypnotised person may be able to solve mental problems of great difficulty which are beyond the range of his normal powers.   Again, stupor, unlike hypnosis, cannot be originated, guided, or terminated at will.   Further, hypnosis does not arise from pathological changes in the brain and its blood-vessels, nor has it a fatal termination.

(III.) **Látah.**—X talks of látah as if it were a disease, though, as Moll has pointed out, the word " látah " designates the sufferers from the complaint, not the disease itself; but this is a minor matter.   The disease, according to Gilles de la Tourette, is a " *tic* " characterised by certain abnormalities of movement, particularly by the imitation of gestures, and of certain anomalies of speech, such as the use of bad language and the repetition of the last words uttered in the patient's presence.   Bamberger states that violent contractions of the flexors and extensors of the muscles of the leg take place when the patient attempts to stand, and thus a jumping movement is produced.

According to Clifford and Talcott Williams, the condition is latent in the Malay race, and can be produced by startling them and making them jump.   They will then imitate actions which are painful, dangerous, or obscene.   The Malays are a race particular to a fault about all matters of personal modesty; but a látah Malay woman will strip naked in a public place at the casual invitation of a passing stranger.

In attempting to establish an analogy between hypnotism and " látah," X, as usual, states an old fallacy without adducing a single fact in support of it.   His theory is apparently a reproduction of that of Dr. Gillmore Ellis (*The Journal of Mental Science*, January, 1897, p. 32).   Neither writer seems to be aware of the fact that similar views were expressed at an earlier date by several Continental observers, and their unsoundness demonstrated by Moll and others.

The fallacy appears to have arisen from untrained and superficial observation.   Thus, it has been noticed that both the látah Malay and the hypnotised person imitate gestures ; the conditions, therefore, are assumed to be similar.   The circumstances, however, under which they do so are widely different.   The moment a " látah " is startled he will at once imitate any gesture made before him by any one.   He will also mimic the swaying motion of wind-shaken boughs as readily as the actions of a human being (Clifford).   No verbal suggestion is necessary.   On the other hand, hypnotised subjects never copy movements made before them unless they have been trained to do so, and then only the movements of the hypnotiser. Again, hypnotised persons, even despite energetic suggestions, will not imitate actions which involve real danger, actual indelicacy, or obscenity, nor do they make use of bad language. Further, the hypnotic subject, unlike the látah, does not hop about like a kangaroo the moment you startle him. Finally, hypnosis can be terminated at will, but the disease from which the látah suffers is uncontrollable and frequently incurable.

Other writers besides X have attempted to establish a connection between hypnosis and many and widely differing diseased conditions. In every instance the fallacy has been due to the imperfect observation of some isolated hypnotic phenomenon. Benedikt's theory is fairly characteristic of this class. In his view of hypnosis, its numerous, varied, and complex mental and physical conditions are ignored, and it is simply classified as an artificially induced catalepsy ; because in hypnosis the muscles can be rendered rigid by suggestion.

Such theories have the merit of simplicity, and possess the additional advantage that they can be made without careful observation or prolonged study. What should we think, however, of the observer who described normal human life as simply an artificially induced sneeze, because the act of sneezing could be readily evoked by the presentation of a pinch of snuff!

We can produce paralysis, stammering, or pain by suggestion, but hypnosis itself is none of these things. Moll points out that it is illogical to call hypnosis a disease because morbid imitations of it are to be found. Yawning itself is not a disease, although attacks of it occur which are morbid in character. Thus, we are no more justified in inferring that the hypnotised subject suffers from hysteria because he can imitate its symptoms, than in concluding that an actor is mad when he portrays insanity. Further, hypnosis—subject to the limitations already referred to—is entirely under the control of the operator, or of the subject himself ; but there is no disease which can be originated, guided, and terminated at a moment's notice.

Moll also draws attention to the fact that these physiological theories frequently contradict each other. Thus, Rieger and Conrad regard hypnosis as an artificial mania, while Meynert maintains that it is an experimentally produced imbecility—two

forms of mental disease which are utterly dissimilar. Semal and
Hack Tuke also called hypnosis an artificially induced insanity.
We might, says Moll, call hypnosis an insane condition, if we
also regarded sleep and dreams as such. When psychologists
wish to discover analogies to mental disorders they always have
recourse to dreams; but no one maintains that in order to lose
our sanity it is only necessary to go to sleep. Two conspicuous
characteristics of hypnosis are suggestibility and the fact that the
state can be terminated at will; but we do not find these united
in mental disorders or in neuroses. While physiologists fail to
consider what an enormous influence an idea, aroused, for
example, by the word "Awake!" exercises, their theories will
ever remain unsatisfactory. We ought, Moll continues, to set our
faces decidedly against the way in which certain physiologists
juggle with words, as if the enigmas of consciousness were child's
play to them. When Mendel, speaking of the phenomena of
hypnosis, explains that we have to do with a strong stimulation
of the cerebral cortex, and Ziemssen declares the exact contrary,
i.e. that the cerebral cortex is too little stimulated, and the sub-
cortical centres too much, we are startled at such contradictions,
and can only hope that in the future less will be asserted and
more proved.

THE SECONDARY OR SUBLIMINAL CONSCIOUSNESS THEORY.

Within recent times another theory has arisen. This, instead
of attempting to explain hypnotism by the arrested action of
some of the brain centres which subserve normal life, would do
so through the arousing of certain powers over which we normally
have little or no control. This theory appears under different
names, "Double Consciousness," "*Das Doppel-Ich*," etc., and the
principle on which it depends is largely admitted by science.
William James, for example, says: "In certain persons, at least,
the total possible consciousness may be split into parts which
coexist, but mutually ignore each other."
    The clearest statement of this view was given by the late
F. W. H. Myers; he suggested that the stream of consciousness
in which we habitually lived was not our only one. Possibly
our habitual consciousness might be a mere selection from a

✓multitude of thoughts and sensations—some at least equally conscious with those we empirically knew. No primacy was granted by this theory to the ordinary waking self, except that among potential selves it appeared the fittest to meet the needs of common life. As a rule, the waking life was remembered in hypnosis, and the hypnotic life forgotten in the waking state: this destroyed any claim of the primary memory to be the sole memory. The self below the *threshold* of ordinary consciousness Myers termed the "subliminal consciousness," and the empirical self of common experience the "supraliminal." He held that to the subliminal consciousness and memory a far wider range, both of physiological and of psychical activity, was open than to the supraliminal. The latter was inevitably limited by the need of concentration upon recollections useful in the struggle for existence; while the former included much that was too rudimentary to be retained in the supraliminal memory of an organism so advanced as that of man. The recollection of processes now performed automatically, and needing no supervision, passed out of the supraliminal memory, but might be retained by the subliminal. The subliminal, or hypnotic, self could exercise over the nervous, vaso-motor, and circulatory systems a degree of control unparalleled in waking life.

He suggested that the *spectrum of consciousness*, as he called it, was indefinitely extended at both ends in the subliminal self. Beyond its supraliminal physiological limit lay a vast number of complex processes belonging to the body's nutrition and well-being. These our remote ancestors[1] might possibly have been able to modify at will, but to us they seemed entirely withdrawn from our sphere of volition. If we wished to alter them we must do so by drugs and medicaments, whether the body to be treated was our own or another's.

At the superior or psychical end the subliminal memory included an unknown category of impressions, which the supra-liminal consciousness was incapable of receiving in any direct fashion, and which it must cognise, if at all, in the shape of messages from the subliminal consciousness. Myers arranged hypnotic phenomena into three divisions:—

---

[1] It is to be noted that Myers used the term "ancestors" somewhat loosely. It is not clear in the present instance whether he meant remote *human* ancestors, or some lower form of animal life.

(1) The Great Dissociative Triumph of Hypnotism, namely, the inhibition of pain under conditions of nerve and tissue with which it was usually inevitably connected.

Here, psychologically, the whole interest lay in the question whether pain was suppressed together with sensations of every kind, or whether other sensations persisted, pain alone being inhibited. Our ancestors,[1] Myers suggested, had already attained to a rough practical knowledge of this distinction. They knew that if you stunned a man by a blow he would not feel the pain for some time. Also, that if you ran pins into particular parts of a witch's body she, although perfectly awake and conscious of other sensations, would feel no smart.

The second of these discoveries was the more important. By stunning your enemy you only proved that vital functions could continue unimpaired, notwithstanding that the brain's action was so far disturbed that all consciousness was temporarily abolished. By pricking the witch in her " marks "—now called hysterical analgesic zones or patches—you proved that pain was a dissociable accident of organic injury ; that other sensations might persist, and that of pain alone be in some way inhibited. The insensitiveness to pain which ran wild in hysteria was now being directed into useful channels by " hypnotic suggestion." Some *intelligence* was involved in a suppression thus achieved ; for this was obtained, not, as with narcotics, by a general loss of consciousness, but by the selection and inhibition, from amongst all the percipient's possible sensations, of disagreeable ones alone. This was not a mere anæsthetisation of some particular group of nerve-endings, such as cocaine produced : it involved the removal also of a number of concomitant feelings of nausea, exhaustion, and anxiety, which were not always directly dependent on the principal pain, but needed, as it were, to be first subjectively distinguished as disagreeable before they were picked out for inhibition. This freedom from pain was obtained without either deadening or dislocating the general nervous system, with no approach either to coma or to hysteria. The so-called hypnotic trance was not necessary : sometimes the pain could be prevented by " post-hypnotic " suggestion destined to fulfil itself after the

[1] *I.e.* Comparatively recent human ancestors.

awakening; and, if there were trance, this was often no mere lethargy, but a state fully as alert and vivid as ordinary waking life.

Myers argued from this that it was plain that hypnotic analgesia thus induced was by no means a mere ordinary narcotic —not a fresh specimen of familiar methods for checking pain, by arresting all conscious cerebration. It was a new departure; the first successful attempt at dissociating forms of sensation which, throughout the known history of the human organism, had almost invariably been found to exist together.

(2) **The Associative or Synthetic Triumphs of Hypnotism, namely, the production and control of organic processes which no effort of the ordinary man could set going or in any way influence.**

Hypnotic analgesia, Myers said, might be classed with equal justice as a dissociative or as an associative act. The sensations were severed from the main supraliminal current, and thus far the act was dissociative. The group itself, however, had to be formed, and the more complex it was the more this involved some associative act. Inhibition of all the pain consequent on an operation was in reality a complicated associative process. It involved (*a*) the singling out and fitting together of a great number of sensations which had the one subjective bond of being disagreeable; and (*b*) the inhibition of all of them, which thus left the supraliminal consciousness in perfect ease.

In further illustration of the associative powers of hypnotism, Myers referred to alterations in the pulse, the secretions, excretions, etc.; he also cited Delbœuf's case of two symmetrical burns on the same subject, one of which ran the ordinary course of inflammation, while in the other the morbid action was arrested by suggestion (p. 84).

(3) **The Intellectual or Moral Achievements of Hypnotism.**

These, like the others, were based upon physiological changes, but presented problems still more profound. The removal of the craving for alcohol and morphia, the cure of kleptomania, bad temper, excessive indolence, etc., were all cited by Myers as illustrating the moral and psychological changes which suggestion could effect.

Volition, etc.—According to Myers, the hypnotic subject was not a maimed and stunted normal individual, but one who, while he had gained increased power over his own organism, had not at the same time lost his volition, or the mental and moral qualities which had formerly distinguished him. He admitted that there was some difficulty in explaining hypnotic obedience; but held—justly, as we have seen—that this would be refused when the act suggested was contrary to the subject's moral nature. He believed that a complete comprehension of the suggested act existed in the subliminal strata, and that, when great need arose, the subliminal self would generally avoid compliance, not necessarily by awakening the organism into ordinary life, but by plunging it into a hysterical access or into a trance so deep that the unwelcome order lost its agitating power. The moral tone of the somnambule was, in Myers' opinion, the precise opposite of the drunken condition. Alcohol, by paralysing first the higher inhibitory centres, made men boastful, impure, and quarrelsome. Hypnotisation, apparently by a tendency to paralyse lower appetitive centres, produced the contrary effect. The increased refinement and cheerfulness of the developed somnambule were constantly noticed.

The Possible Source or Origin of Hypnotic Control over Intimate Organic Processes.

Myers asked whether we could find anything in our ancestry which suggested to us these internal powers of modifying circulation, quickening cell-proliferation, and altering trophic processes in unknown ways. He admitted that the analogies to which we could appeal were vague and remote, yet he said we could point to the general fact that, in man and the higher animals, an increase in the power of modifying the action of the organism, as a whole, had evidently been purchased by a decrease in the power of modifying its internal parts or constituent elements. The self-shaping powers of the amœba, the self-regenerating powers of the worm or crab, died gradually away into the comparative fixity of the organism of the higher mammalia.

It was possible, he thought, that this fixity was more apparent than real. "We may," he said, "regard the human organism as an aggregation of primitive, unicellular organisms, which have divided their functions and complicated their union in response to the demands of the environment, and along such lines of evolution as were possible to the original germ. It is possible, too, that all these processes—beginning with the amœboid movements of the primitive cell—were accompanied by a capacity of retaining the impress of previous excitations, a rudimentary memory which at first constituted all the consciousness which our lowly ancestors [1] possessed. And further, as evolution went on, and more complex operations were developed, while the primitive processes of cell-change became stereotyped by long heredity, the memory which represented these earlier changes sank to a low psychical depth, became subliminal, and could no longer be summoned by voluntary effort into the supraliminal sequence of conscious states. How do we know that any psychical acquisition is ever wholly lost? or even that a memory is the weaker because it has sunk out of voluntary control? It may be possible, by appropriate artifices, to recall primeval memories, and to set in motion any physiological process which could at any moment of our ancestral history have been purposely, however blindly, performed."

In justice to Myers, however, it must be admitted that he was doubtful whether all hypnotic phenomena could be explained by the above theory. Thus, he asked: Do not the moral and psychological achievements of hypnosis represent a point *beyond* that to which such analogies can carry us? These changes must, he said, of course, rest on a physiological basis; but that basis implies a well-developed human brain. The knowledge of cortical centres, which must somewhere exist to make such changes possible, can scarcely have been inherited from pre-human ancestors. Nothing, perhaps, in the whole inquiry is of deeper interest than the possibilities thus dawning upon us of disentangling, from the cerebral labyrinth which represents a man's tastes and character, the special brain processes which stand for some special temptation—say, those which represent the reaction of his organism to alcohol. What is the hidden process that to one patient makes brandy as nauseating as it is to a cat—that in another patient makes the morphia craving as impossible as it is to a rabbit?

[1] *I.e.* the original germs of evolution.

Hysteria, a Disease of the Subliminal Self.

Myers did not consider the subliminal self free from disturbance and disease any more than the supraliminal. Subliminal disturbances, he said, were likely to arise and make themselves felt in the supraliminal being. "How shall we distinguish," he asked, "these subterranean from the superficial storms? How shall we recognise, for instance, a disturbance of the 'hypnotic stratum'—as we may style, for convenience' sake, that group of potential perceptions and reactions which are readily evoked in a suitable subject by the hypnotic trance? It would be absurd to attempt to explain *ignotum per ignotius*, the ætiology of disease by its relation to hypothetical strata of the subliminal self. But one remark I must make, since, crude as it may be, it offers at least a chance of light upon a subject at present hopelessly confused.

"I say, then, that our most plausible conception of a morbid disturbance of the hypnotic self is a derangement of functions or capacities which are habitually observed in the hypnotic state, and in that alone. I should say that the reason for so referring the source of such derangement would be increased if the subject were, when hypnotised, aware of the exciting external cause of such derangements, and capable of modifying them in a way impossible to him in waking life.

"Now it is a striking characteristic of the hypnotic self that it can exercise over the nervous, the vaso-motor, the circulatory systems a degree of control unparalleled in waking life. . . . Are we aware in practice of any malady or group of maladies in which these functions, these capacities, are the subject of special disturbances? Are there anæsthesiæ appearing, shifting, and disappearing as rapidly as the suggested anæsthesia of hypnotism? Are there anomalous vaso-motor disturbances which seem to follow the patient's mere caprice?

"The reader will answer with the word *hysteria*. And, meaningless or misleading though that term be, it is in fact our first and obvious reply. Not indeed all, but almost all, the phenomena which can be induced by suggestion in the hypnotic state occur spontaneously in hysterical patients.

"But this will not complete our answer. From the point

of view of our present analogy, the *differentia* of hysteria will be simply an irrational self-suggestion in regions beyond the power of the waking will—a morbid or uncontrolled functioning of powers over the organism which affect profounder modifications than the empirical self can parallel. Thus the production of patches of anæsthesia or analgesia is a characteristically hysterical symptom, and it implies a power of modifying the sensibility to touch or pain which we cannot imitate under ordinary conditions."

"But when hysteria is thus regarded, it is seen that several other maladies fall under the same category; '*attaques de sommeil*,' 'association - neuroses,' '*Zwangsvorstellungen*,' and a host of monomanias, show a similarly morbid functioning of precisely that class of powers which hypnotism exhibits to us in harmless or beneficent operation. They are self-suggestions of an irrational and hurtful kind. They are diseases of the hypnotic stratum. Hypnotism is not a morbid state; it is the manifestation of a group of perfectly normal, but habitually subjacent powers whose beneficent operation we see in cures by therapeutic suggestion, whose neutral operation we see in ordinary hypnotic experiment, and whose diseased operation we see in the vast variety of *self-suggestive* maladies.

"I would offer this view to the consideration of those who justly realise the close connection between hypnotism and hysterical phenomena, but mistakenly endeavour to force all the hypnotic phenomena into the hysterical category.

"M. Babinski, for instance, argues as follows on behalf of the Salpêtrière view that all hypnotic subjects are hysterical. The Nancy subjects, he says, although asserted by Nancy doctors to be non-hysterical, yet show in the hypnotic trance phenomena which we observe elsewhere in hysteria alone. For that reason they must, in effect, be hysterical. This, surely, is to reason in a somewhat obvious circle; and those who, with the great majority of competent judges, are convinced that non-hysterical persons may most assuredly be nevertheless hypnotisable, must seek some other explanation for the similarity of phenomena in the two states. That explanation I have here attempted to give by suggesting that hysteria (and many cognate troubles) should rather be said to fall under hypnotism, than hypnotism under hysteria. Those self-suggestive troubles exhibit the disordered working of a stratum of the self which is *per se* as normal and as essential to man's completeness as any other, and which surpasses the superficial stratum in the degree of power which the will informing it can exercise over the organism."

To those who, without stigmatising either hypnotism or subliminal manifestations in general as necessarily *morbid*, are yet disposed to style them *abnormal*, and to regard them as a mere curiosity, which can never be closely inwrought with human progress, Myers had a further word to say.

The "normal" man was likely, he thought, to become as question-begging an individual in physiological as the "natural man" in theological treatises. What *is* man's nature and what *is* man's "norm"? If the question were asked in regard to some lower animal type the answer would be a comparatively easy one. But man's end and aim are not so simple as a rabbit's; he must choose between ideals; he must pursue the higher objects, even to some sacrifice of the lower. Thus we should hesitate to assume that Brigham Young had fulfilled man's end and aim more successfully than Sir Isaac Newton.

Myers suggested that psychological experiment was still at much the same point as was medical experiment in the days of Hippocrates; that though we attempted to describe and analyse the psychical nature with which we had to deal, we had scarcely yet invented any instruments for probing or artifices for modifying it. Not only so, but the very idea of trying to modify our psychical selves by deliberate scientific experiment was as foreign and unacceptable to most men, as the idea of modifying his death-rate by sanitation was to the African savage.

Just as the scientific discoveries of such men as Pasteur and Lister had increased our power of checking or curing disease from the physical side, in a manner and to an extent which was not dreamt of by the earlier physicians, so Myers thought it was possible that in hypnotism we might find a somewhat similar power of influencing psychical conditions.

After criticising adversely the theories of Mesmer, Heidenhain, Charcot, Bernheim, and others, Myers said :—" It is, therefore, as it seems to me, in a field almost clear of hypothesis that I suggest my view that a stream of consciousness flows on within us, at a level beneath the threshold of ordinary waking life, and that this consciousness embraces unknown powers, of which these hypnotic phenomena give us the first sample."

THEORY OF THE LATE PROFESSOR DELBŒUF.

In many respects Delbœuf's views closely resembled those of Myers. Thus, Delbœuf believed that suggestion was not only capable of inhibiting sensations of pain intimately associated with organic injury, and of modifying or arresting various morbid nervous conditions which arose more or less directly from it; but was also capable of influencing the organic changes which, under ordinary circumstances, would have resulted from the injury itself. In support of this theory, he cited numerous interesting cases, of which the following are examples :—

One of his subjects had her fingers accidentally severely crushed; suggestion at once stopped the pain, and the healing process was exceptionally rapid. Another subject had a considerable portion of her thumb cut off. The following day, after a sleepless and painful night, she was unable to use her hand. Suggestion entirely removed the pain, and the wound healed with unusual rapidity.

On June 15th, 1886, a strong young peasant woman was shot in the back with a revolver. All attempts to extract the bullet failed; and during several days her recovery seemed more than doubtful. When Delbœuf saw her, on June 26th, all immediate danger had disappeared; but she was extremely feeble, and could hardly sit up for half an hour a day in an arm-chair. She had frequent attacks of shivering, followed by profuse perspiration. She could only take liquid nourishment, and this was rarely retained. She also suffered greatly from insomnia, and from persistent pain in the abdomen. The bowels were constipated, and defecation and micturition were painful. The wound was kept open with antiseptic dressings. She was hypnotised on June 26th, and the process was repeated the following day. Improvement was immediate and marked: she was able to retain solid food, pain disappeared, and the action of the bladder and bowels became normal. By June 30th, she was able to stand and walk, and to do light work, such as sewing or knitting. A few days later, she was again hypnotised, and at once recommenced

her ordinary domestic occupations. The wound healed rapidly
and she shortly afterwards took another situation. There was no
relapse.

Delbœuf's most striking case, that of the two symmetrical
burns, has already been described (p. 84).

In Delbœuf's opinion, the persistent belief that one was
suffering from disease might sometimes ultimately cause disease;
and, in the same way, the conviction that a morbid condition did
not exist might contribute to its disappearance. He considered
that the organic changes that followed such an injury as we
have described in the case of J. (p. 84) were not alone due to
the injury itself, but were also partly caused by the subject's
consciousness of pain. The absence or presence of pain might, to a
greater or lesser extent, influence vaso-motor conditions. On the
one hand, organic injury, unassociated with pain, might not be
followed by congestion, inflammation, or suppuration; while in an
identical injury, accompanied by pain, these conditions might be
present. The consciousness of pain, in addition to being sometimes responsible for morbid changes at the site of injury, might
also help to spread them to other parts more or less remote; and
thus, when pain was removed or relieved, this really meant the
disappearance or decrease of one of the factors in the organic
malady.

According to Delbœuf, experiments like these led us to suppose that the action of the moral on the physical might be almost,
if not quite, equal to that of the physical on the moral. Hence
it followed that the idea of absence of mischief might bring
about, or at least favour, a cure. How, asked Delbœuf, are we to
explain the mechanism of this inverse action of the moral on the
physical? The action of organs which are dependent upon the
sympathetic system cannot be modified voluntarily by the will;
the unstriped muscles, the vaso-motors, the glands, act without
the intervention of the cerebral hemispheres.

The following was his explanation: In the lower forms of life
the animal was just as conscious of what was taking place in its
interior as it was of what was happening at its periphery. With
the progress of development, however, its attention would be
directed more or less exclusively, on the one hand, to the organs
which placed it in direct relationship with the external world,
and warned it of the passing of outside events of importance to

its existence and well-being; on the other, to the means of attack or defence, which it learnt to use from day to day with greater certainty and vigour. At the same time, the cares of the interior would be got rid of more and more completely, and would be confided to a servant who had been trained to look after them, and whose zeal could be depended upon. In a highly developed animal such as man, the importance of conscious life distracted the attention from the phenomena of vegetative life : the continual obligation to provide for the necessities of existence absorbed the will, while the mechanical regularity with which internal organs acted rendered conscious attention regarding them unnecessary. In ordinary life our attention was mainly concentrated on the external world, the principal source of our pleasures and our pains ; and our will was devoted to perfecting our means of attack and defence. The rapid changes of external phenomena masked the regularity of internal phenomena, which took place habitually without our knowledge. The care of the vegetative life had been handed over by the will to nervous mechanisms which had learnt to regulate themselves, and which in general fulfilled their task to perfection. Sometimes the machine went wrong, and intervention became desirable. The power which formerly voluntarily regulated it had, however, dropped out of the normal consciousness; and, if we desired to find a substitute for it, we must turn to hypnotism. In the hypnotic state the mind was in part drawn aside from the life of relation, while at the same time it preserved its activity and power. Voluntary attention could be abstracted from the outer world, and directed with full force upon a single point ; and thus the hypnotic subconsciousness was able to put in movement machinery which the normal consciousness had lost sight of and ceased to regulate. It might then be able to act, not only on the reflexes, but on the vaso-motor system, on the unstriped muscles, on the apparatus of secretion, etc. If a contrary opinion had till now prevailed, this was because observation had been exclusively directed to the normal exercise of the will. The will could, however, in the hypnotic state, regulate movements which had become irregular, and assist in the repair of organic injury. In a word, hypnotism did not depress, but exalted the will, by permitting it to concentrate itself upon the point where disorder was threatened.

2 B

THEORY OF PROFESSOR BEAUNIS.

Somewhat similar views are also expressed by Professor Beaunis. The cerebral activity, at a given instant, he says, represents a collection of sensations, ideas, and memories. Of those some alone become sufficiently conscious to enable us to perceive them clearly and precisely, while the remainder pass without leaving durable traces. In a series of cerebral acts a certain number of intermediate links frequently escape us, and it is probable that the greater number of mental phenomena take place without our knowledge. Sensations to which we do not pay any attention may nevertheless excite cerebral action, and originate, without our knowledge, ideas and movements of which we afterwards become conscious. Our brain acts without our knowledge, with an activity of which we are unable to form an idea ; and the facts of consciousness are only feeble fugitives from this mysterious work. Hypnotic phenomena, Beaunis thinks, afford examples of this subconscious cerebration.

Beaunis' description of subconscious mental activity so closely resembles the theories of the late Professor W. B. Carpenter that I now give an account of these, in justice to the earlier writer.

CARPENTER'S UNCONSCIOUS CEREBRATION.

According to Carpenter, much of our intellectual activity—both reasoning and imaginative—was essentially *automatic*, and might be described physiologically as the *reflex action of the Cerebrum*. There was, he said, a further question, namely, whether this action might not take place *unconsciously*. The view had been held by German metaphysicians, from Leibnitz onwards, that the mind might undergo modifications, without being itself conscious of the process until the *results* presented themselves to the consciousness, in the new ideas, or new combinations of ideas, which the process had evolved. This "Unconscious Cerebration," taking place in the higher sphere of cerebral activity, had its exact parallel in such automatic acts as those of walking, when the latter occurred while the attention was uninterruptedly diverted from them.

Each of the nervous centres had an independent "reflex" activity of its own, sometimes "primary" or "original," sometimes "secondary" or "acquired"; while our *consciousness* of its exercise depended upon the impression which it made upon the Sensorium, which was the instrument alike of the external and of the internal senses. Regarding, therefore, all the automatic operations of the mind as "reflex actions" of the Cerebrum, there was no more difficulty in comprehending that such reflex actions might proceed without our knowledge—their results being evolved as *intellectual products*, when we became conscious of the impressions transmitted along the "nerves of the internal senses" from the Cerebrum to the Sensorium—than there was in understanding that impressions might excite muscular movements through the "reflex" power of the Spinal Cord, without the necessary intervention of sensation. "In both instances," Carpenter said, "the condition of this mode of unconscious operation was that the *receptivity* of the Sensorium should be suspended *quoad* the changes in question, either by its own functional inactivity, or through its temporary engrossment by other impressions."

As an example of this form of unconscious mental activity, Carpenter cited the *spontaneous* remembrance of some name, phrase, occurrence, etc., which we had been previously vainly trying to recollect. It was important to note, he said, that the lost name suddenly flashed into our consciousness, either when we were thinking of something altogether different, or when we had just awakened out of profound sleep. In the first case the mind might have been entirely engrossed in the meantime by some quite different subject of contemplation, and we could not detect any link of association whereby the result had been obtained, notwithstanding that the whole "train of thought" which had passed through the mind in the interval might be most distinctly remembered. In the second case, the missing idea seemed more likely to present itself when the sleep had been profound than when it had been disturbed.

Carpenter cited various authorities and examples in illustration of the above phenomenon. Of these the following are the more interesting: Miss Cobbe said we often "ransack our brains" to find some lost name, etc., and, failing to do so, we at last turn our attention to other matters. By and by, when, so far as consciousness goes, our whole minds are absorbed in a

different topic, we exclaim, "*Eureka!* the word was so and so."
So familiar is this phenomenon, that we are accustomed in
similar straits to say, "Never mind; I shall think of the missing
word by and by, when I am attending to something else"; and
we deliberately turn away, just as if we possessed an obedient
secretary whom we could order to hunt up the missing word
while we occupied ourselves with something else. The more
this common phenomenon is studied, the more the observer of
his own mental processes will be obliged to concede, that, so
far as his own conscious self is concerned, the research is
made absolutely *without him.* He has neither pain, pleasure,
nor sense of labour in the task, and his conscious self is
all the time suffering, enjoying, or labouring on totally different
ground.

In speaking of the same phenomenon, the late Dr. Oliver
Wendell Holmes said the idea we were seeking comes all at once
into the mind, delivered like a prepaid parcel laid at the door of
consciousness, like a foundling in a basket. How it came there,
we do not know. The mind must have been at work, groping
and feeling for it in the dark; it cannot have come by itself.
Yet, all the while, our consciousness, *so far as we were conscious of
our consciousness,* was busy with other thoughts.

Carpenter said that he was in the habit of trusting to this
method of recollection. He found he was much more likely to
recover lost memories in this way, by withdrawing his mind from
the search when it was not quickly successful. It was better to
give himself up to some other occupation, rather than to induce
mental fatigue by continued unsuccessful efforts.

In further confirmation of the above theory, Carpenter cited
the phenomena observed with "talking tables" and "planchettes."
Here, ideas which had passed out of the *conscious* memory sometimes expressed themselves in *involuntary muscular movements,* to
the great surprise of the individuals executing them. Generally
the answers given in this way only expressed the ideas consciously
present to the minds of the operators. True answers were, however, sometimes given to questions as to matters of fact, notwithstanding that there might be entire ignorance (proceeding from
complete forgetfulness) of those facts, or absolute disbelief in the
statement of them. These results, which were falsely attributed
to "spiritual" agency, were really due to the revival of lost

impressions, which now disclosed their existence through the automatic motor apparatus.

Carpenter also asserted that there were cases in which two distinct trains of mental action were carried on simultaneously— one *consciously*, the other *unconsciously;* the latter guided the movements, which might express something quite unrelated to the subject that was *entirely* and *continuously* engrossing the attention. In support of this he quoted the following passage from Miss Cobbe :—

"Music-playing is of all others the most extraordinary manifestation of the powers of unconscious cerebration. Here we seem not to have one slave, but a dozen. Two different lines of hieroglyphics have to be read at once, and the right hand has to be guided to attend to one of them, the left to another. All the ten fingers have their work assigned as quickly as they can move. The mind, or something which does duty as mind, interprets scores of A sharps and B flats and C naturals into black ivory keys and white ones, crotchets and quavers and demi-semiquavers, rests, and all the other mysteries of music. The feet are not idle, but have something to do with the pedals, and, if the instrument be a double-action harp (or an organ), a task of pushings and pullings more difficult than that of the hands. And all this time the performer, the *conscious* performer, is in a seventh heaven of artistic rapture at the results of all this tremendous business, or perchance lost in a flirtation with the individual who turns the leaves of the music-book."

Carpenter also received from a distinguished prelate the following account of his own frequently repeated experience of another form of unconscious cerebration :—

"I have for years been accustomed to act upon your principle of 'Unconscious Cerebration,' with very satisfactory results. I am frequently asked, as you may suppose, to preach *occasional* sermons; and when I have undertaken any such duty, I am in the habit of setting down and thinking over the topics I wish to introduce, without in the first instance endeavouring to frame them into any consistent scheme. I then put aside my sketch for a time, and give my mind to some *altogether different subject ;* and when I come to write my sermon, perhaps a week or two afterwards, I very commonly find that the topics I set down have *arranged themselves,* so that I can at once apply myself to develop them on the plan in which they present themselves before me."

In the following example, given by Wendell Holmes, the individual was *conscious of the flow of an undercurrent* of mental action, although this did not rise to the level of distinct ideation :—
A business man, who had an important question under consideration, gave it up for the time as too much for him. Immediately after having done so he was conscious of an action going on in his brain, which was so unusual and painful as to excite his apprehensions that he was threatened with paralysis, or something of that sort. After some hours of this uneasiness, his perplexity was all at once cleared up by the solution of his doubts coming to him—worked out, as he believed, in that obscure and troubled interval.

According to Wendell Holmes, it is doubtful whether the persons who think most—that is, have most conscious thought pass through their minds—do most mental work. The tree you plant, he said, grows while you are sleeping. So with every new idea that is planted in a real thinker's brain : it will be growing when he is least conscious of it. An idea in the brain is not a legend carved on a marble slab : it is an impression made on a living tissue, which is the seat of active nutritive processes. Shall the initials I carved in bark increase from year to year with the tree, he asked, and shall not my recorded thought develop into new forms and relations with my growing brain ?

Carpenter believed that the same mode of unconscious action had a large share in the process of *invention*, whether artistic or poetical, scientific or mechanical. When inventors were brought to a stand by some difficulty, the tangle was more likely to unravel itself if the attention was completely withdrawn from it, than by any amount of continued effort. They kept the desired result strongly before their attention in the first instance, just as we did when we tried to recollect something we had forgotten, by thinking of everything likely to lead to it; but, if they did not succeed, they then put the problem aside for a time, and gave their minds to something else. Later, just what they wanted " came into their heads."

Remarks.—The " subliminal " or " secondary consciousness " theory presents many points for consideration; of these the following are the more important :—

(I.) The Hypnotic Powers and the Conditions more immediately associated with them.

The special point of interest in the cases cited as illustrating the powers of the hypnotic state is the supposed mental condition of the subject. The immediate origin of hypnotic phenomena depended, according to Myers, upon a *voluntary* alteration in the arrangements of ideas. The introduction of the term *voluntary*, with, at the same time, the recognition that all the subject's attention was not requisite for the production of any solitary hypnotic phenomenon, formed an important distinction between this theory and some of those we have already considered.

With regard to Bernheim's theory, when discussing those of the Nancy school, I raised the following, amongst other, objections :—

(a) The hypnotic condition cannot be called one of mono-ideism, because many phenomena can be evoked at the same time.

(b) It cannot be explained by the concentration of the attention upon a single point, because, again, many phenomena can be evoked simultaneously.

(c) It is not due to arrested or impaired volition, as we have shown (1) that the subject can resist the suggestions of the operator; and (2) he can in cases of self-hypnosis voluntarily create the phenomena for himself.

(d) It cannot be explained by "suggestion" alone, as this was merely the artifice used to excite the phenomena.

Despite these objections, one must admit that certain of the phenomena described by Myers, which are also cited by others as illustrating the theory of monoideism, possess one important point in common, namely, a change in the arrangement of ideas. If, for example, a hypnotised subject, supposed to be under the influence of his operator, sees a hallucinatory cat, and a self-hypnotised subject successfully suggests one to himself, the phenomenon is practically identical in both instances. The only difference is the explanation of its origin. Bennett believed that the hypnotised subject saw a hallucinatory cat because the genesis of his ideas was not interfered with, but only their voluntary synthesis. Thus, the operator was able to suggest the remembrance of a cat; but the subject, owing to the involuntary arrest of certain mental powers, failed to understand that it was only a remembrance, and believed in its reality. In Myers' opinion, the subject, instead of having lost the power of voluntary synthesis of ideas, had acquired an increased power of voluntary association and dissociation of ideas. The remembrance of the image of a cat had received hallucinatory vividness, not because the subject was unable to check it from lack of voluntary synthesis of ideas, but because he had elected to allow it to become vivid by voluntarily inhibiting the appearance of all ideas which would have interfered with its clearness, while, at the same time, he had associated with it ideas connected with the remembrance of formerly seen cats.

Bernheim, as we have seen, attempted to explain the phenomena of hypnosis by the *involuntary* concentration of the attention on one point. According to Myers, the mental changes which took place were not only voluntary but varied ones; and thus, if the phenomena were due to the subject's attention, he must have acquired the power not only of turning it upon one point, but upon several points simultaneously.

The inhibition of sensory impressions in hypnosis presents a certain analogy to what is found in the normal state. The student at his books, who wishes to carry on his work without disturbance, may gradually train himself to be unconscious of external sounds. He teaches his attention to concentrate itself upon the problem before him, and to disregard more and more the noises which might distract him. So also, in looking into a microscope with one eye, he may train himself to keep the other eye open, and at the same time to become unconscious of the objects within its field of vision. Here, both the hypnotised and non-hypnotised subject are producing voluntary changes in their attention. Important points of difference, however, exist between the two.

(1) The student does not disregard auditory or visual impressions the first time he tries to do so. On the contrary, prolonged training is often necessary for him to obtain this power; and frequently he is unable to acquire it. In the deeply hypnotised subject, on the other hand, the power can be developed by a single suggestion, and with almost absolute certainty.

(2) In the normal subject the inhibition of the sensory impressions is associated with concentration of the attention upon something else. The moment the student closes his books he

becomes conscious, for example, of the organ-grinder under his window, of whose presence he was ignorant a moment before. The instant the attention ceases to be directed to the object under the microscope, the brain becomes conscious of the impressions received through the other eye. With the hypnotised subject the condition of the attention is extremely variable. You may find absence of painful sensations at the very moment that you direct the subject's attention to the fact that you are piercing his flesh deeply with a needle. Again, you may find increased sensory perceptions of the two points of a compass, when you have engaged his attention in the attempted solution of a mental problem. This inhibition of sensory impressions by the normal subject might, perhaps, be justly regarded as an acquired automatic act, but it is an automatism which only acts properly when the attention is voluntarily concentrated on something else. At first the student's attention must have been consciously divided between the problem contained in his book, and the process of inhibiting the sensory impressions. In the hypnotised subject, the inhibitory act, seeing that it has been performed without previous training, cannot be regarded as completely analogous to the acquired automatic inhibitory act of the normal subject. It can also be performed without conscious concentration of all the attention in another direction. We must not conclude, however, that the hypnotic act is not associated with a concentration of *some* of the attention, merely because (a) the subject is attending to something else at the same time, and (b) because he is not conscious of attending to the particular act itself. It is possible that the hypnotic act may have been performed by means of a subconscious concentration of attention, which existed in some lower hypnotic substratum of the personality.

(II.) Moral and Volitional Conditions.

The views of Myers practically agree with those I have expressed in discussing the question of so-called automatism. I have rarely, however, myself seen subjects try to escape objectionable commands in the manner in which he described it, although several instances of this kind have been recorded by Professor Beaunis and others. In one of these cases the subject refused to awake after a disagreeable post-hypnotic suggestion had been given. Another, under similar circumstances, rather than fulfil the suggestion, passed from the "alert" to the "deep" stage of hypnosis.

(III.) Hysteria.

Myers' theory that hysteria is a disease of the hypnotic substratum is an extremely ingenious one, and is the only reasonable explanation of the resemblance between certain hypnotic and hysterical phenomena with which I am acquainted. As we have seen, those who believed that hypnosis and hysteria were identical stated that the hysterical alone could be hypnotised. On the other hand, those with wider experience have successfully demonstrated that the hysterical are generally, if not invariably, the most difficult to influence. Of this fact Myers' theory possibly affords an explanation. May not the difficulty of inducing hypnosis in the hysterical—of making one's suggestions find a resting-place in them—be due to the fact that the hypnotic substratum of their personality is already occupied by irrational self-suggestions which their waking will cannot control?

(IV.) The Evidence for the Existence of a Subliminal Consciousness.

The subliminal consciousness theory is so interesting and important that I propose to refer at some length to the phenomena that might be cited as evidence in its favour; and also to discuss the attempts to explain these phenomena in other ways. Before doing so, however, I wish to draw particular attention to one extremely important point—namely, the varying significance given to the term "secondary consciousness" by different authorities. Thus, some regard the condition simply as a substratum of the personality; while others consider the phenomena to be so striking and distinct as to entitle them to be considered as forming a secondary *personality*. The former view is the one I hold, and I propose later to give my reasons for adopting it.

The facts in favour of the existence of a secondary consciousness may be divided into three groups :—(*a*) Those arising from, or more or less closely associated with, morbid states. (*b*) Those occurring in normal waking or sleeping life. (*c*) Those arising spontaneously, or as the result of suggestion, in the hypnotic condition.

(*a*) Phenomena arising from, or more or less closely associated with, Morbid States.

To those who have not studied hypnotic phenomena this group is practically the only one that is recognised. The cases comprised under it differ widely. At its lower end, so to speak, are included those in which the patients, after a seizure of some sort, perform certain acts of which their ordinary consciousness is ignorant. These vary from purposeless automatic acts to thefts committed with more or less skill or cunning, and, apparently, are neither recalled in the normal state nor in subsequent attacks. At the highest end of the group we find Félida X,[1] whose case differs in many respects from these. Indeed, it is doubtful whether many of the former can be justly cited as cases of double consciousness, and this point will be again referred to, when summarising and contrasting the different groups.

The following are illustrative cases :—

(1) Louis V.—This young man presented two distinct states, differing from each other mentally, morally, and physically. In the primary state he was docile and intelligent, while sensibility and movement were normal. In the secondary he was violent, vicious, and less intelligent; and presented hysterical contractures. Each state was completely independent of the other, and possessed absolutely distinct memories. ("The Life History of a Case of Double or Multiple Personality," by A. T. Myers, M.D., *Journal of Mental Science*, January, 1886; "Les Variations de la Personnalité," par MM. Bourru et Burot, *Revue de l'Hypnotisme*, 1887, p. 193.)

(2) Dr. Rieger (*Der Hypnotismus*, 1884, pp. 109-115) cites a case of frequently recurring attacks of secondary consciousness in an epileptic. In the normal condition his character was orderly; but this state alternated with others during which he would leave his house for weeks at a time, and lead the life of a thief and

[1] Pp. 385-6.

vagabond; sometimes being sent to prison, sometimes to asylums. In his primary condition he had no memory of the acts for which he had been punished.

(3) Dr. Lewis C. Bruce (*Brain*, 1895, vol. xviii. p. 54) gives an account of an asylum patient who not only showed two separate and distinct states of consciousness, but in whom also the right and left brain alternately exerted a preponderating influence over the motor functions. At one time he was ambidextrous and only understood English, at another he was left-handed and spoke Welsh.

The account of the following case is condensed from the notes supplied me by Dr. Albert Wilson, of Leytonstone, who also kindly permitted me to see the patient :—

(4) Mary W., born October, 1882, had, in April, 1895, an attack of meningitis associated with influenza. During the third and fourth weeks of the illness there was high temperature with delirium bordering on mania; and she called people snakes and did not recognise her friends. In the fifth week, during convalescence, her character changed; and she began to give those around her names which were not their own : thus, her father was " Tom "; her mother, " Mary Ann," etc. About the sixth week attacks of secondary consciousness appeared; the patient would suddenly turn a somersault on the bed, and then assume a new character—returning suddenly to the normal and resuming what she had been occupied with before the attack. At first the seizures lasted from ten to fifty minutes, but increased to hours, days, and weeks as the time went on. The secondary self knew nothing of the primary one, and *vice versâ ;* further, the secondary self had apparently lost much of the knowledge the primary self had acquired. Thus, in the second state the patient did not know what her legs and arms were, and was childish in her talk. She could write her name, however, but this she did backwards, beginning at the tail of the last letter and writing quickly from right to left—not mirror-writing.

After a few months the periods of normal life became shorter, and in place of one secondary stage various others showed themselves from time to time. Of these there were sixteen in all, termed by Dr. Wilson stages *a, b, c, d,* etc. In each stage the patient remembered what had happened during previous attacks of the same stage, but knew nothing of what had occurred in any of the other stages; while the primary consciousness remembered events in the normal life alone, and knew nothing regarding the incidents which happened in any of the numerous other stages.

At the end of a year the normal condition rarely appeared, and then only as a flash—sometimes coming to the surface for five or ten minutes, sometimes only for a few seconds.

The following states were noted, most of them being named by the patient herself:—

(*a*) The patient called herself "Thing"; she was vacant, knew nothing of her past life, and could not stand.

(*b*) Called herself "Old Nick," and was passionate and mischievous.

(*c*) Here there was catalepsy with deaf-mutism, but the patient wrote down all she wanted.

(*d*) In this stage the patient had forgotten not only the incidents of normal life, but apparently also much of the general knowledge acquired during it. In writing, she spelt backwards in the manner already described.

(*e*) A stage characterised by terror.

(*f*) Here the patient called herself "Good thing," and was docile, but usually without power in her feet or hands; this stage, however, was quite distinct from (*a*).

(*g*) The patient now called herself "Pretty dear," was sweet and amiable, but could not write or spell.

(*h*) Called herself "Mamie Wud"; in this state she recalled the events of childhood better than when awake, but was unable to remember anything about her illness.

(*i*) This stage was somewhat like (*d*); when in it the patient knew nothing, and thought she was just born.

(*k*) Here, the patient called herself "Old Persuader," and asked for a stick to strike people with, if they would not do what she wished.

(*l*) She called herself "Tom's darling," and was apparently a nice child.

(*m*) In this stage she asserted that she had "no name," and was violent and unkind.

(*n*) She called herself "The dreadful wicked thing," threw her slippers into the fire in a temper, etc.

(*o*) In this stage she called herself "Tommy's lamb," and was blind and idiotic.

(*p*) In December, 1896, a further stage developed, which lasted till February, 1897. In it the patient constantly repeated the word "picters," and drew beautifully; she even did so when she was prevented from seeing the paper on which she was drawing. The original self was unable to draw. During this stage the pupils were dilated and reacted feebly to light, while the patient was apparently insensible to sound.

As time went on, the patient, when in abnormal stages, began to have some idea of what had taken place in her ordinary life; when in the latter condition, however, she still had no recollection of anything that had happened in any of the abnormal stages. In July, 1898, she passed into a condition more closely resembling the normal one; she was still, however, childish, and called herself "Critter Wood."

In the spring of 1900, five years after the commencement of her illness, she had apparently settled down into stage (*g*), but had been taught that Mary W., not "Pretty dear," was her name. She was a fine, healthy, well-developed girl, who helped in the house and was anxious to learn typewriting in order to keep herself. Her character, however, differed slightly from her original one, and she was still somewhat childish at times.

In another group of cases the secondary state, while markedly inferior to that particular individual's primary one, finds its counterpart in degenerate states which are not necessarily insane.

(5) Of this the following case, recorded by "Dagonet" (G. R. Sims) in the *Referee*, January 31st, 1897, is an example:—One night Mr. Sims received a message from the master of a workhouse, to the effect that the police had brought a man to the Infirmary whom they had found insensible in the street, apparently suffering from drink. A letter, signed by Mr. Sims, was in his pocket. Mr. Sims knew him as a professional man in a good position. Next day he was conscious, but absolutely denied his identity. He said he was a street musician, and that his cornet had been stolen during a row in a public-house where he was playing. He, returned to his lodgings as soon as he was discharged from the Infirmary, and told his landlady he thought he must have had a fit and fallen down in the street, for he was bruised and ached all over, but did not remember anything about it. Exclusive of the time passed in the Infirmary, he had been absent from his lodgings for a week, but maintained that he had

only left the house that morning. A few days later he fulfilled an important professional engagement. All went well for some time; then he again suddenly disappeared. Search was made for him, and he was eventually found playing a cornet outside a public-house in Camden Town. Addressed by his proper name, he made no sign, and when questioned asserted that he had been an itinerant musician for the last fifteen years. To-day Mr. —— is again living an ordinary respectable professional life, and has not the slightest knowledge of his periodical lapses into another personality—that of a street musician. His name is well known to all who are familiar with music and the drama.

In another group, the secondary state, instead of being one of obvious mental disorder, differs little in intelligence and volition from the primary one. The following are examples :—

(6) Ansel Bourne, an itinerant preacher aged 61, residing at Greene, Rhode Island, suddenly disappeared. In spite of the publicity which the newspapers gave to the fact and the efforts of the police to find him, he remained undiscovered for two months. He then found himself at Norristown, Pennsylvania, where for the previous six weeks he had been keeping a small variety store under the name of A. J. Brown, appearing to his neighbours and customers as a normal person. When his normal consciousness returned, he was extremely alarmed to find himself in an unknown situation, with absolutely no memory of his surroundings or of the incidents which had taken place from the date of his disappearance. (*Proceedings of the Society for Psychical Research*, 1891, p. 22.)

(7) Emile X., barrister, sometimes passed without loss of consciousness into a secondary condition which lasted from a few minutes to several days. During it he led an active life which apparently did not differ from his normal one. The state always terminated suddenly, and the ordinary consciousness retained no recollection of what had just passed. After one attack, which lasted three weeks, he came to himself a hundred miles from home. (Dr. Proust, Professor of Hygiene at the Hôtel Dieu, Paris, *Revue de l'Hypnotisme*, March, 1890.)

(8) Mr. N., aged 32, educated, consulted Forel, and told him the following story. He stated that he had been living for some weeks in Zurich and had vague recollections of arriving there after a long voyage. Recently he had read two newspaper articles describing the sudden disappearance from Australia of a Mr. N.,

and he felt that he was the person referred to, although at the same time it seemed impossible that this could be true. N. entered the Burghölzli Asylum for treatment and was hypnotised by Forel, who succeeded in restoring his lost memory by suggestion, and thus obtained an account of his doings from the time he had left Australia. There was no reason, pecuniary or moral, for his disappearance. He recovered under Forel's treatment. [" Ein Fall von temporäner, totaler, theilweisse retrograder Amnesie (durch Suggestion geheilt)" von M. Naef, Voluntärarzt an der Heilanstalt Burghölzli," *Zeitschrift für Hypnotismus*, 1897, p. 321.]

(9) The following[1] is the most recent example I have been able to trace of the group we are considering :—On April 16th, 1900, George Ridderband, aged 19, a law student and the son of a well-known lawyer, suddenly disappeared from his home in New York. No reason, except that he had been studying hard for an examination, was discovered for this either at the time or afterwards. His parents put the matter in the hands of the police. On April 21st, the lad walked into a police station and told the following story. Five days previously he suddenly found himself walking in the street, but neither knew who nor where he was, nor could he recall anything as to his past life. Since then he had been wandering about, struggling in vain to revive his lost memories, keeping meanwhile a diary of his proceedings. He asked if any one corresponding to him had been advertised for as missing, and the sergeant recognised him as the lost George Ridderband. He was taken home and placed under medical care. At first he did not recognise any of his relatives, but a week later his memory commenced to return ; he was still, however, unable to account in any way for his disappearance.

In another section of this group, the secondary state, from a physical, moral, and intellectual point of view, is superior to the primary one. The following are examples :—

(10) A girl, aged 18, healthy, but quiet and somewhat stupid in character, swallowed some *Unguentum Lyttæ*. After the acute symptoms of poisoning passed off, a cutaneous hyperæsthesia of the head and morbid sensitiveness to sound remained. She had frequent attacks of temporary insensibility, and passed alternately from her ordinary mental condition to a secondary one, and from this in its turn back again to the normal one. In the

---

[1] From the *New York Herald*.

secondary state she was excitable : her conversation was lively and spirited, and she was intellectually superior to what she was in the primary condition. The memories of the two states were absolutely distinct : the primary self knew nothing of the second-ary one, the secondary self nothing of the primary one. ("Case of Double Consciousness," by Thomas Mayo, M.D., F.R.C.S., *London Medical Gazette*, New Series, vol. i. 1845, p. 1202.)

(11) Mary Reynolds, a dull and melancholy young woman, was found one morning in a profound sleep, from which it was impossible to arouse her. After twenty hours she awoke, but her disposition was absolutely changed, and she had no memory of her past. She was now cheerful, buoyant, sociable, and merry ; but did not recognise her friends, and had lost the power of reading and writing. Five weeks later, she passed into the primary state ; again became dull and melancholy, and remembered nothing of her secondary condition. After the lapse of a few more weeks, she again passed into the secondary state following a profound sleep, and took up her new life precisely where she had left it. The memories of the two states were absolutely distinct : in the first she remembered former primary states, but these alone; in the second she only remembered former secondary states. These alterations of consciousness continued for fifteen years, then finally ceased, leaving her permanently in the second state. In this she remained without change for the last twenty-five years of her life. ("Case of Mary Reynolds," by Dr. Weir Mitchell, *Trans. of the College of Physicians of Philadelphia*, April 4th, 1888.)

(12) Félida X, aged $14\frac{1}{2}$, without known cause, though some-times under the influence of emotion, had attacks of sharp pain in both temples, followed by a state of profound stupor, which lasted ten minutes. She then spontaneously opened her eyes and appeared to awake, but in reality passed into a condition of secondary consciousness. This lasted for an hour or two, then the stupor and sleep reappeared, and she passed into her ordinary state. The secondary state differed markedly from the primary one. In the latter she was a miserable, querulous, hysterical invalid ; and remembered nothing of her secondary life, which was superior, both intellectually and physically, to the primary one. Here she was gay, active, and intelligent; and remembered not only all the events which had taken place in former attacks of secondary consciousness, but also those of normal life. As

2 c

time went on, the frequency of the secondary attacks became greater and their duration longer, till, at the age of 24, they commenced to exceed the periods of normal life. But from 24 to 27 years of age she remained in the normal state. After this the secondary attacks became more and more frequent, and finally almost completely occupied her entire existence. In 1875, Félida, who was then 32 years of age, told Azam that she still suffered from attacks associated with loss of memory. These so-called " attacks," however, were simply lapses from her secondary consciousness into her ordinary primary one. Thus, once when returning from a funeral, she felt her attack, *i.e.* her normal state, come on. She became unconscious for a few seconds without her companions noticing it; then awoke in the primary state, absolutely ignorant of the reason for which she was in a mourning coach. Accustomed to these accidents, she waited till, by skilful questions, she was able to grasp the situation, and thus none of those present knew what had happened. Later she lost her sister-in-law after a long illness, and, during a relapse into the normal state, knew nothing about the death, and only guessed at it from the fact that she was in mourning. In the earlier periods the transition from one state to another was marked by a stage of more or less prolonged unconsciousness. As time went on this diminished, and, finally, the loss of consciousness became so brief that Félida was able to disguise it. In 1887, when Azam published the account of the case, Félida was 44 years of age, and her lapses into normal life had become more and more rare. (*Hypnotisme, double conscience, et altérations de la personnalité*, par le Dr. Azam. Paris, 1887. J. B. Ballière et Fils.)

In 1888, Dr. Ladame, of Geneva, communicated a somewhat analogous case to the *Société Médico-Psychologique*, which had been cured by suggestion.

Spontaneous somnambulism affords another example of Group (a). In volition and consciousness are to be found the main differences between it and induced somnambulism. The hypnotic subject knows what he is doing and why he does it, and can reject disagreeable suggestions. Unless specially trained, he usually only acts in response to influence from without—influence more or less directly transmitted to him by the suggestions of others. The spontaneous somnambule, on the contrary, acts his own dreams. His hallucinations sometimes excite criminal acts; and authentic cases are recorded in which spontaneous somnambules have committed murder, under the delusion that the person attacked was a wild beast or a burglar. Spontaneous somnambulism, properly speaking, is a neurosis; and, as Hack Tuke pointed out, in its severest forms it approaches perilously near epilepsy, while the condition of mental automatism which sometimes succeeds epileptic fits closely resembles that of the sleepwalker. Yellowlees looks upon spontaneous somnambulism as a form of insanity, and terms it *somnomania*. He holds that the sole difference between it and insanity or epileptic violence is that it occurs during sleep, and involves only a temporary arrest of volition, instead of the more prolonged loss of control which results from organic mischief.

(b) Facts in support of a Secondary Consciousness drawn from Normal Waking or Sleeping Life.

Here the evidence is not so clear as in the preceding section, but, without the hypothesis of a secondary consciousness, it is difficult to explain phenomena such as the following :—

(1) *Time appreciation in cases such as those about to be cited.*

Dr. George Savage possesses the power of awaking at a given hour, and has tested it on several occasions. The following is an example :—One day, having to catch an early train, he determined to awake at 6 A.M., and slept soundly without awaking until the exact time. The seven following mornings he awoke exactly at 6 A.M., notwithstanding that he went to bed at different hours and there was no necessity for early rising. This involuntary repetition of self-waking at unusual times also occurred when he was roused by others at abnormally early hours. Thus, when in the Alps, if he were called at 2 or 3 A.M., he would certainly awake spontaneously at the same hour next morning, even if he had been much fatigued by climbing. Dr. Savage states that the accuracy of the time of awaking in these instances has puzzled him greatly.

The following is Professor Marcus Hartog's own account of his case :—

"When I was a student, under 17, I found I could, sleeping soundly, awake at any given hour I had set myself overnight. The peculiarity of such awaking was that it was always sudden and complete, not preceded by a period of broken sleep, nor accompanied by the drowsiness of an ordinary unprepared awaking. If I found that it was needless to get up I soon fell asleep again, and then had the ordinary drowsy awaking, often oversleeping myself. This faculty has persisted with me.

"Again, without previous training, between the ages of 20 and 25, on three distinct occasions I had to nurse friends, when I had to administer food and medicines at regular intervals, attending also to their necessities as they arose. The last occasion extended over, I think, three weeks. On each occasion the facility and manner of awaking completely and suddenly was exactly the same as for early rising, whether at the stated hour or at the least stir of the patient. On lying down to rest again and closing my eyes, I seemed to see a gradually widening vista, and as my eyes diverged I fell asleep; the time occupied could not have been more than a quarter of a minute, though I felt wide awake at the moment of closing my eyes. My sleep on these occasions was singularly, if not absolutely, dreamless, though I was under the greatest mental anxiety while awake."

In Professor Hartog's case the awaking at fixed hours was never involuntarily repeated, *i.e.* as regards the awaking at repeated intervals. Sometimes, however, when he set himself to awake at a fixed time in the morning, this was repeated for several days, as in Dr. Savage's case.

Here no ordinary physiological explanation is possible; and, while the ordinary consciousness was asleep, an intelligence of some kind must have watched the passage of time.

(2) *The recollection of forgotten facts without the association of ideas connected with normal memory.*

Every one, I think, must recall instances similar to those described by Carpenter, in which he has tried to remember a forgotten name, and, after having failed to recall it by every device imaginable, has at last put the problem on one side in disgust and turned his attention to other things. Later, the forgotten name rises into consciousness with a suddenness which is startling, and no association of ideas can be discovered to account for its appearance.

(3) *The execution of mental work, which the ordinary consciousness had failed, or neglected, to perform.*

My personal experiences afford examples of this quite as striking as those cited by Carpenter. Thus, when I began to speak in public, I wrote my lectures beforehand and committed them to memory. Later, I confined myself to jotting down the various headings, and to recalling mentally the different facts I wished to group around them. I then dismissed the subject from my mind. As soon as I began to speak, the lecture unrolled itself, as it were : sentences appeared to spring unbidden to my lips, and were uttered with greater ease and fluency than those which had formerly been carefully committed to memory. If the lectures had to be published, they were written after delivery ; and though I was able to reproduce their substance, I was always conscious that I failed to do so as to their exact form.

Further, after a time, either from increased confidence in my own powers or from the fact that I was overworked, the ordinary waking-self kicked more and more at the task demanded of it. In consequence of this, the secondary self received less carefully prepared information ; but, despite this, it continued to do its work equally well.

Since I left college I had done no literary work of any kind until I began to write on hypnotism, and my earlier efforts were difficult and painful. In every instance I began by collecting an over-abundant supply of information, and then had difficulty both in grouping and expressing it. I frequently spent hours in painful thought, with no more apparent result than the writing of a few lines ; and even these often failed to satisfy me. Gradually, however, I came to rely more and more on the secondary self. When I encountered a difficulty, I recalled as clearly as I could the facts I wished to express, then put the matter on one side. A day or two later, I often was able to dictate to my secretary for hours at a stretch. Not only so, but the work was characterised by marked absence of effort, and accompanied by a distinct feeling of detachment, and even of surprise. The moment before a sentence was uttered, I could not have told what it was likely to be. Further, the memory of what I dictated in this way soon sank below the level of ordinary consciousness. If I read it a few weeks later, it appeared to be the work of some one else, and I could not trace the association of ideas which must necessarily have been connected with its execution.

Where the aid of the secondary self had not been evoked, and the work had been done at the first attempt, consciously and laboriously, I could always afterwards recall, more or less perfectly, the steps of reasoning, association, etc., which had been connected with my work.

(4) *The so-called inspirations of genius.*

According to Myers, works of genius, instead of being the result of an " infinite capacity for taking trouble," were due to the intelligent action of a secondary consciousness. The labour was performed in a " subterranean workshop," as it were, and then presented in completed form to the normal consciousness. The latter not only believed that it had done the work itself, but thought that this had been performed instantaneously.

This view practically reproduced that of Carpenter as to the origin of what he termed *invention.* The invasion of the *inspiration* into the normal consciousness is often sudden and startling. While the subject of it undoubtedly believes that he, *i.e.* his ordinary waking self, originated it, he, at the same time, often acts as if it were something unconnected with his usual stream of consciousness. He feels that the inspiration may escape him, and with feverish haste tries to record it with pen, pencil, or brush.

(c) HYPNOTIC PHENOMENA WHICH APPARENTLY SUPPORT THE THEORY OF A SECONDARY CONSCIOUSNESS.

These are too numerous to be recounted in detail, and it might even be claimed that every deeply hypnotised subject shows evidence—if in memory-changes alone—of the existence of a secondary consciousness. In the waking state he can recall nothing of what has happened in profound hypnosis; but when hypnotised he not only remembers the events of previous hypnoses, but also all that his ordinary memory can recall of waking life, and even, in addition, much that it has forgotten.

The time appreciation experiments already reported (pp. 119-133) furnish one of the most striking instances of double consciousness with which I am acquainted. Further, the fact that nothing could be recalled by the ordinary hypnotic self regarding calculations which must inevitably have been made in some form of hypnosis, apparently showed that the subject possessed a third substratum of the personality. This view is also held by William James, who wrote me as follows :—

"Miss D.'s case is most extraordinary. I agree entirely with you that a 'third self' must be involved, but what such a third self in its totality may signify, I haven't the least idea."

The dressmaking problem, with its solution in the hypnotic state (p. 320), is also an interesting example of the spontaneous action of the hypnotic self. Further, it illustrates experimentally the probable origin of the inspirations of genius, and the way in which they reach the normal consciousness. Miss D. in her waking state was striving after a result which she could not obtain, just as an inventor or artist might have done. Later, when she was again in the waking state and thinking of something else, the solution of the problem came suddenly into her mind. She thought she had solved it there and then. Questioning in a subsequent hypnosis, however, quite accidentally revealed the following facts :—

First, she had worked out the problem when profoundly hypnotised, her condition at the time resembling deep sleep.

Secondly, on awaking she knew nothing of what she had done, and it was only after the lapse of some hours that the uprush into the ordinary consciousness occurred.

Thirdly, this uprush brought with it no knowledge of its origin, *i.e.* her waking self neither knew then nor afterwards whence the *inspiration* had been derived.

Fourthly, when again hypnotised she recalled that the problem had been present in her mind during hypnosis. She also remembered having solved it, and that her primary consciousness was ignorant of the fact. Further, she also knew the exact moment at which the uprush had taken place, and was evidently amused by the primary consciousness having claimed as its own the work done by the secondary one.

The phenomena of automatic writing, of which examples have already been cited (pp. 139-141), show not only that a secondary consciousness exists, but also that it may be in action simultaneously with the normal one.

The following cases also apparently afford evidence of the existence of two or more sub-conscious states.

(1) Sarah L. was the first person in whom I found any evidence of so-called multiple personality; and, when she came under my notice over twelve years ago, I knew nothing of the literature of the subject. In the normal state she was quiet, respectful, and somewhat shy, and retained this character when I hypnotised her. She was a profound somnambule; in waking life she knew nothing of the events of hypnosis, but in hypnosis could recall all the memories of the normal state as well as the incidents of hypnotic life. Her surgical and medical history has already been given (No. 6, pp. 161-2, and No. 25, pp. 197-8), and the reader is now referred to it in order to show the genuine and profound character of the hypnosis.

Before coming under my care, Sarah L. had been hypnotised and exhibited by a stage performer; and, some time after the events just recorded, her mother told me that Sarah occasionally hypnotised herself, and that the condition then differed markedly from the one I induced. After some coaxing, the girl consented to hypnotise herself, and went through the following performance:—First, she closed her eyes and appeared to pass into a lethargic state; then a few minutes later awoke with a changed expression: instead of having a shy and modest air, her eyes sparkled and she looked full of mischief. In place of addressing me as " Sir "—she had formerly been a servant of mine, and an extremely respectful one—she put her hand on my arm and said in a familiar way, " I say." She then began to ask me impertinent questions about the persons she had seen at my house, and to criticise them in a particularly free and sarcastic fashion. The performance was so interesting and amusing that I got her to hypnotise herself on a good many occasions. The same phenomena always appeared; she invariably became familiar, inquisitive, and sarcastic; while her highest praise for any one she approved of was conveyed in the words, " She'll do." Other facts were noticed and reported to me by her mother. Thus, sometimes when Sarah hypnotised herself, she would remember that her mother owed her a few coppers and insist upon having them at once. If they were refused, she would take them by force:

to this, however, her mother lent herself. The girl would then generally go out and buy oranges, and, on her return, eat them all herself: this selfishness was quite out of keeping with her normal character. Sometimes when her mother asked her to do work that was distasteful to her, such as blacking the grate, she would induce self-hypnosis with profound lethargy, and remain apparently deeply asleep for hours. I had never taught her to hypnotise herself, nor, so far as I could learn, had this been done by any one else. During this third stage—which was one of self-hypnosis—she remembered everything that had happened in previous conditions of this kind, and also the events of the normal state and those of ordinary hypnosis; but the waking consciousness and the ordinary hypnotic one knew nothing of the events of this third state. After I had observed the condition for some time, I concluded that it was not likely to be beneficial to the subject, and suggested during ordinary hypnosis that she should lose the power of creating it. The suggestion was successful and the condition never reappeared.

(2) Pierre Janet has been fortunate in finding several subjects who apparently possess so-called multiplex personalities, and has published full and interesting accounts of their cases. Amongst these that of Léonie ——, is, I think, one of the most striking. This subject, Madame B., aged 45, possessed, according to Pierre Janet, three distinct and well-marked personalities, viz.: Léonie I.; the Léonie of normal life, a serious and sad peasant woman, calm, slow, gentle, and timid. Léonie II.; Léonie in the ordinary hypnotic state, a gay, noisy, restless being, given to irony and bitter jesting: who describes her visitors in an impertinent fashion, and apes their airs and graces. Léonie II. refuses to identify herself with Léonie I., and calls the latter a stupid woman.

Madame B., *i.e.* Léonie I., has had attacks of spontaneous somnambulism since she was three years old, and from sixteen upwards has been frequently hypnotised by various people. Now, when Léonie II. is called to the front, she knits together the events of her spontaneous and induced somnambulistic states, and forms the history of her life from them; the memories of waking life are not forgotten, but these are ascribed to Léonie I.

When Léonie II. is hypnotised more deeply, a third personality appears, Léonie III., who is grave, serious, slow in speech

and movement. This Léonie separates herself both from Léonie
I. of waking life, and the Léonie II of the ordinary hypnotic
state. The former she describes as a good, but rather stupid
woman, and the latter as crazy. "Fortunately," she says, 'there
is nothing of me in either of them." Léonie I. knows herself
alone; Léonie II. knows herself and Léonie I., while Léonie III.
not only knows herself, but also the two others. Léonie I. is
embarrassed and ashamed when Léonie II.'s friends, who are
strangers to her, speak to her in the street. Léonie II. spontaneously writes letters, which Léonie I. finds and destroys, as she
does not understand them. Afterwards Léonie II. hides her
letters where she knows Léonie I. will never look for them.
Léonie II. visits places where Léonie I. has never been, then disappears and pushes Léonie I. to the front, leaving her frightened
by her strange surroundings, etc.

(3) In "An Experimental Study of Visions" (*Brain*, 1898)
Dr. Morton Prince records some interesting experiments which he
made with Miss X, a patient who suffered from hysterical
neurasthenia. Miss X was easily hypnotised and at first passed
into the ordinary "deep" stage, then, when ordered to sleep more
profoundly, a fresh condition developed, which differed both from
that of waking life and from ordinary hypnosis. According to
Dr. Prince, these stages formed three distinct personalities, viz :—

X, I. The Miss X of ordinary waking life, who is reserved,
morbidly conscious, self-contained, serious, deferential, and
dignified.

X, II. The Miss X of the primary hypnotic condition, who
is sad, serious, and apparently weak and suffering.

X, III. The Miss X of the secondary or deeper hypnotic
state, who is flippant and jovial, free from all physical infirmities,
full of fun and reckless.

X, I. remembers the events of waking life alone and knows
nothing of X, II. and X, III. : while X, II. remembers all that has
passed in previous primary hypnotic states, also all that X, I. can
recall, and in addition some other events of waking life which X,
I. has forgotten.

X, III. remembers all the events of the secondary or deeper
hypnotic stages, as well as everything X, I. and X, II. can recall.
In addition, she can describe incidents in the past life of X, I.
that are lost to the memory of the latter, and can thus explain

much that the waking personality is at a loss to account for. She knows all about many of the little absent-minded doings of X, I.; and does not hesitate to voluntarily tell of them, although X, I. is morbidly and unnecessarily reserved about her whole life.

Dr. Prince made this tripartite personage look into a globe, which took the place of the ordinary glass ball used in crystal gazing, and describes the visions which the different personages saw. The following is one of the most interesting of these :—

X, III. was the personality in action and voluntarily related the following incident, telling it with much gusto as a joke against Miss X (X, I.), whom she talked of as " She " :—" ' She ' received a letter from a photographer yesterday. ' She ' put it into her pocket, where ' She ' had some bank-notes. Then, as ' She ' walked along, ' She ' took out the money and tore it to pieces, thinking it was the letter. ' She ' threw the money into the street." In response to questioning, X, III. repeated the words of the photographer's note and counted mentally, with some difficulty and concentration of thought, the amount of money. X, III. said " She " was absent-minded, and thinking of something else when " She " tore up the money. Hypnosis was now terminated and the ordinary personality X, I. appeared, who, in reply to questions, stated that she had received a letter from her photographer which she had torn up, and that she had the bank-notes in her pocket. She was asked to show them, and produced the letter. This surprised her, but she thought she must have left the bank-notes at home and could not believe she had destroyed them. The notes were undoubtedly lost, and an account of the occurrence, similar to that given by X, III., was obtained by making Miss X (X, I.) look into the globe and suggesting that she should see what had really happened. Here, apparently, the ordinary hypnotic state, namely X, II., was induced by indirect suggestion and fixed gazing; and the vision appeared in response to the suggestions of the operator.

" Crystal gazing," the method employed by Dr. Prince, is not really necessary for the production of hypnotic visions ; it simply acts by presenting a point upon which the suggested memories are concentrated and rendered, as it were, objective. Any memory which exists in the hypnotic consciousness can be evoked by suggestion without the crystal. Under ordinary circumstances the hypnotic subject rarely visualises his memories, but when he looks into the crystal, this acts as a suggestion that he should see with his eyes what has happened. I have frequently made similar experiments with hypnotic subjects, and in place of the crystal made them look at the top of my stethoscope, which answered equally well.

Gurney stated that he had experimentally demonstrated the existence of positive and distinct stages of memory within the conscious portion of the hypnotic trance. The subjects of these experiments were first hypnotised lightly, and something was told them which they were asked to remember. Deeper hypnosis was then induced, when the subject was asked what it was that he had just been told; it was then found that he neither remembered what had been related to him, nor even the fact that he had been told anything at all. While in this deep stage, which Gurney termed *B*, some new incident was related to the subject which he was again asked to remember. He was then recalled to the lighter stage, termed *A* by Gurney, and asked to repeat what he had been told: he had forgotten what he had heard a few minutes before in stage *B*, but repeated instead what had been told him in the earlier stage *A*, in which he now again found himself. Brought once more to *B*, he similarly remembered what he had been told in that state, while he was again completely oblivious of what had been impressed upon him in *A*. On awaking, he retained no memory of anything that had been told him in either stage.

Many cases, of which the following is an example, were cited by Gurney to illustrate these alterations in hypnotic memory:—

(4) S., a young man living at Brighton, was told in state *A*, the lighter stage of hypnotic trance, that the pier-head had been washed away, and in state *B*, the deeper stage of trance, that an engine boiler had burst at Brighton station and killed several people. He was then brought from stage *B* back again to *A*, when he recalled all that had been told him about the accident to the pier. Hypnosis was again deepened; stage *B* appeared, and the following conversation took place between the operator and the subject:—

Operator. " But I suppose they will soon be able to build a new one."

Had the pier been present in S.'s mind, this remark, said Gurney, would naturally have been taken to refer to it, as it had formed the subject of conversation only a few seconds before. S., however, at once replied : " Oh, there are plenty on the line" —meaning, plenty of engines.

Operator. " The pile-driving takes time, though."

S. " Pile-driving ? Well, I don't know anything about engines myself."

The subject was now brought back to stage *A* and the conversation continued :—

Operator. " If they have plenty more, it does not matter much."

S. " Oh, they can't put it on in a day ; it was a splendid place."

Operator. " Why, I am talking about the engine."

S. " Engine ! What, on the pier ? I never noticed one there."

Here the subject's mind had obviously again reverted to what had been told him in stage *A*.

In the above case, as in all others of a like nature cited by Gurney, the normal self knew nothing of stages *A* and *B*, and these knew nothing of each other.

Remarks.—The importance of memory in relation to subconscious states is insisted on both by William James and Myers. According to the former, the theory of "double consciousness" is only, after all, a development of what is found in Locke's famous chapter on " Identity and Diversity : " namely, that personality extended no further than consciousness, and that there would be two different persons in one man, if the experiences undergone by that man fell into two groups, each gathered into a distinct focus of recollection. Further, says James, " it must be admitted that, in certain persons at least, the total possible consciousness may be split into parts which coexist, but mutually ignore each other and share the objects of knowledge between them, and—more remarkable still—are complementary."

Myers held that the formation of a secondary chain of memory was the fundamental point in hypnosis. This chain of memory was essential to the grouping of the various acts which manifested the secondary consciousness. This classification excludes, and I think justly so, some of the cases cited by some authorities as examples of double consciousness. Amnesia, even when associated with alterations in character, does not constitute double consciousness. If it did, the bather who had forgotten the number of his machine and lost his temper might be described as a case of secondary personality.

It must be admitted, however, that the phenomena just cited as affording evidence for the existence of a secondary consciousness are explained in other and even widely differing ways. Most of the discussion has centred round the phenomenon of time appreciation, with its attendant calculations, and to this I now propose to refer.

THEORETICAL EXPLANATIONS OF TIME APPRECIATION IN HYPNOSIS.

Delbœuf, as we have seen, pointed out that the terminal days in Beaunis and Liégeois' experiments fell on easily recognised dates, with which the subjects were acquainted. These experiments, he said, did not show, as they were supposed to do, that somnambules possessed the power of counting days, but only that they were able to retain a given date. To remove this objection, his suggestions were made in minutes, and the majority of mine were given in a similar, but even more complicated, form. In explaining the phenomenon, therefore, we must take into account not only the appreciation of the passage of time, but also the feats of memory and arithmetical calculation which sometimes exceeded the subject's normal powers.

Bernheim's Theory.

This is mainly based upon the supposed occurrence of self-hypnosis in somnambules and the existence during that condition of a peculiar mental concentration, with subsequent revival of hypnotic memories. According to Bernheim, conscious mental activity exists both in sleep and in hypnosis. During sleep we are conscious that our mind thinks and works, just as the hypnotic somnambulist knows what he is doing; but the form of consciousness differs from that of waking life. In both sleep and hypnosis concentration of the nervous force upon the suggested idea is the characteristic phenomenon. This continues to exist, although dream succeeds dream in sleep, and varying suggestions are instantly executed in hypnosis : the nervous concentration has only changed its object, the focus shifted its place.

According to Bernheim, if an individual goes to sleep determined to awake at a given hour, his attention is fixed upon this idea, and he thinks about it voluntarily and consciously all night. When he awakes, he believes he does so spontaneously, since the conscious thoughts of sleep are forgotten. Finally, he says, the lost memories of hypnosis may be revived by chance association of ideas, like forgotten impressions of the waking state, and also in other ways, and therefore the memory of the suggestion has not been latent all the time. In support of this he cites :—

First: Experiments.—Two subjects, who had received deferred suggestions, when hypnotised and questioned in the interval, stated that during natural sleep they had once dreamt of what had been suggested during hypnosis.

Secondly : Certain general observations as to the mental condition in somnambules.—The memory, he says, of what has taken place during hypnosis depends upon the psychical concentration already referred to; every time this is reproduced, the lost memory is revived. Somnambules pass easily and spontaneously from the normal to the hypnotic state; they then become self-absorbed and concentrated, and recall the operator's suggestions. They know when these should be executed, and take their measures accordingly. They reinforce the idea of not forgetting them, just as a person in natural sleep determines not to miss the hour set for awaking. Although the suggestion may have been present in their minds the greater part of the day, they forget it if we divert their attention from themselves by speaking to them. By doing this we have disturbed their psychical concentration—drawn their cerebral activity from the inside to the outside—and produced another state of consciousness in which the memory of the suggestion is lost, the memories of the second or hypnotic state being effaced in the first or normal one.

In consequence of this, when the somnambule carries out a suggestion, he believes that the idea has newly and spontaneously dawned in his mind—"*He no longer remembers that it is a memory.*" Thus, in Bernheim's opinion, a deferred suggestion is no more difficult to explain than one executed immediately on awaking.

Three points are involved in Bernheim's theory :—

(1) *Nervous concentration and its relationship to hypnotic memory.*

Bernheim's theories as to nervous concentration, etc., have already been discussed (pp. 339-45), and their fallacies pointed out.

(2) *Admitting that hypnotic memory is associated with this psychical concentration, the evidence in favour of the frequent and spontaneous occurrence of the latter is far from convincing.*

Granting that two subjects had *once* dreamt of a suggestion during natural sleep, this does not justify the conclusion that somnambules pass easily and spontaneously from the normal to the hypnotic state. Further, although the memories of hypnosis whether self-induced or not, are lost on awaking, these can be easily evoked by questioning in subsequent hypnoses. If, therefore, subjects passed spontaneously into the hypnotic state, and thought about the suggestions, they could be made to recall the fact that they had done so. Despite this, Bernheim's generalisations are founded on the two dreams just cited ; and he has apparently made no attempt to discover the actual mental conditions involved, although he might easily have done this by means of the simple method of interrogation in subsequent hypnoses.

(3) *Granting both the points in dispute, i.e. the psychical concentration and its spontaneous occurrence, the difficulty is still unsolved.*

If no trace of the hypnotic memory remains in the normal state, what advantage does the normal consciousness obtain from the unknown or forgotten fact that the hypnotic consciousness recalled the suggestion at some time before the date fixed for its fulfilment ?

Beaunis' Objections.

Beaunis also raises many objections to Bernheim's views. Thus, while admitting the influence of attention and concentration upon the production of certain hypnotic phenomena, he holds that these are insufficient to explain deferred suggestions. They may account for a hallucination realised immediately on awaking, but not for one that has been retarded for several days. Here the subject was unconscious of the suggestion until the hallucination appeared at the hour fixed, and it is absurd to suppose that all this time he was under the influence of a dominant idea. Bernheim's experiments, therefore, do not settle the question. Granting that the subject dreamt of the suggestion in normal sleep two days before it fell due, it is still necessary to explain how it was carried out at the time fixed. The suggestion, it is true, now involves a shorter period of time, *i.e.* two days instead of the original number; but this, while reducing the extent of the problem, still leaves it unsolved.

Beaunis disputes Bernheim's assertion that those who wish to awake at a given hour think of this all night, for, he says, if this were true, they would afterwards remember having done so. Dreams which have passed rapidly through the brain can often be recalled in every detail: we should, therefore, be able to remember still more vividly the ideas upon which our attention has been constantly fixed. Further, he states that some people always know what o'clock it is, and, if suddenly asked, are able to give an exact reply, no matter how much their attention may have been concentrated on other things. Had they consciously noted the passage of time, they would afterwards be able to recall having done so. This, however, is not the case, and they are unable to explain how the feat was performed.

Finally, in contradistinction to Bernheim, Beaunis justly points out that important differences exist between the modes in which the lost memories of the waking state, and those of hypnosis, are revived. The former may be recalled at any time by a chance association of ideas: for example, things long forgotten may be remembered on hearing the name of some one we knew in childhood. The lost memories of hypnosis, however, possess the distinctive and essential characteristic that they cannot be revived by a chance association of ideas, and are, therefore, fundamentally different from those of the waking state. The hypnotic suggestion is only realised at the hour fixed, and cannot take place before, even when associations occur which would have restored lost normal memory. Thus, if it is suggested to *A* that he is to do something at the expiration of ten days, when he

2 D

hears *B* cough three times; *B's* signals, if given at any time before the day fixed, produce no response, although they inevitably do so when the appropriate time arrives.

Beaunis' Theory.

Beaunis attempts to explain the phenomenon of time appreciation by the existence in the human organism of a subconscious physiological power of time measurement. The phenomenon of deferred suggestion, he says, is analogous to that of awaking at a fixed hour from normal sleep; and both may be explained by the existence of a sort of mental mechanism, arranged like an alarm-clock, to produce a movement at a fixed hour. The brain, as already stated, is a machine which acts without our knowledge, with an activity we are unable to estimate; and the things of which we are conscious only feebly represent this mysterious work. The power of appreciating time, rudimentary (or, rather, atrophied) in the civilised man, is well developed in the savage and lower animals. Thus a dog, accustomed to go out with his master at a certain hour, will show that the time has arrived by expressive pantomime, should his master delay a little in getting ready for his walk. In Beaunis' opinion, the measurement of time by somnambules is an act of subconscious cerebration.

Paul Janet's Objections.

Janet grants that an image of which one is unconscious may exist in the memory; and, further, that it can be revived, even at a fixed date, if the operator associates the suggestion with some definite sensation, as, for example, the sight of a particular person. He cannot, however, understand the return of the lost memory at a fixed day *without* other association than the numeration of time. Thirteen days, for example, do not represent a sensation, but form an abstraction. The carrying out of a suggestion, therefore, at the expiration of such a period presupposes the existence of a subconscious power of measuring time—an entirely unknown faculty. Up to this everything could be explained by the law of association of ideas; but here we make a sudden jump, and the thread of analogy is completely broken. No association can explain the subconscious counting of thirteen days, and the " suggestion theory " breaks down here.

Beaunis' Reply.

A day is not an abstraction. The idea of a day represents a series of definite impressions, the result of external agencies, such as light, temperature, etc., which produce in our organism different kinds of reactions. Animals know exactly the hour at which they are habitually fed, and an attack of fever returns at the same hour each day, or every other day, for weeks; this indicates that the measurement of time is not an abstraction, but has its roots in the very life of the organism. The periodicity of days, weeks, months, and seasons corresponds to periodic organic variations, which under certain circumstances may acquire sufficient intensity to constitute a sort of "subconscious faculty for measuring time," although the word "faculty" is a little too philosophic a term for an organic aptitude of this kind.

REMARKS.—Beaunis' explanation assumes (1) the existence of a subconscious faculty for measuring time, and (2) its applicability to the cases in question.

(1) *The Subconscious Measurement of Time.*—According to Beaunis, time appreciation is highly developed in savages, while certain civilised persons can awake at a given hour, and others always know what o'clock it is. In support of this, however, he does not cite a single example or experiment. Let us take the simplest case, *i.e.* awaking at a given hour. Many persons, it is true, believe that they can do this: usually, however, the self-waker only shows the power of giving himself a lighter sleep than usual; he awakes several times during the night, and in the end does not always hit the exact hour. On behalf of the Society for Psychical Research, several persons, who believed they possessed this power of self-waking, tested it in a rigorously scientific manner. The results were disappointing. One experimenter only succeeded on 2 occasions out of 17, and one of these was his usual hour of awaking; another was successful in 5 times out of 29, but on 3 of these he awoke at other hours as well; while the third was right 2 out of 13 times; and the fourth only succeeded in 4 instances out of 46.

Since I became interested in time appreciation, many people have assured me that they could awake at any given hour. None of them, however, were able to experimentally reproduce the alleged phenomenon, while the cases of Savage and Hartog, already referred to, are the only genuine ones I know of. If, however, the faculty were as universal as Beaunis asserts, there would be no employment for the professional "knockers up" of manufacturing districts.

The "fever" argument is also fallacious; it is the parasitic malarial micro-organisms which manifest periodicity, not their human hosts.

(2) *The Applicability of Beaunis' Theory to the particular Cases in question.*—The experiences of Savage and Hartog [1] undoubtedly show that certain persons can awake at a given hour. The existence of such a faculty as a rare occurrence in the normal state, does not, however, explain why it is almost universal among hypnotic somnambules: to invoke it is an attempt to explain the little-known in terms of the less-known; and the analogy, even if successfully established, does not solve the problem, but adds another to it. Granting that the uncivilised man possesses some natural power of marking the passage of time, it would be of little use to him in cases such as those described by Delbœuf and myself. If he cannot count above five, how is he to bring his powers to bear on a suggestion which starts from, say, 3.15 P.M. yesterday, and is to terminate in 40,845 minutes?

Delbœuf's Theory.

Delbœuf first pointed out that his subjects in the normal state were unable to make the necessary calculations involved in his time experiments. As the latter were successful, this showed, he said, that the subjects when hypnotised had an idea of the passage of time, and subconsciously calculated when the suggestions fell due. Apparently they possessed a sort of mechanism like an alarm-clock, which they set to go off at a fixed time.

Edmund Gurney's Objections to the Theories of Delbœuf and Beaunis.

According to Gurney, commands to be fulfilled at a particular date involved the reckoning of time. This was usually assumed to be physiological. Thus, Delbœuf believed that the subject calculated when the order fell due, and said to himself: "I shall fall into a trance at such and such a moment, and then perform the act." The subject set his organism like an alarm-clock for a

[1] Pp. 387-8.

given time ahead : his mind, relieved of responsibility, then went off duty till the suggestion fell due, when it was aroused by its own automatic machinery, the action resembling the running down of an alarm-clock. Gurney asserted that hypnotic subjects never formulated their orders in this way, and that Delbœuf's explanation was pure guesswork, unsupported by fact.

Further, he said, even if we granted the purely physiological hypothesis for cases of short duration—where the idea of the time fixed could be easily grasped, and thus the setter of the alarm-clock knew exactly what he was about—it would be a very different thing to extend it to others where the command had been executed after the lapse of months.

Gurney, like Delbœuf, drew a distinction between commands to be carried out at a specific date, such as New Year's Day, and those where a length of time alone was named, as in the direction to do something " on the sixty-ninth day from this." In the former instance, the brain might at once register the date along with the order, and the arrival of the former would thus suffice to arouse the latter. A length of time could not be registered in this way. Its termination, till reckoned by the calendar, was quite indefinite ; and when the particular day arrived it conveyed nothing likely to revive the suggestion—it carried no more *sixty-ninthness* about it than any other day.

Gurney considered that Beaunis' explanation did not fully meet Janet's objection that such a length of time—*i.e.* sixty-nine days—was simply an abstraction. Admitting that " a day " was a sufficiently familiar and definite unit to present a concrete character—that it represented a series of conscious reactions— and further, that there were periodic organic changes which extended over weeks and months, this did not prove that " the measurement of time was not an abstraction, but had its roots and conditions in the very life of the organism." It did not follow that " sixty-nine days " were concrete in character because this was the case with " one day," and, further, the organic con- ditions associated with established physiological periods were absent from these other periods, suddenly and arbitrarily fixed by human volition. *The vital processes were as unable to make a time calculation of this kind as a school-boy's digestion to work out a proposition of Euclid.* Such time measurement was not a function of animal life ; its result was not an inevitable bodily

state, but a needless act.   It depended—not on progressive
changes in the stomach or blood—but on an original course of
cerebration taking place in the higher tracts of the brain, initiated
by an impression, that of the command, which had a distinct
psychical side.

According to Gurney, the passage of time must be registered,
looking at it from the brain side alone, not by general gradual
change, but by a series of specific changes corresponding to the
days and units of measurement; and this was the only kind of
cerebral process capable of clearly differentiating the case from
that of ordinary physiological time reckoning.   Further, unless
cerebral events such as were normally correlated with the ideas
" sixty," " sixty-one," " sixty-two," etc., really took place, how
could the gulf be spanned with precision ?   Any other kind of
change would not know when to stop, or how to associate a point
it had reached with the order given long before.   Granting that
these specific brain-changes took place, was it not reasonable to
suppose that their mental correlate existed ; and that, hidden
from our view, there was an actual watching of the course of
time ?   This hypothesis, he said, went a long way towards
removing Paul Janet's difficulty—from this point of view his
" unknown faculty " resolved itself into a known one, working in
the normal way, but below the surface of ordinary consciousness.

Gurney's Theory.

As we have seen, the carrying out of a post-hypnotic command
several thousand minutes after awaking can neither be explained
by any ordinary physiological power of appreciating time, nor by
a supposed spontaneous rehypnosis with temporary revival of
memory.   The feat, according to Gurney, could only be performed
as the result of the intelligent action of a secondary consciousness,
which watched the time as it passed just as the ordinary one did;
and, when the correct time arrived, pushed the ordinary consciousness on one side, took its place, and carried out the
command.   In Gurney's opinion, the mental conditions involved
in the execution of post-hypnotic commands varied widely in
different cases.   Of these the following are examples :—

(1) A subject was told to do something ten minutes after she
awoke.   On awaking, she looked at the clock until the expiration

of the time, then executed the order. In this case the subject was conscious of having consulted the clock, and afterwards—apart from any question of the revival of hypnotic memory in post-hypnotic states—remembered having done so.

(2) A subject was told to do something five minutes after he awoke. Immediately on awaking, he looked at the clock, and continued to do so at intervals, talking naturally meanwhile to those present. At the end of five minutes he executed the order. Afterwards, he neither recollected looking at the clock, nor carrying out the command.

This case appeared to occupy an intermediate position between No. 1 and the others about to be cited.

(3) A subject was told that on the thirty-ninth day from then he was to execute a post-hypnotic suggestion. He had no memory of the command when awake, and no reference was made to it until March 19th, when he was suddenly asked, during hypnosis, how many days had elapsed since it was given. He instantly replied, " Sixteen," and added that there were twenty-three more to run. Both statements were correct.

(4) Another subject was told on March 26th, that he was to do something on the 123rd day from then. On April 18th, he was rehypnotised and asked if he remembered the order. He at once replied, " Yes, this is the twenty-third day; a hundred more." Further questioning made it clear that every few days the command occurred to his mind, and that he calculated how many days had passed and how many more had to elapse. His waking memory retained no recollection of the original suggestion, nor was it aware of the memories and calculations which he had described when hypnotised.

In the two last cases the watching was undoubtedly wholly of an internal kind, and although obviously accompanied by consciousness, was afterwards entirely forgotten.

REMARKS.—The experiments — as also those described in Groups 3 and 4, Automatic Writing, pp. 139-141—showed, according to Gurney, that the hypnotic substrata included higher psychical functions than mere random spurts of memory—to wit, processes of deliberate reckoning and reflection, which it would be almost impossible to conceive as having only a physiological existence. In No. 4,[1] the order itself was remembered and

---

[1] *I.e.* in No. (4) just cited, not Group 4.

realised by the secondary consciousness, while the primary consciousness was wholly without knowledge of it. In Gurney's opinion, these so-called automatic writings, in most cases at all events, were intelligent, and involved mentation. When a statement was made which the subject was told he was afterwards to record in writing, the performance might possibly be regarded as an exclusively automatic one, due to a "setting of the organism." Sometimes, however, the impression was made without a hint as to the future—without the faintest suggestion that it would afterwards produce any result whatever. Yet, in the midst of quite irrelevant surroundings and experiences, the phenomenon appeared, as soon as the opportunity of "automatic" representation arose. Here the organism could not have been specially set for the effect. Further, if we regarded the action as purely automatic, we should be compelled to concede a singular power to hypnotic impressions, viz. that of storing up energy in the brain which would work mechanically outwards along the motor nerves, as soon as the act of writing was sufficiently easy for the muscles. Moreover, memory on rehypnotisation afforded strong evidence of mentation. Not only did the subject remember the original idea conveyed to him, and the fact that he had written something, but also the exact words he had used to convey his conception of the impression. Surely this indicated an intelligent apprehension of the words. We have seen that the memory of these so-called automatic acts could be recalled in hypnosis, while others, in addition, indicated the existence of a hypnotic memory superior to the normal one, since the facts recorded had occurred at an early period of the subject's life and had long been forgotten.

Granting the existence of a secondary consciousness, how far does this explain all the phenomena we have been considering ?

The facts just cited—and these might be supplemented by many more—apparently indicate not only that a secondary consciousness exists, but also that it can act simultaneously with, and independently of, the primary one. Even, however, if we grant the existence of a secondary consciousness, this does not explain all the phenomena of time appreciation and arithmetical calculation that we have been considering.

Obviously, if the intelligence of the secondary consciousness were at all comparable to that of the primary one, it would not be difficult for it to calculate the arrival of the 39th or the

123rd day from any given date. In Gurney's cases, it apparently performed this feat with ease, and the subject when hypnotised could recall the manner in which it had been accomplished.

Here the secondary consciousness apparently acted in just the same way as the primary one might have done under similar circumstances; having to execute an order on the 39th day from a given date, it recalled the fact from time to time, and noted how many days had passed and how many had to come. Many of the experiments I have cited, notably the more complicated ones executed by Miss D., present more difficult problems; and by none of the theories already considered can these be properly solved. Bernheim's explanation, as we have seen, is in opposition to observed facts, while Gurney's objections to that of Beaunis apply with even greater force to my cases. Thus, if there is little analogy between ordinary physiological periods of time, and, for example, 39 days chosen suddenly and arbitrarily by human volition, the analogy is still less between the former and, say, 40,845 minutes.

Further, the secondary consciousness theory, while it affords a reasonable explanation of the way in which Gurney's subjects carried out their suggestions, fails to account for much that is important in the cases of time appreciation I have cited. The following are the principal points which demand explanation :— (1) The want of hypnotic memory as to the manner in which the suggestions were carried out. (2) The fact that the suggestions not only involved feats of arithmetical calculation and memory far beyond the subjects' normal powers, but also in some cases beyond their ordinary hypnotic ones. (3) The difference in the nature of the time appreciation required in Gurney's cases and in those cited by me.

(1) *The want of hypnotic memory as to the manner in which the suggestions were carried out.*

According to Bernheim, the hypnotic subject is conscious in all stages; and all the memories of hypnotic life, which are lost on awaking, can be restored by suggestion or other means. This statement is not absolutely correct. Hypnotic life, it is true, is more conscious than the normal one, and lacks the prolonged and regularly recurring periods of unconsciousness represented in the latter by sleep. Sometimes, however, deeply hypnotised subjects receive impressions and even perform acts of which they are unconscious :—

(*a*) Thus, where anæsthesia has been induced for surgical purposes, the subjects can recall nothing of the operations, either when awake or in subsequent hypnoses. Generally speaking, however, present forgetfulness does not prove past unconsciousness. When we find, however—in the instances where analgesia and hyperæsthesia have been simultaneously excited—amnesia as to certain sensations, associated with hyperæsthesia as to others, we have reasonable grounds for inferring that the sensations which cannot be recalled never occurred, and thus could not be present to consciousness. This view is further strengthened by the fact that the operations were characterised by absence of shock, persistence of analgesia after awaking, and unusual rapidity of healing.

(*b*) If a subject is told to be unconscious of everything until aroused by the operator, he will, if neither questioned nor touched, take no notice of what is said or done around him, while suggestion, in subsequent hypnoses, often fails to revive any memory of what has taken place.

(*c*) If a simple movement is suggested, of which volition does not disapprove, it may after a time become automatic : *i.e.* after having been frequently consciously and voluntarily performed, it may be executed unconsciously, as a genuine automatic act, in response to the habitual stimulus which has excited it. Here, again, the lost memory cannot be recalled by suggestion in subsequent hypnoses.

With the exception of examples of the three classes just cited, the acts of hypnotic life are performed consciously, and can be recalled by suggestion in subsequent hypnoses. Further, since the hypnotic memory is more exact and far-reaching than the normal one, the absence of memory as to given circumstances of hypnotic life *other than those just cited* is markedly suspicious. These suspicions are deepened when the forgotten act is analogous to those invariably remembered by the hypnotised subject. Gurney's subjects easily remembered their calculations as to the days that had passed, those that had to come, and the terminal time of the experiment. In some instances, when the arithmetical problems involved were simple, Miss O.[1] recalled in subsequent

[1] See pp. 134-9.

hypnoses the fact that she had calculated the terminal time of the suggestion, and had set herself to carry it out at the appointed hour. This, by the way, Gurney asserted hypnotised subjects never did. When the experiments became more complicated, Miss O. ceased to do this, and then, like Miss D.,[1] was unable to revive in hypnosis the slightest trace of memory as to the manner in which the suggestions had been carried out: they could then recall no calculations and no time-watching, no foretelling of the terminal time, and no recognition of it when it arrived. Yet, from what we know of hypnotic memory, it is impossible to doubt that, if calculations and observations of this kind had been made by the subjects, they would have been able to have remembered them when again hypnotised.

(2) *The fact that the suggestions not only involved feats of arithmetical calculation and memory beyond the subjects' normal powers, but also in some cases beyond their ordinary hypnotic ones.*

Delbœuf pointed out that his subjects in the normal state were unable to make the necessary calculations involved in his time experiments; therefore, the success of these experiments, he said, demonstrated that the subjects when hypnotised had an idea of the passage of time, and subconsciously calculated when the suggestions fell due. Experiments made in hypnosis, however, showed that the subject was quite incapable of calculating even much simpler problems than those involved; and, although this fact was recorded by Delbœuf himself, he apparently entirely missed its significance.

When my subject, Miss D., was asked to calculate in hypnosis the time that the suggestions would fall due, she was wrong in the first nine instances, her errors frequently being extremely gross ones. Again, unless specially asked to do so, the secondary consciousness, apparently, made no calculations at all. The time appreciation, however, could not be carried out independently of such calculations—obviously the subject could not perform an act at the expiration of 40,845 minutes unless she—or some "self" or "consciousness" within her—knew the terminal time this represented.

Further, in Miss D.'s case, the hypnotic memory was apparently incapable of retaining the complicated series of figures

[1] See pp. 119-89.

which were read to her. When she was questioned about them
in subsequent hypnosis, but before the fulfilment of the suggestions, she always recalled that the latter had been made, but
rarely correctly remembered their details—her recollection being
less and less distinct in proportion to the time which had elapsed
since they had been received.

(3) *The difference in the nature of the time-appreciation required
in Gurney's case and in those cited by me.*

There is a marked difference between the recognition of a
particular day on its arrival, and the last minute in such a series
as 40,845. A secondary self or intelligence, which can count
the days that have passed and those that have to come, and
refreshes its memory by doing this every night, could have no
difficulty in recognising the terminal day. The varying impressions from the external world, which tell us that a new day has
dawned, would be received as freely by the secondary as by the
primary consciousness; and all that the former would have to do
would be to associate them with the calculation it had made the
previous night that the next day would be the suggested one. In
my cases the problem was a widely different one. Granting that
some intelligence worked out the arithmetical portion and
determined that the suggestion fell due, for example, at 3.25 P.M.,
a fortnight later, the determination of the arrival of that particular
moment differs widely from the recognition of the dawning of a
given day. Admitting that some intelligence, equal to the
primary one, tried to determine when this moment arrived,
circumstances, often specially arranged, added to the difficulties of
the task. In some instances, for example, Miss D. was in a
darkened room for several hours before the suggestion was
executed, and absolutely without any of the ordinary methods of
determining the time. Even if she knew what o'clock it was
when she entered the room at noon, how could she determine
when it was 3.25 ?

The general conditions of memory, then, in reference to the
experiments I have cited, apparently show that the ordinary
secondary consciousness of hypnosis—or at all events such manifestations of it as Gurney describes—did not participate in them at
all. Further, the feats in calculation and memory were beyond the
power of that consciousness; we have no evidence of the secondary

consciousness carrying out time appreciations comparable to those involved in these particular cases. Some intelligence, however, must have made the arithmetical calculations, and, further, corrected them when they were erroneously worked out by the secondary consciousness, as revealed by my questions in hypnosis. "Something" also must have remembered the complicated series of figures and the varying results of the calculations, and also, in some fashion, noticed the time as it passed, and connected this with the date given as the result of the calculations involved in the suggestions. Could the problems have been worked out by a third consciousness acting independently of the other two? The theory that a multiple as well as a secondary consciousness exists is not a new one, although, as far as I know, it has not yet done duty in explaining the phenomenon of time appreciation.

Multiple Personalities in Relation to Time Appreciation and Calculation.

Miss D., as we have seen, wrongly calculated in hypnosis when a complicated time suggestion would fall due; notwithstanding this, the suggestion was carried out correctly in the waking state. The subject, however, was unable to recall, when again hypnotised, that she had corrected the original erroneous calculation; while at the same time no recollection either of the original suggestion, or of the erroneous calculation and its subsequent correction, existed in the normal waking consciousness. The results of the time appreciation and calculation, presumably due to a third consciousness, appeared as a sudden uprush into whatever personality—waking, sleeping, or ordinary hypnotic—happened to be present at the moment. When the ordinary hypnotic consciousness had been asked to make the necessary calculations, and did so erroneously, the third consciousness ignored these mistakes and did its work correctly. Further, the passage of the message from the third to the second consciousness seemed to make a particularly strong impression upon the latter, or to leave, for some time at all events, the door of communication open between the two. Thus, the second consciousness, which had forgotten the details of the suggestion before these were carried out, could recall them accurately for some time after they had been executed.[1]

[1] See p. 188.

Further, in the experiments cited, we notice (1) that the ordinary hypnotic consciousness possessed no recollection of having made the calculations necessary for finding out the terminal time, and (2) could not recall any form of time-watching. Further, the ordinary hypnotic memory was incapable of retaining the complicated series of suggestions : it remembered they had been made, but could not recall their details. Thus, hypnotic forgetfulness was not only manifested in reference to acts which might possibly be regarded as automatic ones inherited from some ancestral type, but was also shown in regard to others of an entirely different nature, and which cannot possibly have arisen in this way. Obviously some of these phenomena cannot be regarded as hereditary automatic acts of the hypnotic state; nor as analogous to normal automatic ones, seeing that they had not been previously performed in the hypnotic condition. The simultaneous appearance in hypnosis of a greater number of phenomena (regarding them from their physical side only) than can be manifested in waking life, may possibly be explained by the existence of several subconscious states. The normal attention, apparently, cannot attend to so many things at once as the hypnotic. Now, as we have seen, certain of these hypnotic acts, seemingly performed unconsciously, really demand intelligent attention : not only did they require it in the past, but, as they are neither inherited nor acquired automatic acts, they obviously require it in the present. The evidence in favour of several subconscious states is further strengthened by the fact that these intelligent hypnotic acts to which we have just referred are sometimes performed without any feeling of effort. But, as Ribot says : "Every one knows by experience that voluntary attention is always accompanied by a feeling of effort, which bears a direct proportion to the duration of the state and the difficulty of maintaining it."

Granting that one or more subconscious states exist in the human personality, and that hypnotic phenomena owe their origin to the fact that we have by some means or other succeeded in tapping them, two questions still remain :—

First, let it be supposed that I possess a friend called "Brown," who is usually, physically and mentally, an ordinary individual ; from time to time, however, he manifests an extraordinary increase of physical powers. Still more rarely, again, he displays a range of mental powers of which he had formerly given no indication.

I ask for an explanation : I am told that "Brown," as I know him best, is indeed "Brown"; but that his increased physical powers are due to the fact that when he shows them he is "Jones," and his increased mental ones to the further fact that he is then "Robinson." Granting that the phenomena afford evidence of three separate personalities, I cannot accept this explanation as a solution of the problem in its entirety. I want to know, first, how "Jones" and "Robinson" acquired their powers, and, secondly, what has been done to or by "Brown" to enable their powers to be evoked.

Myers' explanation, or at all events part of it, was that these powers were a revival of those formerly possessed by some lower ancestral type. He frankly admitted, however, that the analogies to which we could appeal were certainly vague and remote, and that to find them we must leave the higher mammalia and descend to the crab, worm, or amœba. As we have seen, Delbœuf's theory was practically a similar one.

Is it reasonable, however, to suppose that the hypnotic powers, regarded as a whole, existed in some lower ancestral type ?

Granting that a limited analogy exists between lower animal types and hypnotised subjects, as to their power of influencing certain physical conditions, it would, I think, be impossible to establish an analogy between the mental and moral powers of the latter and those of the savage or lower animal. For example, the subject who suddenly developed increased arithmetical powers was not likely to have derived them from some savage ancestor who was unable to count beyond five, or from some lower animal, presumably ignorant of arithmetic. Again, the same subject *when hypnotised* spontaneously solved a difficult problem in dressmaking. The power of correctly designing a garment, in accordance with the passing fashion of the present day, could hardly have been derived from some woad-stained ancestor, or lower animal form. Further, the increased modesty of the hypnotised subject, his greater power of controlling or checking morbid passions or cravings, does not find its counterpart in the savage or the ape.

Myers admitted that the argument from analogy was weakest when we considered the mental and moral powers of hypnosis. But if it is the essential characteristic of the subliminal state that the "spectrum of consciousness" is extended at both its physiological and its psychological ends, surely an explanation is equally necessary of both these extensions. A theory in itself imperfect becomes still more so, when every fact that is supposed to establish the extension of one end of the spectrum renders the extension of the other still more difficult to explain.

If we admit that hypnotic powers are derived from some lowly non-human type, is their easy recovery probable?

I have seen cases in which all the phenomena characteristic of deepest hypnosis could be readily evoked, *absolutely without training*, within a couple of minutes of the commencement of the process employed for the induction of the primary hypnosis. If any of these were derived from amoeba, worm, or crab, the rapidity with which they were aroused was surely surprising.

Is it likely that the hypnotic powers should have been lost in development?

Some of the powers of the hypnotic state are said to have dropped out of the supraliminal consciousness in the process of evolution, as their association with it had become unnecessary in the struggle for existence. It must be noticed, however, that many of these powers have not only ceased to be employed automatically or unconsciously, but also have sometimes apparently disappeared altogether; and, until hypnosis was induced, no means existed by which the supraliminal consciousness could evoke them. Now, the powers which the hypnotic self possesses are so numerous, varied, and frequently so essential for the comfort or well-being of the individual, that it is difficult to conclude that development is responsible for their loss! Take, for example, the power of inhibiting pain. Granting that some lower type possessed it—a fact difficult to prove—when and why was this important power dropped? In this over-civilised age, we appear to have abandoned some of the powers of the subliminal self just at the very moment when we most require them; as is shown by the complaints about street noises and the manners of children. In many instances, at all events, the supraliminal self is sadly embarrassed by the fact that it cannot perform that feat, so easy to the subliminal one, of shutting out undesired sensations of sound; and can, in consequence, neither work by day nor sleep by night.

What is the connection between hypnotic methods and the production of hypnotic phenomena?

To this I think no reasonable answer has been given.

Personally, I can see no logical connection between the acts of fixed gazing, of concentration of attention, or of suggested ideas of drowsy states, and the wide and varied phenomena of hypnosis. Hypnotic phenomena do not appear spontaneously, and some of the methods described must have been employed in each case before primary hypnosis was induced. But I cannot conceive the idea that such methods explain the phenomena.

Shock, hysteria, etc., are said to be the origin of the phenomena of multiple personalities in cases unassociated with hypnotism, but these terms explain nothing. We know little of the essential conditions associated with these morbid states, nor why they should produce an apparent severing of the personality in some instances and not in others.

Pierre Janet's Theory.

According to Pierre Janet, the presence of the secondary self is always a symptom of hysteria ; the essential fact about hysteria being its lack of synthetising power, and the consequent disintegration of the field of consciousness into mutually exclusive parts. Further, the primary and secondary consciousnesses added together never exceed the normal total consciousness of the individual.

Here the generalisation is certainly far too wide. Doubtless many cases of secondary consciousness correspond with Janet's description ; others, however, present conditions which are its exact opposite. Thus, while hysteria is a prominent symptom in cases of *spontaneous* " secondary consciousness," it is, on the other hand, not necessarily connected in any way with its " hypnotic " forms. Thousands of healthy men, absolutely devoid of any trace of hysteria, have been hypnotised ; while hysteria itself, instead of favouring the induction of hypnosis, renders it more difficult.

Further, on the relation between the severed personalities and the normal total consciousness, William James justly points out that many instances have been noted in which the secondary self is more highly developed than the primary one—it knows, for example, all that the ordinary self. ever knew, and also much that it had either forgotten or never known. Dr. Prince's case [1] is a typical example of this. Here, the third personality not only knew all about her own life and that of the secondary personality,

[1] Pp. 394-5.

but also could recall (*a*) all that the normal personality could remember, and, further, (*b*) many things that the primary personality had known, but forgotten, as well as (*c*) acts which the normal self had performed automatically or absent-mindedly, and which had only aroused normal consciousness partially, if at all. (*d*) Finally, the third personality recalled events which had occurred in the delirium of fever—things which the primary self was absolutely ignorant of, and indeed had never known.[1]

Remarks.—None of the theories we have been examining can be considered satisfactory. No revival of powers supposed to be possessed by lower animal forms can possibly explain the entire range of hypnotic phenomena; neither, again, can they be accounted for by an interrupted connection between the nerve-cells, nor by that elastic term "hysteria." Gurney's theory—that the secondary consciousness calculates and watches the time just as the primary one might do—is satisfactory for those instances in which it has been proved that this has occurred. It fails, however, when we attempt to apply it to those instances in which the proof was absent, and in which the feats in calculation and time appreciation were beyond the powers of the secondary self.

As the secondary self is often intellectually superior to the primary one, though we do not know why, we might be inclined to admit, although equally without reason for it, that the third self transcends the second one. As all the selves inhabit one body, and as the secondary and tertiary ones have presumably access to all the information which reaches the primary, are we to suppose that they have proved the apter scholars? It seems more than fanciful to imagine that while the school-boy's ordinary self was learning his lessons, a second boy was peering over his shoulder, as it were, and doing the work still better. What must we say, however, to the idea of a third boy learning along with Nos. 1 and 2, and surpassing both of them?

Even granting that a third self exists, and that it possesses powers superior to those of the second one, we are not yet at the end of our difficulties, for the examples of time appreciation we have been discussing present problems still more complex than those with which Gurney had to deal. As we have seen, there is a marked difference between knowing a particular day on its

---

[1] In Félida X's case, the secondary personality, which arose *spontaneously*, was markedly superior to the primary one (pp. 385-6).

arrival, and recognising which is the terminal one amongst a long series of minutes. For example, suppose that a suggestion to be fulfilled in 40,845 minutes fell due at 3.15 this afternoon, and that—from 12.20 P.M. of the same day—the subject of it remained in a room where she was deprived of all ordinary means of determining the passage of time. We have seen that the ordinary hypnotic self was frequently unable to make the necessary calculations involved in the problem. Now, granting that the subject's third personality was able to do so, and had actually calculated 3.15 as the terminal time, and further, that this self had noted the time on entering the room and calculated that 2 hours and 55 minutes had to expire before the suggestion fell due, and even admitting that this third self was able to impart this information to the primary consciousness and to enlist its aid in the attempt to hit upon the exact moment, viz. 3.15, the question still remains, how was this done ?

According to William James, our usual time appreciations—minutes, hours, and days—have to be conceived symbolically and constructed by successive mental additions. To realise an hour, we must count "now!" "now!" "now!" indefinitely. Each "now" is the feeling of a separate bit of time, and the exact sum of the bits never makes a very clear impression on our minds. We have no sense for "*empty time*," and have to subdivide the time by noticing the sensations; after we have received a certain number, our impression of the amount told off becomes quite vague, and our only way of knowing it accurately is by counting, noticing the clock, or some other symbolic conception. Our estimation of the length of time varies from many causes. A time full of interesting experiences seems short in passing, but long when looked back upon ; time empty of incident is long in passing, but seems short in retrospect. Time passes quickly when we are so occupied with what is happening as not to notice the time itself. When we do nothing and feel but little we grow more and more attentive to the passage of time. The length of a watched minute seems incredible because the attention is devoted to the feeling of the time itself, such attention being capable of extremely fine subdivision. In conclusion, James says, "We are constantly conscious of a certain duration—the specious present—varying in length from a few seconds to probably not more than a minute, and that this duration (with its content perceived as having one part earlier and the other later) is the original intuition of time. Longer times are conceived by adding, shorter ones by dividing, portions of the vaguely bounded unit, and are habitually thought by us symbolically. Kant's notion of *intuition* of objective time as an 'infinite necessary continuum' has nothing to support it. The *cause* of the intuition which we really have cannot be the *duration* of our brain processes or our mental changes. That duration is rather the *object* of the intuition which, being realised at every moment of such duration, must be due to a permanently present cause. This cause—probably the simultaneous presence of brain processes of different phase—fluctuates; and hence a certain range of variation in the amount of the intuition, and its subdivisibility, accrues."

Further, "the direct *intuition* of time is limited to intervals of considerably less than a minute. Beyond its borders extends the immense region of *conceived* time, past and future, into one direction or another of which we mentally project all the events which we think of as real, and form a systematic order of them by giving to each a date."

If we accept James' explanation as to the methods by which time appreciations are carried out—and I know of no other more plausible—the time appreciations of Miss D. seem still more remarkable and inexplicable.

While I have endeavoured to show that the theories as to the origin of so-called secondary and multiple personalities are entirely inadequate, both as to the states themselves and to their phenomena, *I have no theory of my own to bring forward in substitution for these.* The fresh facts I have cited, although interesting, only add to the complexity of the problems we have to solve. As William James truly says, these manifestations of the "hidden self" are immensely complex and fluctuating things, which we have hardly begun to understand, and concerning which sweeping generalisation is sure to be premature. Meanwhile, he adds, a comparative study of subconscious states is of the most urgent importance for the comprehension of our nature.

At the beginning of this chapter I drew attention to the fact that so-called hypnotic phenomena might be divided into two apparently well-defined groups. I now propose to discuss the second of these :—

GROUP II.

Therapeutic Results, when these occur in conditions unassociated with clear and unmistakable Symptoms of Hypnosis.[1]

As already stated, many intermediate stages are to be observed between the second group, and that which we have recently been discussing, *i.e.* hypnotic somnambulism. For the sake of convenience and clearness, I propose to disregard the links which connect the two groups, and to limit myself to the consideration of the therapeutic phenomena which have apparently been produced by "suggestion" alone.

The cases drawn from *my own practice*, cited in the chapters on " Hypnotism in Surgery " and " Hypnotism in Medicine," were selected for the following reasons :—

(1) As I wished to give striking examples of the therapeutic powers of hypnotism, I practically cited successful cases alone.

(2) As I desired to show that the curative results of hypnotic treatment were often lasting, I selected those cases in which I had been able to trace the after-history.

(3) For the sake of increased evidential value, I confined myself to instances where the patients had been seen by other medical men, both before and after hypnotic treatment.

The question of the depth of the hypnosis, or even whether hypnosis had been induced at all, was not taken into consideration. I now propose to repair this omission, and to divide all the cases cited into two classes :—

(*a*) Those in which genuine hypnosis was induced.

(*b*) Those in which the characteristic phenomena of hypnosis were absent.

After having made this division, I will discuss the mental and physical conditions which were apparently present in the second class.

I. SURGICAL CASES.

Profound hypnosis was induced in all the surgical cases reported from my own practice, the only apparent exception being that of Mrs. —— (No. 8). In this instance it is true that

[1] It is to be noted that this Group is invariably included in all general statistics as to "Suggestibility," *i.e.* all patients who have responded to *curative suggestions* are therein assumed to have been *hypnotised.*

the patient appeared to be awake. She had, however, been deeply hypnotised on former occasions, and her condition during operation was really one of hypnosis, although this had been so modified by training as to make it resemble the waking state.

II. MEDICAL CASES.

1 A. *Grande Hystérie.*—In Case No. 1, the only one fully recorded, there were no symptoms of hypnosis.

1 B. *Monosymptomatic Hysteria.*—In Nos. 6, 7, 8, and 9 hypnosis was induced, while in Nos. 5 and 10 it was apparently absent.

1 C. *Ordinary Hysteria.*—In Nos. 20, 21, 22, 24, 25, and 29 hypnosis was induced, while in Nos. 23, 26, 30, and 31 it was absent.

1 D. *Mental Troubles of a Hysterical Nature.*—None of my cases in this group, *i.e.* Nos. 32, 33, 34, 35, 36, 37, as well as the unnumbered case following No. 37, presented symptoms of hypnosis.

2. *Neurasthenia.*—In Case No. 40 hypnosis was induced; in Case No. 41 hypnosis was apparently absent.

3. *Insanity.*—In No. 46 hypnosis was induced.

4. *Dipsomania.*—In Nos. 56 and 61 hypnosis was induced, while in Nos. 57, 58, 59, 60, 62, and 63 it was apparently absent.

5. *Morphinomania.*—In No. 65 hypnosis was induced, while in No. 64 it was apparently absent.

6. *Vicious and Degenerate Children.*—In Nos. 68, 69, 71, and 72 hypnosis was induced; in Nos. 70 and 73 it was apparently absent.

7. *Obsessions.*—In Nos. 80, 81, and 85 hypnosis was induced; in Nos. 82, 83, 84, and 86 it was absent.

8. *Epilepsy.*—In No. 94 hypnosis was induced; in No. 95 it was absent.

9. *Chorea.*—In No. 99 hypnosis was induced.

10. *Stammering.*—In Nos. 101 and 102 hypnosis was apparently absent.

11. *Sea-sickness.*—In Nos. 103 and 104 hypnosis was induced.

12. *Skin Diseases.*—In Nos. 109 and 110 hypnosis was induced.

Thus out of the above fifty-nine illustrative *medical* cases twenty-eight were hypnotised, and thirty-one presented no symptoms of hypnosis.[1] Further, though many of the latter were cases of grave and long-standing illness, yet in some instances the recovery was extremely rapid. Was their recovery due to hypnotic influence or simply to " suggestion," more or less closely associated with emotional conditions? This question is an extremely difficult one to answer. On the one hand, the conditions regarded as characteristic of hypnosis were wanting. Thus :—

(1) In most instances, owing to muscular spasm or mental unrest, concentration of attention was absent, and there was repose of neither mind nor body.

(2) There was no involuntary closure of the eyes.

(3) In a few instances the patients became drowsy, but this resembled the drowsiness of normal life, and was not followed by amnesia.

On the other hand, the evidence as to the results being due to " suggestion " alone is by no means convincing. Thus :—

(1) The patients were actually subjected to one or other of the usual methods of inducing hypnosis. Fixed gazing (except in cases of convulsions and the like), monotonous passes, and suggestion were all employed.

(2) Suggestion in ordinary life, apart from profound emotional states, rarely produces curative results such as those described.

(3) Many of the patients were absolutely incredulous as to their receiving benefit from the treatment.

(4) Others approached the subject with an open mind, but few, if any, had profound faith in it.

(5) In most instances, suggestion had already been unsuccessfully employed, and sometimes so even when associated with profound emotional states.

While I am quite willing to admit that I cannot demonstrate that the cases in question were hypnotised, I find it equally difficult to believe that their recovery was due to suggestion alone. For, as just stated, suggestion had already played an important part in their treatment, and entirely with negative results.

Thus, for example, in Case No. 1, the blisters which were applied to the limbs to render muscular movement painful were so many indirect suggestions.

---

[1] *I.e.* despite the fact that these patients all underwent hypnotic treatment, none of them presented *unmistakable* symptoms of hypnosis.

In No. 10, the patient had firmly believed that a certain doctor could cure him, but this self-suggestion had produced no result.

In No. 23, the patient had received varied and forcible suggestions; for instance, she was told that the application of Pacquelin's cautery was certain to cure her. Despite this, it had no effect; but suggestions, *when associated with hypnotic methods*, were at once responded to.

No. 31 is particularly interesting. The patient, a well-known scientific man, had systematically tried to influence himself by suggestion, but without success. After three hypnotic sittings, he not only recovered from his insomnia, but also acquired the power of self-suggestion. He could prevent sea-sickness and arrest the pain of organic disease, even although this power had not been suggested to him by me.

In Nos. 58 and 59, two typical cases of dipsomania, the patients had undoubtedly received frequent and forcible suggestions from their friends and relatives, but, despite this, suggestion produced no result until associated with hypnotic methods.

In most of the other cases cited suggestion had already played a part, but in none had it produced the slightest effect.

Taking all the above facts into consideration, while I am not prepared to assert that the cases in question were genuinely hypnotised, I find it equally difficult to believe that the curative results were due to suggestion alone. It is possible that, owing to the methods employed, some change was produced in the patients' organism which rendered them more susceptible to the influence of suggestion than they had previously been in the normal state. Further than that I have nothing to say, for I am ignorant both as to the exact nature of the change in question, and of the reason why hypnotic methods should have evoked it.

CHAPTER XIII.

THE SO-CALLED DANGERS OF HYPNOTISM.

I HAVE purposely refrained from discussing the risks of hypnotic practice until theory had been dealt with. For the question whether danger exists depends mainly upon the evidence which can be adduced in favour of hypnotic automatism. As we have seen, however, automatism cannot be regarded as the essential characteristic of the hypnotic state.

Braid did not believe that hypnotic practice was dangerous, and his views have already been stated (pp. 292-3).

Personally, I have never seen a single hypnotic somnambule who did not both possess and exercise the power of resisting suggestions contrary to his moral sense.[1] Despite this, I can conceive the possibility that, under certain circumstances, hurtful suggestions might be made with success. If a subject believed that hypnosis was a condition of helpless automatism, and that the operator could make him do whatever he liked, harm might result, not through the operator's power, but in consequence of the subject's self-suggestions.

The cases in which it has been "clearly proved" that hypnotism has done undoubted harm are neither numerous nor important. Charcot, and other members of the Salpêtrière school, asserted that hysterical symptoms sometimes appeared after the attempted induction of hypnosis. That such phenomena occurred with them is not surprising, when one considers the nature of the patients and their surroundings, and the violent and startling methods sometimes resorted to. Charcot also recorded one or two instances where the employment of hypnotism for stage purposes had produced bad effects.

It is to be noted that Bernheim, who still believes in the

---

[1] This statement includes also all the slighter forms of hypnosis.

possibility of suggested crime, admits that no single instance of genuine hypnotic crime has yet been proved, and asserts that in the "classical" cases, copied from one author to another, the subjects had really not been hypnotised at all. Even if one admitted that hypnotism was not free from danger, the same thing could be said of other methods of treatment.[1] The points to be considered are the nature of the risks, and whether these are capable of being minimised or eliminated. The opponents of hypnotism, however, instead of discussing these points calmly, have sometimes attacked hypnotism on account of its alleged dangers in a manner which they themselves would be the first to recognise as unfair if applied to any other branch of science.

For example, in the *Revue Médicale de l'Est*, February 1st, 1895, Bernheim records the only case, as far as I know, in which death followed hypnosis induced by a medical man. The patient suffered from phlebitis, accompanied by severe pain; and to relieve this, Bernheim hypnotised him. He died two hours afterwards, and *post-mortem* examination showed that death was due to embolism of the pulmonary artery. The case is referred to in the *British Medical Journal*, and though it is admitted that the occurrence was nothing more than an "unlucky coincidence," it is stated, at the same time, that "it is at least arguable that the psychical excitement induced by the hypnotising process may have caused a disturbance in the circulatory system, which had a share in bringing about the catastrophe." Bernheim has hypnotised over 10,000 hospital patients; sometimes this would be done for the relief of pain associated with inevitably fatal maladies, and, therefore, the matter for surprise is that death has not more frequently occurred during, or shortly after, the induction of hypnosis. The majority of fatal illnesses receive medical treatment: it would, then, according to the theory of the *British Medical Journal*, be justifiable to argue that the administration of drugs "may have had a share in bringing about the catastrophe." Certainly their use is likely to be attended with more physical and psychical excitement than is involved in the hypnotising processes in vogue at Nancy.

Such arguments against hypnotism are dangerous and apt to provoke unpleasant replies. For example, Moll, in speaking of

[1] A medicine given to relieve insomnia sometimes produces a "drug-habit"; treatment by *suggestion*, however, does not give rise to a "hypnotic-habit."

certain hostile criticisms, said: "If Professor —— had shown the same scepticism when the tuberculin craze excited all Germany, much injury to science and to his patients would have been prevented. The wantonness with which at that time the lives of many were staked will remain as a lasting blemish upon science; and it cannot be denied that the excessive use of tuberculin was the cause of the untimely death of many human beings. In ordinary life, one would describe such a proceeding as an offence against the person, of which the issue was death. I cannot admit that there is a special law for clinical professors, and that when they have, in such a manner, hastened the death of a human being, another expression should be used."

Articles upon hypnotism by X, which appeared in the *Journal of Mental Science,* have already been referred to. His statements as to its dangers show evidence, I am afraid, of too hasty generalisation, as well as of misquotation. Thus, in referring to my address to the Psychological Section of the British Medical Association at Edinburgh,[1] he says: "The bold attempt of Dr. Milne Bramwell to prove that there are no drawbacks to the therapeutic use of hypnotism is, however, a challenge which should be promptly met." Now I have never, either in writing or speaking, asserted that there were no drawbacks to the therapeutic use of hypnotism, but, on the contrary, have constantly pointed out that such existed. For example, in this country hypnotism is rarely resorted to until other remedial measures have failed, and this greatly decreases its chance of success. Further, I have never denied that hypnotism, through ignorance or malice on the part of the operator, might be so misused as to do harm; this risk, however, is not only grossly exaggerated, but falls far short of that associated with ordinary medical treatment.

What I really said was totally different, namely, that, as far as my experience went, the employment of hypnotism by medical men acquainted with the subject was devoid of danger. In support of this, I cited Forel's assertion that he, as well as Liébeault, Bernheim, Wetterstrand, van Eeden, de Jong, Moll, and the other followers of the Nancy school, had never seen a single instance in which mental or physical harm had been

<hr>

[1] Sixty-sixth Annual Meeting of the British Medical Association. See the *British Medical Journal,* September 10th, 1898, pp. 669-678.

caused by hypnotism. No complete record of their cases has been published, but the number certainly exceeds fifty thousand. On October 15th, 1898, Forel informed me that he still held this opinion, and had never observed even the slightest inconvenience from hypnotic practice. Further, I have watched the work of nearly all those cited by Forel, and have seen nothing opposed to his statement.

I could add many names to Forel's list, but will content myself by quoting two in this country, choosing them for their connection with asylum practice.

In 1890, Dr. Percy Smith and the late Dr. A. T. Myers published an account of the hypnotic treatment of twenty-one insane patients in Bethlem Hospital. I am authorised by the former to state that no harm was done.

I have also Dr. Outterson Wood's permission to state that, while he acted as Honorary Secretary to the British Medical Association Committee for the Investigation of Hypnotism, he performed many experiments, and arrived at the following conclusions with regard to hypnotism :—(1) Its phenomena were genuine. (2) It was of distinct therapeutic value. (3) Its use in skilled hands was absolutely devoid of danger.

My position might be attacked in two ways : (A) by attempting to prove mal-observation ; (B) the facts being granted, by showing that they did not warrant the conclusions drawn from them. These, the only two points at issue, X entirely ignores. He says : "Very many observers have seen cases in which hypnotism has been followed by very definite and distinctly evil results. Many instances of this kind have been recorded, and good service would be done by their collection and tabulation, as a check to future assertions of this kind." Granting that this be true, what connection has it with the point in dispute ? If a group of surgeons performed a certain operation fifty thousand times without a death, would they not be justified in inferring that in their hands, at all events, it was devoid of danger ? Would their position be weakened by the " collection and tabulation " of the failures of others ?

Still there remain for discussion the hypnotic dangers referred to by X, namely (1) evil results recorded by other observers, and (2) those occurring in his own practice.

(1) Harm reported by Others.

As regards this group, X does not cite a single authority or case; surely the "collection and tabulation" to which he refers should have been done beforehand, and the results presented in such a way as to enable one to judge of their value as evidence.

I have investigated every case brought to my notice where hypnotism was stated to have done harm, and in none has the charge been proven. The two following may serve as a commencement of the "collection" X is desirous of making:—

(A) A patient, suffering from torticollis, who had been under my care for a few weeks, shortly afterwards underwent a surgical operation; an important blood-vessel was accidentally cut, and about ten days later she died from secondary hæmorrhage. I was informed that the surgeon asserted the hæmorrhage and death were due to the fact that the patient's constitution had been weakened by hypnotism. If this were true, the relatives felt that they had contributed to the death by permitting the patient to try hypnotic treatment, and I was asked whether I could in any way reassure them. This I had little difficulty in doing. I informed them (a) that hypnotism did not weaken the constitution; under its influence Esdaile had reduced the mortality in the removal of the tumours of elephantiasis from 50 to 5 per cent, and my own operative cases had all done well. (b) Even granting that hypnotism could weaken the constitution, it was unreasonable to suppose that its influence had spread from the patient to the surgeon, and thereby caused him to accidentally cut a blood-vessel. (c) I mentioned the not unimportant fact that I had absolutely failed to hypnotise the patient.

(B) In April, 1897, a medical acquaintance told me I must alter my views as to the dangers of hypnotism, because by its means, M., a Swiss medical man, had seduced eleven young female patients, and had in consequence been condemned to five years' imprisonment. One of the victims, I was told, had committed suicide, and before doing so, had left a written statement of the fact that she had been seduced through hypnotism. Further, I was informed that these statements were confirmed by ample official evidence. This I asked to see, and received what was described as "the official testimony from Dr. Calonder, of the *Advokaturbureau* in Chur, where the case was tried, stating that hypnotism had been abused in this shocking betrayal." My colleague continued, " I could also forward you the four German newspapers sent me ; but as they contain no details which I have not already given you, you probably would not care to have them."

The following is a translation of the document in question :— " In reply to your favour of the 26th inst., I hasten to inform you that, at the trial of Dr. M., no support was found for the assertion that he had employed hypnotism in the treatment of his patients. —(Signed) Dr. Calonder."

I asked for the German newspapers, and found that in the account of the trial hypnotism was not even mentioned. I then laid the matter before Professor Forel, of Zurich, who replied as follows :—" Dr. M. has never hypnotised a patient. The question was not raised at the trial, and no one suggested that he had employed hypnotism. The entire history is an English invention. In Zurich no one has spoken or written of hypnotism in con- nection with Dr. M. He is a throat specialist—an ordinary erotic pig, and has long been known as such. I have written to the Judge of the Supreme Court who tried Dr. M., and he has sent me a written statement which confirms mine; this I now enclose so that you may have a trustworthy document." Pro- fessor Forel's letter and that of the Judge are still in my possession. They describe Dr. M.'s methods of seduction, but as these have nothing to do with hypnotism, and are not particularly suitable for publication, I refrain from quoting them.

(2) X's Cases

X says that in his special department, presumably asylum practice, the evils consequent on hypnotic influence are grave, and that the few cases in which it seemed desirable to induce hypnosis were, in the end, apparently deteriorated in mental condition, and that the conservation of mental power, so urgently indicated, was, in fact, endangered. From this he concludes that hypnosis involves a weakening of the power of self-control, and " is, indeed, a shunting on one of those side tracks of disordered mental function of which insanity is the terminus." Here I may point out :—

(1) No figures are given, and the word "few" is an in- definite one.

(2) The disease from which the patients suffered is not stated, nor the absolutely essential information given whether it was one likely to end in mental deterioration apart from the treatment.

(3) If X found that hypnotic treatment produced grave evils in every instance in which he employed it, the fact that he continued to use it in other cases, besides the first one in which it had done harm, certainly demands explanation.

(4) X gives no detailed account of his cases, and thus the dangers to which he refers are based more upon assertion than upon evidence which might be examined and judged.

(5) It is to be noted, too, that X regards hypnosis as a condition analogous to hysteria, stupor, and látah. As already pointed out, this view is an entirely erroneous one. Thus, if X evoked these conditions in his patients by artificial means, the idea that these states had anything to do with hypnosis cannot be entertained for a moment. At the same time, if he actually succeeded in producing the symptoms of hysteria, stupor, and látah in patients who were already suffering from some other form of mental disorder, I can readily believe that this " involved a weakening of their powers of self-control, and was, indeed, a shunting on one of those side tracks of disordered mental function of which insanity is the terminus."

Granting even that mental deterioration actually resulted from X's so-called hypnotic practice, one cannot help feeling that his personal and limited experiments do not warrant the conclusions he draws from them. Fortunately, it is not a recognised principle in medicine that those who fail have the right to cry " Halt !" to the successful !

The commonest examples of the alleged evil results of hypnotic practice are found on examination to be nothing but cases of delusional insanity. A sensational instance of this kind recently went the round of the Continental press. It was asserted that a University professor had hypnotised one of his students and made him the subject of many disagreeable experiments. It was even stated that the former had only escaped conviction by exercising his hypnotic influence over the witnesses, and compelling them to give false evidence. This story was not devoid of foundation. A student had actually brought an action against a professor on the grounds just stated. It was proved in court, however, that the professor had never hypnotised any one, and that the student was suffering from delusional insanity.

From time to time charges of a like nature are made in the police courts, and are the subject of sensational paragraphs in the daily press: sometimes, improbable as it may seem, they are even gravely reproduced in medical journals.

In the insane mind, hypnotism and telepathy are gradually taking the place of electricity, and I frequently receive letters from persons who complain that they are the victims of telepathic persecution. In every instance, however, the writers are obviously insane.

CHAPTER XIV.

Historical.—Looking back on the revival of mesmerism, and on the origin and earlier development of hypnotism, one must admit that these movements were almost entirely due to Elliotson and Esdaile, Braid and Liébeault, all of whom were more or less martyrs to what they believed to be the truth.

Elliotson's researches cost him official position, reputation, fortune, and friends. He never entered University College after the practice of mesmerism had been forbidden within its walls; and from that time (1838) forward, until the Second International Congress of Experimental Psychology was held there in 1892, neither hypnotism nor mesmerism received the slightest recognition by the College. At the latter date, at the request of the late Dr. A. T. Myers, I brought to the Congress several patients who had undergone painless hypnotic operations. When I showed these at two of the meetings, reinducing analgesia and other hypnotic phenomena, history repeated itself. Just as Elliotson's demonstrations excited so much interest that he found he had to move from a smaller to a larger lecture room, so the same thing occurred in my case.

Esdaile's earlier mesmeric work was ignored by the medical authorities, while his later efforts were bitterly opposed. In his case, however, opposition only acted as a stimulus. It impelled him to do more than he had ever intended, and thus brought about his appeal to the Government, which resulted in the establishment of the official mesmeric hospital at Calcutta.

Esdaile was more a surgeon than a man of science, and could not understand why Professor Bennett supported 'hypnotism' at the very time 'mesmerism' was so fiercely attacked. Esdaile had evidently failed to grasp the importance of Braid's views as

2 F

to the *subjective* nature of hypnotic phenomena, and said he would willingly have called his operations 'hypnotic,' if he had known that a change of title was all that was necessary in order to insure their recognition.

Esdaile's later days were certainly saddened by the treatment he received, and he naturally asked what he had done to deserve it. He pointed out that he had remained poor for the sake of mesmerism, and had also saved thousands of human beings the pain which, until then, had invariably been associated with surgical operations. This, in itself, surely did not justify his being considered as an outcast from his profession.

Braid, who was essentially open-minded, and inspired with the truest scientific spirit, eagerly seized upon all fresh facts, and altered his theories in accordance with them. He not only invented the terminology we still use, but even, at a later date, rejected it as misleading.

Although Braid believed that hypnotic suggestion was a valuable remedy in functional nervous disorders, he did not regard it as a rival to other forms of treatment, nor wish in any way to separate its practice from that of medicine in general. He held that whoever talked of a "universal remedy" was either a fool or a knave : similar diseases often arose from opposite pathological conditions, and their treatment ought to be varied accordingly. He objected to being called a hypnotist ; he was, he said, no more a 'hypnotic' than a 'castor-oil' doctor.

Liébeault was rather neglected than abused. Although Elliotson had many followers, and Braid obtained a certain amount of scientific recognition, Liébeault, like Esdaile, worked alone. If he were mentioned at all, a thing which rarely happened, it was only as a fanatic or a madman.

Methods of inducing Hypnosis, Susceptibility, etc.—The various methods of inducing the hypnotic state, as well as the causes which apparently influence susceptibility to hypnosis, have already been discussed in detail. The principal points which ought to be kept in mind are :—

(1) That there is as yet no satisfactory explanation why hypnosis should be evoked by the methods employed.

(2) That the varying susceptibility to hypnosis is equally difficult to understand. We do not yet know why identical

methods should produce hypnosis in one instance, and have apparently no effect in another.

(3) That it is equally unexplained why susceptibility to curative suggestions should obviously be developed in patients who have undergone hypnotic methods of treatment, but in whom hypnosis has not manifestly been evoked.

The Experimental Phenomena of Hypnosis.—Many of the phenomena which are stated to occur in the hypnotic condition are undoubtedly genuine, and their existence has been confirmed by careful and repeated experiment. Others, such as the production of blisters and changes of temperature by suggestion, must be rejected : there is, as far as I am aware, no trustworthy evidence as to their occurrence.

Hypnotism in Medicine.—It is difficult to estimate the exact value of hypnotism in comparison with other forms of treatment. There are, however, one or two broad facts which ought to be kept in mind :—

(1) Hypnotism, as already pointed out, is not a universal remedy. It is simply a branch of medicine, and those who practise it sometimes combine it with other forms of treatment. Thus, in some instances it is difficult to say what proportion of the curative results were due to hypnotism, and what to other remedies.

(2) On the other hand, many cases of functional nervous disorder have recovered under hypnotic treatment after the continued failure of other methods. The cases already cited illustrate this. Many of the patients had long suffered from serious illness, while in most instances several years have now passed without relapse.

Further, the diseases which frequently respond to hypnotic treatment are often those in which drugs are of little or no avail. For example, what medicine would one prescribe for a man who, in the midst of mental and physical health, had suddenly become the prey of an obsession ? Such patients are rarely insane : they recognise that the idea which torments them is morbid ; they can trace its origin and development, but yet are powerless to get rid of it. In a recent case, the patient [1] gave the following account of his illness. He was upset, he said, by some trouble of a sentimental nature, and went to Paris for a day or two's change. There he saw a play in which insanity

---

[1] This patient recovered after a week's hypnotic treatment.

was skilfully portrayed by one of the actors. Immediately afterwards the laughter and gestures of his friends appeared insane in character, and he awoke the next night with the feeling that he himself was going mad. From the intellectual side he knew his friends were not insane, and did not believe that he was likely to become so; but the obsession was ever present. In cases of this kind hypnotism frequently yields good results; and, until I began hypnotic practice, I had no conception of the number of people whose lives were made miserable by morbid ideas. Sometimes these take the form of undefined dreads, and are associated with neurasthenia; at other times some particular obsession dominates the patient's whole life.

(3) In estimating hypnotic results, it must not be forgotten, too, that the majority of cases treated in this way are extremely unfavourable ones. Since I came to London, patients have rarely been sent to me when they first fell ill, and with most of them every other form of treatment had been tried before hypnotism was resorted to. As the value of hypnotic treatment and its freedom from danger become more fully recognised, it will doubtless be employed in earlier stages of disease. When that day comes the results ought to be still more striking.

(4) Above all else, it should be clearly understood that the object of all hypnotic treatment ought to be the development of the patient's control of his own organism. As already pointed out, many illnesses represent the culminating point in a life which has been characterised by lack of discipline and self-control. While attention is given to physical culture, the emotional side is too often neglected; but much disease would be prevented if we could develop and control moral states just as an athlete does physical ones.

The so-called Dangers of Hypnotism.—I have little to add to what has already been said as to the dangers of hypnotism. Although I am willing to admit that it is possible that harm may be done through the mismanagement of hypnotic cases, I have personally seen no evidence of this either in my own practice or in that of others. Further, I have never seen even the slightest bad effect follow carefully conducted hypnotic experiments. For several years Sidgwick, Gurney, Myers, and others experimented regularly on the same group of male subjects, and the latter suffered neither at the time nor afterwards.

There remains the further question as to the risks which may be encountered by those who embark on hypnotic practice. These have practically ceased to exist. It is true that an attempt was made in 1893 to discredit hypnotism by drawing attention to the fallacious nature of Luys' experiments and theories, but, as already stated, his experiments had long ceased to interest real students of hypnotism. At the present day the treatment of hypnotism by the profession is not only fair but generous.

Hypnotic Theories.—The views of the mesmerists and those of the Salpêtrière school have ceased to interest scientific men. All theories which attempt to find a general explanation of hypnotic phenomena in a physiological or a psychological inhibition, or in a combination of the two, will doubtless suffer a similar fate. The increased volition and intelligence, which are frequently observed in the " alert " stage of hypnosis, can be explained neither by an arrested action of the higher nervous centres nor by a hypothetical automatism. Further, subjects can be taught to hypnotise themselves, and can then induce the state and its phenomena at will. In such cases it is absolutely impossible that the phenomena can be due to the suspension of the subject's volition, or to the operator's supposed power of controlling him.

If the subliminal consciousness theory does not satisfactorily explain all the problems of hypnosis, we are at all events indebted to it for a clearer conception, not only of the condition as a whole, but also of many of its component parts.

The following points in this theory seem most worthy of notice :—

(1) That the essential characteristic of the hypnotic state is the subject's far-reaching power over his own organism.

(2) That volition is increased and the moral standard raised.

(3) That the phenomena of hypnosis arise from, or at all events are intimately connected with, voluntary alterations in the association and dissociation of ideas.

(4) Subliminal or subconscious states are more clearly defined than in previous theories.

(5) Myers' theory [1] closely resembles Braid's latest one. The

[1] At the Meeting of the British Medical Association, Edinburgh, 1898, Myers by special request, gave an account of his hypnotic theories to the Psychological Section. See *British Medical Journal*, Sept. 10th, 1898, p. 674.

existence of alternating consciousnesses was not only recognised
by Braid, but was also regarded by him as explanatory of certain
hypnotic phenomena.

The appreciation of time, with its accompanying necessary
calculations, and the solution in hypnosis of the 'dressmaking
problem' (p. 320), are phenomena which have an important
bearing on hypnotic theory.   Doubtless Carpenter would have
regarded the latter as a case of "unconscious cerebration."   The
so-called secondary self, however, was quite conscious that it had
solved the problem ; and, when hypnosis was again induced, was
able to give an account of the occurrence, and to tell when the
knowledge it had elaborated was received by the ordinary self.

While the phenomena of hypnosis show that consciousness
can be split up into two or more well-defined parts, this does not
justify us in concluding that distinct *personalities* may exist in
the same human being.   To the physiologist, at all events,
something more is necessary than evidence of alternating groups
of memories and changes of temper.   To put the matter
crudely, the phenomena we term mental are dependent on the
life and activity of the organ which we call the brain.   All the
physical part of the mechanism is enclosed in one skull, and the
varying psychical manifestations are associated with the changes
that take place therein.   It is doubtless true that an individual
may receive impressions which do not arouse consciousness at
the time, and that these may be the starting-point of mental
processes of which he only afterwards becomes conscious through
their results.   In hypnosis, too, he may do mental work of which
he is conscious in that condition, and of which he may yet know
nothing in the normal state.   Through accident or disease he
may become amnesic, aphasic, or both; or he may revive
memories long lost to his normal consciousness.   All these
varying psychical conditions, however, have their physical
correlative; they correspond to changes which have taken place
in that particular individual's brain.   However great may be the
alterations in consciousness, however marked the changes in
character, we cannot get away from the fact that these are
dependent on the one brain the individual was born with, and
the changes that one brain has undergone in subsequent life.
'John Smith' does not cease to be 'John Smith' when he is
hypnotised, nor when he becomes insane.

If Braid and Myers have done much towards giving us a clearer idea of the hypnotic state, they have also added to the difficulties of explaining it. A conception of hypnosis which limited its manifestations to simple automatic movements was comparatively easy to explain. The hypnotic subject who, while he has not lost the physical and mental powers of his waking condition, has acquired new and far-reaching ones, presents a very different problem. But normal life contains many problems, both physiological and psychological, which are yet unsolved, and some—such as the causal connection between mental and physical states—which are apparently insoluble; and while this is so, it would be unreasonable to expect a complete explanation of that still more complex state—the hypnotic. Further observation, however, is always giving us clearer insight, if not into the central problem itself, at all events into the phenomena that characterise it. What increased practical advantage this may give us in curing and preventing disease, alleviating pain, giving sleep, and improving moral states, time alone will show.

CHAPTER XV

REFERENCES.

FRENCH.

FROM THE *REVUE DE L'HYPNOTISME*, vol. i. 1887-88 to vol. xv. 1900-01.

ARTIGALAS et RÉMOND, Drs. Vol. vi. p. 250. " Note sur un cas d'hémorrhagies auriculaires, oculaires et palmaires provoquées par la suggestion."

BECHTEREW, Dr. (St. Petersburg). Vol. xiv. p. 89. " La suggestion hypnotique et le traitement de l'onanisme." " Sur les obsessions et les illusions importunes."

Vol. xiv. p. 155. " L'importance de l'hypnotisme et de la suggestion dans le traitement de l'alcoolisme."

BÉRILLON, Dr. EDGAR. Vol. i. p. 218. " Guérison par suggestion post-hypnotique d'une habitude vicieuse datant de dix ans."

Vol. ii. p. 59. " Les applications de l'hypnotisme au traitement des enfants vicieux."

Vol. ii. p. 169. " De la suggestion et de ses applications à la pédagogie."

Vol. ii. p. 176. " Tics nerveux traités par suggestion."

Vol. iv. p. 35. " Valeur de la suggestion hypnotique dans le traitement de l'hystérie."

Vol. iv. p. 153. " Les applications de la suggestion à la pédiatrie et à l'éducation mentale des enfants vicieux ou dégénérés."

Vol. iv. p. 336. " Neurasthénie grave traitée avec succès par la suggestion hypnotique."

Vol. v. p. 97. " Les indications formelles de la suggestion hypnotique en psychiatrie et en neuropathologie."

Vol. vi. p. 165. " Ataxie locomotrice traitée avec succès par la suggestion hypnotique."

Vol. vi. p. 269. " Méchanisme des phénomènes hypnotiques provoqués chez des sujets hystériques."

Vol. vii. p. 129. " Le traitement psychothérapeutique de la morphinomanie."

Vol. vii. p. 177. " Vomissements incoercibles de la grossesse traités avec succès par la suggestion."

Vol. viii. p. 15. " Onychophagie. Hystéro - épilepsie. Guérison rapide par la suggestion."

Vol. viii. p. 90. " Habitudes vicieuses associées chez une petite fille.— Onanisme et onychophagie, traités avec succès par la suggestion."

Vol. viii. p. 241. "Les phobies neurasthéniques envisagées au point de vue du service militaire."

Vol. viii. p. 359. "Le traitement psychique de l'incontinence nocturne d'urine."

Vol. ix. p. 28. "Le traitement de la morphinomanie." (Discussion by TANZI, etc.)

Vol. ix. p. 33. "Phobies neurasthéniques envisagées au point de vue professionel."

Vol. ix. p. 90. "Cri hystérique datant de trois mois guéri en une seule séance par la suggestion."

Vol. xii. p. 167. "Les principes de la pédagogie suggestive." (Giving list of his articles.)

Vol. xiii. p. 102. "De l'emploi de la suggestion hypnotique dans l'éducation des épileptiques."

Vol. xiii. p. 245. "Mal de mer et vertiges de la locomotion."

Vol. xv. p. 84. "Mélancholie traitée avec succès par la suggestion hypnotique."

BÉRILLON et DARIER, Drs. Vol. xiii. p. 179. "Strabisme avec diplopie guéri par la suggestion hypnotique."

BERNHEIM, Prof. Vol. i. p. 129. "De la suggestion envisagée au point de vue pédagogique."

Vol. ii. p. 138. "Sur un cas de régularisation des règles par suggestion."

Vol. xii. p. 137. "A propos de l'étude sur James Braid par le Dr. Milne Bramwell et de son rapport lu au Congrès de Bruxelles."

BESSE, Dr. Vol. iii. p. 213. "Troubles hystériques traités par l'hypnotisme."

BEZANÇON, Dr. (Paris). Vol. i. p. 150. "Diarrhée provoquée par suggestion chez une hystérique hypnotisable." (Also three teeth extracted during hypnotic anæsthesia.)

BOUFFÉ, Dr. Vol. xiii. p. 76. "La suggestion hypnotique comme traitement de l'onychophagie. Quelques réflexions sur ce syndrome considéré comme tare de dégénérescence."

BOURDON, Dr. Vol. iii. p. 141. "Jalousie morbide compromettant la vie, guérie par la suggestion."

Vol. vi. p. 358. "Applications variées de la suggestion chez une hystéro-épileptique."

Vol. viii. p. 59. "Anesthésie chirurgicale par suggestion."

Vol. x. p. 27. "La psychothérapie envisagée comme complément de la thérapeutique générale."

Vol. x. p. 134. "Onychophagie et habitudes automatiques, onanisme, etc., chez les enfants vicieux ou dégénérés."

Vol. xiii. p. 146. "La psychothérapie envisagée comme complément de la thérapeutique générale.

Vol. xiv. p. 145. "L'alcoolisme et le tabagisme traités avec succès par la suggestion hypnotique."

Vol. xiv. p. 176. "Accouchements sans douleurs par la méthode du Dr. Joire. Anesthésie suggestive."

Vol. xv. p. 365. "Applications de la psychothérapie aux neurasthénies graves et anciennes avec complications diverses : phobies, obsessions hypocondriaque, polysarcie, etc."

Vol. xi. p. 268. "Contracture spasmodique de psoas iliaque gauche datant de 4 ans. Guérison en une seule séance."

DÉCLE, CH., et CHAZARAIN, Dr. Vol. ii. p. 144. "Les courants de la polarité dans l'aimant et dans le corps humain."

DÉGA, Mlle. (docteur en médecine, Bordeaux). Vol. xiii. p. 373. "Un cas de spasmes rythmiques hystériques. Guérison rapide par la suggestion hypnotique."

DELBŒUF, Professeur. Vol. vii. p. 200. "Quelques considérations sur la psychologie de l'hypnotisme à propos d'un cas de manie homicide guérie par suggestion."

Vol. ix. pp. 225, 260. "L'hypnose et les suggestions criminelles."

DELBŒUF et FRAIPONT, Profs. Vol. v. p. 289. "Accouchement dans l'hypnotisme."

DIAZ, Dr. A. M. Vol. vi. p. 309. "Quelques faits d'anesthésie chirurgicale sous l'influence de la suggestion."

DOBROVOLSKY, Mlle. Vol. v. pp. 274, 310. "Huit observations d'accouchement sans douleur sous l'influence de l'hypnotisme."

DOMINGOS, Dr. JAQUARIBE (Brazil). Vol. xv. p. 266. "Note sur la guérison d'un cas d'hyperhydrose des mains."

DUMONTPALLIER, Dr. Vol. i. p. 257. "De l'analgésie hypnotique dans le travail de l'accouchement."

Vol. vi. p. 175. "De l'action de la suggestion pendant le travail de l'accouchement."

Vol. vii. p. 173. "Observation de chorée guérie par la thérapeutique suggestive."

Vol. x. p. 21. "Vomissements incoercibles depuis 10 mois, chez une jeune fille de 14 ans. Hystérie. Guérison rapide des vomissements après suggestion hypnotique."

DURAND, Dr. (de Gros). Vol. x. p. 8. "Suggestions criminelles hypnotiques."

Vol. x. p. 161. "L'hypnotisme et la morale."

EEDEN, Dr. VAN. Vol. vi. p. 5. "Les obsessions."

et VAN RENTERGHEM. Vol. ix. p. 161. "Le traitement psychothérapeutique de neurasthénie."

FANTON, Dr. Vol. v. p. 150. "Un accouchement sans douleur sous l'influence de l'hypnotisation."

FAREZ, Dr. PAUL. Vol. xiii. p. 136. "Traitement psychologique du mal de mer et des vertiges de la locomotion (chemin de fer, omnibus, tramway, etc.)."

Vol. xiii. p. 336. "Hypnotisme et sommeil prolongé dans un cas de délire alcoolique."

Vol. xiii. p. 371. "Contre la morphinomanie."

Vol. xiv. p. 53. "Incontinence d'urine et suggestion pendant le sommeil naturel."

Vol. xiv. p. 206. "Hyperhydrose palmaire."

Vol. xiv. p. 296. "Idées délirantes de persécution avec hallucinations auditives et visuelles consecutives à un traumatisme psychique chez un glycosurique. Traitement hypnotique et guérison des troubles mentaux, malgré la persistance de la glycosurie."

FOREL, Prof. AUGUST. Vol. iii. p. 277. "Un cas d'auto-hypnotisation."

FRAIPONT et DELBŒUF, Profs. *See* DELBŒUF

provoqué des états successifs de personnalité chez un hystéro-épileptique."

MARANDON DE MONTHYEL, Dr. E. Vol. xi. p. 289. "Deux cas de fausse grossesse par crainte de la maternité avec rappel immédiat de la menstruation par suggestion à l'état de veille."

MARINESCO, Dr. (Bucharest). Vol. xiv. p. 214. "Un cas d'hémiplégie hystérique guéri par la suggestion hypnotique et étudié à l'aide de la chronophotographie."

MAROT, Dr. Vol. vii. p. 233. "Morphinomanie et suggestion : guérison datant de trois ans et demi."

MAVROUKAKIS, Dr. ANTOINE. Vol. ii. p. 374. "Les neurasthéniques et la suggestion. Agoraphobie traitée avec succès par la suggestion."
Vol. vii. p. 374. "Les neurasthéniques et la suggestion."

MESNET, Dr. Vol. ii. p. 33. "Un accouchement dans le somnambulisme provoqué."
Vol. iv. p. 321. "Autographisme et stigmates."
et ROUX, Drs. Vol. iii. p. 119. "Spasmes de l'urèthre et troubles nerveux."

NEILSON, Dr. HUBERT (Canada). Vol. vi. p. 14. "Le traitement hypnotique de la dipsomanie."

OSGOOD, Dr. HAMILTON (America). Vol. ix. p. 300. "Quatre cas d'eczéma et un de dermatite traités par suggestion."

PAU DE SAINT-MARTIN, Dr. Vol. xv. p. 17. "Thanatophobie, agoraphobie et divers troubles nerveux traités avec succès par la suggestion."
Vol. xv. p. 52. "Orthopédie mentale et morale par suggestion pendant le sommeil naturel."

PRITEL, Dr. Vol. i. p. 157. "Accouchement d'une primipare pendant l'hypnotisme."

PROUST, Prof. Vol. iv. p. 267. "Automatisme ambulatoire chez un hystérique."

RAMEY, Dr. Vol. i. p. 60. "Rétrécissement spasmodique du canal de l'urèthre traité sans succès par l'urèthrotomie interne et guéri par la suggestion hypnotique."

RÉGIS, Dr. Vol. x. p. 321. "Kleptomanie et hypnothérapie."

RÉMOND et ARTIGALAS, Drs. See ARTIGALAS.

RENTERGHEM, Dr. VAN. Vol. vii. p. 215. "Rupture du périnée complète datant de quelques années. Maladie organique du cœur défendant l'emploi du chloroforme pour provoquer l'anesthésie. Opération radicale et sans douleurs notables, sous l'influence de la suggestion sans sommeil."
et VAN EEDEN, Drs. See VAN EEDEN.

RIBOKOFF, Dr. Vol. xiii. p. 127. "Du traitement de l'alcoolisme par la suggestion."

RICHET, Prof. CHARLES. Vol. i. pp. 170, 209. "Les mouvements inconscients."
Vol. ii. p. 208. "Hypnotisme à distance."
Vol. ii. p. 225. "Expériences sur le sommeil à distance."

RIFAT, Dr. Vol. ii. p. 297. "Étude sur l'hypnotisme et la suggestion."

ROUBINOVITCH, Dr. Vol. ii. p. 364. "Le traitement des habitudes vicieuses par la suggestion."

RYBALKIN, Dr. T. Vol. iv. p. 361. "Brûlure du second degré provoquée par suggestion."

SANDBERG, G. (Sweden). Vol. vi. p. 331. "Applications de l'hypnotisme à l'art dentaire."

SCHMELTZ, Dr. (Nice). Vol. ix. p. 47. "Opérations chirurgicales faites pendant le sommeil hypnotique."
Vol. x. p. 120. "Sarcome du testicle gauche opéré pendant le sommeil hypnotique."

SCHRENCK-NOTZING, Dr. VON. Vol. iv. p. 172. "Un cas d'inversion sexuelle amélioré par la suggestion hypnotique."
Vol. v. p. 15. "Remarques sur le traitement de l'inversion sexuelle par la suggestion hypnotique."

SPEHL, Prof. (Brussels). Vol. xi. p. 265. "Épilepsie Jacksonnienne. Traitement par la suggestion indirecte. Guérison."

STADELMANN, Dr. Vol. xiv. p. 330. "Traitement psychique d'un cas de folie délirante (Zwangsirresin)."

TILLAUX, Dr. Vol. iv. p. 26. "Une application chirurgicale, à l'Hôtel-Dieu, de l'anesthésie somnambulique."

TUCKEY, Dr. C. LLOYD (London). Vol. xv. p. 80. "Les indications de l'hypnotisme et de la suggestion dans le traitement de l'alcoolisme."

VALENTIN, Dr. Vol. xi. p. 116. "Du traitement des neurasthénies graves par la psychothérapie."

VLAVIANOS, Dr. Vol. xiii. p. 296. "Du traitement des phobies en général et de l'agoraphobie en particulier."
Vol. xiii. p. 361. "Le traitement de l'alcoolisme par l'hypnotisme."
Vol. xiv. p. 11. "Agoraphobie traitée par la suggestion hypnotique."
Vol. xiv. p. 72. "Tic convulsif du cou et de la tête guéri par la suggestion hypnotique."

VOISIN, Dr. AUGUSTE. Vol. i. p. 4. "De l'hypnotisme et de la suggestion hypnotique dans leurs applications au traitement des maladies nerveuses et mentales."
Vol. i. p. 44. *Observation V.* "Hystérie, folie hystérique. Hallucinations de la vue et de l'ouïe. Idée de suicide. Hémianesthésie et hémi-dyschromatopsie. Traitement par la suggestion hypnotique. Guérison."
Vol. i. p. 161. "Morphinomanie guérie par suggestion hypnotique."
Vol. ii. p. 151. "Observations d'onanisme guéri par la suggestion hypnotique."
Vol. ii. p. 364. "Le traitement des habitudes vicieuses par la suggestion."
Vol. iii. pp. 48, 65. "De la dipsomanie et des habitudes alcooliques et de leur traitement par la suggestion hypnotique."
Vol. iii. p. 130. "Un cas de perversité morale guéri par la suggestion hypnotique."
Vol. iii. p. 353. "Folie lypémaniaque avec idées de suicide datant de 8 ans. Phénomènes choréiques hystériques. Guérison par la suggestion hypnotique."
Vol. ix. p. 22. "Attaques convulsives hystéro-épileptiques. Vertiges suivis de délire et d'hallucinations. Hypnotisme obtenu par le miroir rotatif. Guérison."
Vol. ix. p. 245. "Nicotisme guéri par suggestion."

Vol. x. p. 27. "Hystéro-catalepsie. Difficultés de la suggestion hypnotique tenant à l'absence de l'ouïe et de la vue pendant l'hypnose. Procédé suivi de succès. Guérison de la catalepsie."

Vol. x. p. 341. "Folie lypémaniaque avec hallucinations et idées de persécution, traitée avec succès par la suggestion."

Vol. x. p. 360. "Un accouchement dans l'état d'hypnotisme."

VOISIN, DR. JULES. Vol. ii. p. 242. "Guérison par la suggestion hypnotique d'idées délirantes et de mélancholie avec conscience."

Vol. xv. p. 15. "Orthopédie morale et hypnotisme."

WETTERSTRAND, DR. OTTO G. (Stockholm). Vol. v. p. 141. "Sur le traitement de la morphinomanie par la suggestion hypnotique."

WOOD, DR. EDWARD. Vol. iv. p. 246. "Opération chirurgicale pratiquée dans l'état d'hypnotisme."

FRENCH BOOKS AND PAMPHLETS.

AIMÉ, DR. "De la valeur thérapeutique de l'entraînement suggestif à l'état de veille." *Congrès International de Neurologie.* Bruxelles, 1897.

AZAM, DR. "Note sur le sommeil nerveux ou hypnotisme." *Archives générales de Médecine,* cinquième série, vol. xv. p. 5. Paris, 1860.

"Hypnotisme, double conscience et altérations de la personnalité." Paris, 1887.

BABINSKI, DR. J. "Hypnotisme et hystérie. Du rôle de l'hypnotisme en thérapeutique." Paris, 1891.

BEAUNIS, Prof. H. "Le somnambulisme provoqué." Paris, 1887.

BÉRILLON, DR. EDGAR. "Hypnotisme et suggestion. Théorie et applications pratiques." Paris, 1891.

"Premier Congrès International de l'hypnotisme expérimental et thérapeutique." Comptes rendus. Publiés sous la direction du Dr. Edgar Bérillon. Paris, 1889.

"Les indications formelles de la suggestion hypnotique en psychiatrie et en neuropathologie." Paris, 1891.

BERNHEIM, Prof. "Hypnotisme, suggestion, psychothérapie. Études nouvelles." Paris, 1891.

"L'hypnotisme et la suggestion dans leurs rapports avec la médecine légale." *XII°. Congrès International de Médecine.* Moscou, 1897.

BERTRAND, ALEXANDRE. "Traité du somnambulisme." Paris, 1823.

"Du magnétisme animal en France." Paris, 1826.

BONJEAN, ALBERT. "L'hypnotisme." Paris, 1890.

BRAMWELL, J. MILNE, M.B. "La valeur thérapeutique de l'hypnotisme et de la suggestion." *Congrès International de Neurologie.* Bruxelles, 1897.

BRIAND, DR. "Notes pour servir à l'histoire de la thérapeutique par suggestion hypnotique." *Premier Congrès International de l'Hypnotisme.* Paris, 1889.

BOURRU et BUROT, Drs. "Action à distance des substances toxiques et médicamenteuses." Paris, 1886.

"La suggestion mentale." Paris, 1887.

CHARCOT, DR. J. M. "Œuvres Complètes. Tome IX. Métallo-thérapie et Hypnotisme." Paris, 1890.

CHARPIGNON, Dr. J.   "Physiologie, médecine et métaphysique du mag-
   nétisme."   Paris, 1848.
CROCQ, fils, Dr.   "L'hypnotisme et le crime."   Bruxelles, 1894.
DELBŒUF, Prof. J.   "Une visite à la Salpêtrière."   Bruxelles, 1886.
   "De l'origine des effets curatifs de l'hypnotisme.   Étude de psychologie
   expérimentale."   Paris, 1887.
   "Le magnétisme animal.   À propos d'une visite à l'école de Nancy."
   Paris, 1889.
   "De l'étendue de l'action curative de l'hypnotisme.   L'hypnotisme
   appliqué aux altérations de l'organe visuel."   Paris, 1890.
   "De l'appréciation du temps par les somnambules."   *Proceedings of the
   Society for Psychical Research,* vol. viii. p. 414.
DUMONTPALLIER, Dr.   "De l'action vaso-motrice de la suggestion chez les
   hystériques hypnotisables."   *Gazette des Hôpitaux,* 1885, p. 619.
DUPOTET, M.   "Journal du Magnétisme Rédigé par une Société de Magnéti-
   seurs et de Médecins, sous la direction de M. le Baron Dupotet."
   Vol. iv. 1847, p. 209 ; vol. viii. 1849, p. 66 ; vol. x. 1851, p. 510 ;
   vol. xiv. 1855, p. 400 ; vol. xix. 1860, pp. 62, 105.
DURAND, Dr. (de Gros).   "Cours théorique et pratique de braidisme ou
   hypnotisme nerveux."   1860.
EEDEN, Drs. A. W. VAN RENTERGHEM et F. VAN.   "Clinique de psycho-
   thérapie suggestive."   1887-1889.   Bruxelles, 1889.
   "Psycho-thérapie.   Compte rendu des résultats obtenus dans la clinique
   de psycho-thérapie suggestive d'Amsterdam pendant la deuxième
   période 1889-1893."   Paris, 1894.
FÉRÉ, Prof. CHARLES.   "Sensation et mouvement."   Paris, 1887.
GASCARD, Dr.   "Influence de la suggestion sur certains troubles de la
   menstruation."   *Premier Congrès International de l'Hypnotisme,* p. 182.
   Paris, 1889.
JANET, Prof. PIERRE.   "Les actes inconscientes dans le somnambulisme."
   Revue Philosophique, Mars, 1888.
   "L'automatisme psychologique."   Paris, 1889.
   "État mentale des hystériques."   Paris, 1894.
   "Névroses et idées fixes."   Paris, 1898.
JOIRE, Dr.   "De l'emploi de l'analgésie hypnotique dans les accouchements."
   1898.
JONG, Dr. A. DE.   "Valeur thérapeutique de la suggestion dans quelques
   psychoses."   *Comptes rendus du premier Congrès International de
   l'Hypnotisme expérimental et thérapeutique,* p. 196.   Paris, 1889.
   "Sur les obsessions."   *Deuxième Congrès International de l'Hypnotisme
   expérimental et thérapeutique.*   Moscou, 1897.
   "La suggestion hypnotique dans le traitement de l'alcoolisme et de la
   morphinomanie."   *Idem,* Moscou, 1897.
KRAFFT-EBING, Dr. R. VON.   "Psychopathia sexualis, avec recherches
   spéciales sur l'inversion sexuelle."   Traduit sur la huitième édition
   allemande.   Paris, 1895.
LAFONTAINE, CH.   "Mémoires d'un Magnétiseur."   Paris, 1860.
LIÉBEAULT, Dr. A. A.   "Ébauche de psychologie."   Paris et Nancy,
   1873.
   "Étude sur le zoomagnétisme."   Paris, 1883.

"Le sommeil provoqué et les états analogues." Paris, 1889.

"Monomanie suicide guérie par la suggestion pendant l'état de sommeil provoqué." *International Congress of Experimental Psychology.* Second Session, London, 1882, p. 143.

LIÉGEOIS, Prof. JULES. "De la suggestion et du somnambulisme dans leurs rapports avec la jurisprudence et la médecine légale." Paris, 1889.

LUYS, Dr. J. "Hypnotisme expérimental. Les émotions dans l'état d'hypnotisme." Paris, 1890.

MAGNIN, Dr. PAUL. "Étude clinique et expérimentale sur l'hypnotisme." Paris, 1884.

PERRONNET, Dr. CLAUDE. "Force psychique et suggestion mentale." Paris, 1886.

PITRES, Dr. A. "Des suggestions hypnotiques." Bordeaux, 1884.

RENTERGHEM, Dr. VAN. "Un cas de tic rotatoire (spasmes cloniques idiopathiques des muscles cervicaux), rebelle à toutes les médications instituées—y compris le traitement chirurgical—guéri par la psycho-thérapie." *Congrès de Neurologie.* Bruxelles, 1897.

    et VAN EEDEN. *See* VAN EEDEN.

RICHER, Prof. PAUL. "Études cliniques sur la grande hystérie." Paris, 1885.

RICHET, Prof. CHARLES. "L'homme et l'intelligence." Paris, 1884.

"La physiologie et la médecine." Paris, 1888.

SIMON, Dr. JULES. "Neurypnologie. Traité du sommeil nerveux ou hypnotisme." Traduit de l'anglais par le Dr. Jules Simon. Avec préface de C. E. Brown-Séquard. Paris, 1883.

TARCHANOFF, Prof. JEAN DE. "Lecture des pensées." Paris, 1891.

TOURETTE, Dr. GILLES DE LA. "L'hypnotisme et les états analogues au point de vue médico-légal." Paris, 1887.

"Maladie des tics," p. 585. *Traité pratique des maladies du système nerveux,* par T. Grasset and G. Rauzier : 4me édition, vol. ii. 1894.

VELANDER, Dr. "Un cas de mutisme melancholique guéri par suggestion." *Premier Congrès International de l'Hypnotisme,* 1889, p. 323.

VELSEN, Dr. P. VAN. "À propos d'hypnotisme." 1895.

"L'hypnotisme et la psycho-thérapie."

VOISIN, Dr. AUGUSTE. "Étude sur l'hypnotisme et sur les suggestions chez les aliénés." Paris, 1884.

"De la thérapeutique suggestive chez les aliénés." Paris, 1886.

"Du traitement de l'aménorrhée par la suggestion hypnotique." Paris, 1887.

"Traitement et guérison d'une morphinomane par la suggestion hypnotique." Paris, 1887.

"Traitement des maladies mentales et nerveuses par la suggestion hypnotique." Paris, 1888.

"Les indications de l'hypnotisme et de la suggestion hypnotique dans le traitement des maladies mentales et des états connexes." *Premier Congrès International de l'Hypnotisme,* 1889, p. 147. (Discussion by FOREL, RÉPOUD, and others.) Paris, 1889.

"Traitement de certaines formes d'aliénation mentale par la suggestion hypnotique." *Dritter Internationaler Congress für Psychologie in München,* 1896, p. 380.

2 G

WUNDT, Prof. W. "Hypnotisme et suggestion." Traduit de l'allemand. Paris, 1893.

Congrès International de Psychologie physiologique. Première Session. Paris, 1890. Compte rendu presénté par la Société de Psychologie Physiologique de Paris. Paris, 1890.

Congrès International de Neurologie, de Psychiatrie, d'Électricité médicale et d'Hypnologie. Première Session. Bruxelles, Septembre, 1897. Communications. Paris, 1898.

Deuxième Congrès International de l'Hypnotisme expérimental et thérapeutique. Paris, 1900.

GERMAN.

FROM THE *ZEITSCHRIFT FÜR HYPNOTISMUS*, vol. i. 1892 to vol. x. 1900.

BAUER, Dr. C. Vol. v. p. 31. "Aus der hypnotischen Poliklinik des Herrn Prof. Forel in Zürich."

BERGMANN, Dr. Vol. ii. p. 50. "Ein Fall von Magensaftfluss, geheilt durch hypnotische Suggestion."

BERTSCHINGER, Dr. Vol. vi. p. 355. "Ein Fall von Scorbut und ein Fall von Anämie durch Hypnotismus geheilt."
　　Vol. viii. p. 164. "Psychische Zwangszustände. (*Résumé* of German, French, and English literature on the subject.)

BONJOUR, Dr. Vol. vi. p. 146. "Neue Experimente über den Einfluss der Psyche auf den Körper." (Also in the *Revue de l'Hypnotisme*, vol. xii. p. 79.)

BRÜGELMANN, Dr. WILHELM. Vol. ii. p. 84. "Psychotherapie und Asthma."
　　Vol. ii. p. 300. "Casuistisches." (Asthma.)
　　Vol. v. p. 256. "Suggestive Erfahrungen und Beobachtungen."
　　Vol. x. p. 13. "Zur Lehre von perversen Sexualismus."

BRUNNBERG, Dr. TYKO. Vol. i. p. 434. "Den Hypnotiska suggestionen och dess Anwändung vid Menstruations Rubbningar."

CULLERRE, Dr. Vol. iv. p. 377. "L'incontinence d'urine et son traitement par la suggestion."

DELBŒUF, Prof. Vol. i. p. 46. "Einige psychologische Betrachtungen über den Hypnotismus gelegentlich eines durch Suggestion geheilten Falles von Mordmanie."

DELIUS, Dr. Vol. v. p. 219. "Erfolge der hypnotischen Suggestiv-Behandlung in der Praxis. I."
　　Vol. vii. p. 36. "Erfolge der hypnotischen Suggestiv-Behandlung in der Praxis. II."

DÖLLKEN, Dr. Vol. iv. p. 65. "Beiträge zur Physiologie der Hypnose."

FOREL, Prof. AUGUST. Vol. ii. p. 55. "Die Heilung der Stuhlverstopfung durch Suggestion."
　　Vol. iii. p. 229. "Durch Spiritismus erkrankt und durch Hypnotismus geheilt."
　　Vol. iii. p. 269. "Behandlung eines Falles von Paranoia incipiens (?)."

Vol. iii. p. 270. "2 Fälle von Enuresis, 1 diurna, 1 nocturna."

Vol. x. p. 1. "Bemerkungen zu der Behandlung der Nervenkranken durch Arbeit und zur allgemeinen Psychotherapie."

FREUD, Dr. SIGM. Vol. i. p. 102. "Ein Fall von hypnotischer Heilung nebst Bemerkungen über die Entstehung hysterischer Symptome durch den Gegenwillen."

FRIEDLÄNDER, Dr. Vol. x. p. 17. "Zur kritischen Stellung der sogenannten Erythrophobie und ihrer Behandlung durch Hypnose."

FUCHS, Dr. Vol. viii. p. 373. "Therapie der anomalen Vita sexualis bei Männern mit Berücksichtigung der Suggestiv-Behandlung."

FULDA, Dr. Vol. ii. p. 404. "Morphinismus geheilt durch Hypnose."

GERSTER, Dr. KARL. Vol. i. p. 319. "Beiträge zur suggestiven Psychotherapie."

Vol. iii. p. 206. "Ein Fall von hysterischer Kontraktur."

GRAETER, Dr. Vol. viii. p. 129. "Ein Fall von epileptischer Amnesie durch hypnotische Hypermnesie beseitigt."

GROSSMANN, Dr. Vol. i. p. 71. "Suggestion und Milchsecretion, vorläufige Mittheilung."

Vol. i. pp. 355, 398. "Die Suggestion, speciell die hypnotische Suggestion, ihr Wesen und ihr Heilwerth."

Vol. ii. p. 198. "Die hypnotische Suggestion bei der Reposition und Nachbehandlung von Knochenbrüchen und Verrenkungen."

Vol. iii. p. 76. "Die Erfolge der Suggestionstherapie (Hypnose) bei organischen Lähmungen und Paralysen."

Vol. iii. p. 245. "Zur suggestiven Behandlung der Gelenkkrankheiten mit besonderer Berücksichtigung des chronischen Gelenkrheumatismus und der Gicht."

HASSENSTEIN, Dr. W. Vol. ii. p. 116. "Die Hypnose im Dienste der Säuglingsernährung."

HERZBERG, Dr. Vol. ii. p. 297. "Suggestionstherapie in der Gynäkologie."

HILGER, Dr. Vol. viii. p. 17. "Zur Kasuistik der hypnotischen Behandlung der Epilepsie."

Vol. x. p. 190. "Beitrag zur Frage der Hypnotisirbarkeit."

HILGER und SÄNGER, Drs. Vol. x. p. 223. "Ein Fall von Aphonie nach Laryngofissur geheilt durch systematische Sprachübungen unter Anwendung der Hypnose."

HIRT, Dr. Vol. ii. p. 287. "Ueber die Bedeutung der Verbalsuggestion für die Neurotherapie."

INHELDER, Dr. WALTER. Vol. vii. p. 201. "Ueber die Bedeutung der Hypnose für die Nachtwachen des Wartpersonals."

JONG, Dr. DE. Vol. i. p. 178. "Die Suggestibilität bei Melancholie."

KRAFFT-EBING, Dr. R. VON. Vol. iv. p. 27. "Zur Suggestivbehandlung der Hysteria gravis."

Vol. ix. p. 249. "Ueber Ecmnesie."

LANDGREN, Dr. S. Vol. ii. p. 23. "Offener Brief an Herrn Dr. med. Bingswanger in Kreuzlingen - Konstanz von Dr. S. Landgren, Provinzialarzt in Leksand, Dalekarlien, Schweden."

MARCINOWSKI, Dr. Vol. ix. p. 5. "Selbstbeobachtung in der Hypnose."

MOLL, Dr. ALBERT. Vol. i. p. 107. "Literaturbericht."

MURALT, Dr. Vol. x. p. 75. "Zur Frage der epileptischen Amnesie."

NAEF, Dr. Vol. vi. p. 321. "Ein Fall von temporäner, totaler, theilweise retrograder Amnesie (durch Suggestion geheilt)."

RANSCHENBURG, Dr. Vol. iv. p. 269. "Beiträge zur Frage der hypnotisch-suggestiven Therapie."

RENTERGHEM, Dr. VAN. Vol. iv. p. 333. "Liébeault et son école." (Continued, vols. v., vi., and vii.)

　　Vol. vi. p. 259. "Ein Fall von Muskelkrampf (Tic rotatoire)."

　　Vol. vii. p. 329. "Ein interessanter Fall von spontanem Somnambulismus."

　　Vol. viii. p. 1. "Dritter Bericht über die in der psycho-therapeutischen Clinik in Amsterdam erhaltenen Resultate während den Jahren 1893-1897."

RINGIER, Dr. GEORG. Vol. ii. p. 143. "Ein Fall von hysterischen Mutismus."

　　Vol. ii. p. 317. "Zur Behandlung der Bleichsucht."

　　Vol. vi. p. 150. "Zur Redaction der Suggestion bei Enuresis nocturna."

SÄNGER und HILGER. *See* HILGER.

SCHMIDT, Dr. CURT. Vol. ii. p. 285. "Suggestion und Magenerkrankungen."

SCHOLZ, Dr. i. pp. 172, 187. "Casuistische Mittheilungen über Suggestions-Therapie."

SCHRENCK-NOTZING, Dr. VON. Vol. i. p. 49. "Eine Geburt in der Hypnose."

　　Vol. i. p. 351. "Ueber Suggestion und suggestive Zustände."

　　Vol. ii. p. 1. "Ein Beitrag zur psychischen und suggestiven Behandlung der Neurasthenie."

　　Vol. ii. p. 30. "Die Suggestionstherapie bei krankhaften Erscheinungen des Geschlechtssinnes."

　　Vol. ii. pp. 356, 398. "Suggestion, Suggestivtherapie, psychische Behandlung. Ein kritischer Rückblick auf die neuere Literatur."

　　Vol. iv. p. 209. "Ein experimenteller und kritischer Beitrag zur Frage des suggestiven Hervorrufung circumscripter vasomotorischer Veränderungen auf der äusseren Haut."

SCHUPP, FALK. Vol. iii. p. 46. "Hypnose und hypnotische Suggestion in der Zahnheilkunde."

SEIF, Dr. Vol. ix. pp. 275, 371. "Casuistische Beiträge zur Psychotherapie."

SJÖSTRÖM, Dr. AXEL. Vol. vii. p. 263. "Ein Fall von spontanem Somnambulismus auf hysterischer Grundlage mit schnellster Heilung durch hypnotische Suggestion."

STADELMANN, Dr. Vol. iii. p. 19. "Zwei Fälle von Muskelzückungen bei Anämischen geheilt durch Suggestion nach einmaliger Behandlung."

STEMBO, Dr. Vol. ii. p. 302. "Casuistisches."

TATZEL, Dr. Vol. i. p. 245. "Eine Geburt in der Hypnose."

　　Vol. ii. p. 19. "Drei Fälle von nichthysterischen Lähmungen und deren Heilung mittelst Suggestion."

　　Vol. iii. pp. 260-268. "Fall von hysterischen Anfällen." "Hysterische Krampfe." "Clonischer Krampf der rechten Armmuskulatur." "Clonischer Krampf der Accessoriusmuskulatur." "Traumatische Neurose." "Dipsomanie." "Rheumatismus." "Symptomatische Behandlung bei einem Nierencarcinom."

　　Vol. vii. p. 249. "Die suggestive Behandlung einzelner Formen der Parästhesie der Geschlechtsempfindung."

Vol. vii. p. 257. "Hysterie und Suggestion."

Vol. ix. p. 231. "Eine hypnotische Entfettungskur."

TEUSCHER, Dr. Vol. iii. p. 321. "Ueber suggestiven Behandlung der Kinder."

VOGT, Dr. OSKAR. Vol. vii. p. 285. "Spontane Somnambulie in der Hypnose."

Vol. viii. p. 65. "Zur Methodik der ätiologischen Erforschung der Hysterie."

WETTERSTRAND, Dr. OTTO G. Vol. i. p. 17. "Ueber den künstlich verlängerten Schlaf, besonders bei der Behandlung der Hysterie, Epilepsie und Hystero-Epilepsie."

Vol. ii. pp. 306-312. "Casuistisches."

Vol. iv. p. 8. "Die Heilung des chronischen Morphinismus, Opium- genusses, Cocaïnismus und Chloralismus mit Suggestion und Hypnose (1888-1895)."

BOOKS AND PAMPHLETS.

BAIERLACHER, Dr. EDUARD. "Die Suggestionstherapie und ihre Technik." Stuttgart, 1889.

BENEDIKT, Dr. MORIZ. "Hypnotismus und Suggestion." Leipzig and Vienna, 1894.

BINGSWANGER, Dr. OTTO. "Die Pathologie und Therapie der Neurasthenie." Jena, 1896.

BRÜGELMANN, Dr. W. "Ueber den Hypnotismus und seine Verwerthung in der Praxis." Berlin, 1889.

DESSOIR, Dr. MAX. "Bibliographie des Modernen Hypnotismus." Berlin, 1888. "Das Doppel-Ich." Berlin, 1889. "Erster Nachtrag zur Bibliographie des modernen Hypnotismus." Berlin, 1890.

DUBOIS, Dr. "Correspondenz-Blatt für Schweizer Aerzte." Nos. 10 and 11, 1893.

FOREL, Dr. AUGUST. "Zu dem Gefahren und dem Nutzen des Hypnotismus." *Münchener Med. Wochenschrift.* No. 38, 1889. "Der Hypnotismus, seine psycho-physiologische, medicinische strafrecht- liche Bedeutung und seine Handhabung." Stuttgart, 1891.

HECKER, Dr. EWALD. "Hypnose und Suggestion im Dienste der Heilkunde." Wiesbaden, 1893.

HÜCKEL, Dr. ARMAND. "Die Rolle der Suggestion bei gewissen Erschei- nungen der Hysterie und des Hypnotismus." Jena, 1888.

KRAFFT-EBING, Dr. R. VON. "Eine experimentelle Studie auf dem Gebiete des Hypnotismus nebst Bemerkungen über Suggestion und Suggestions- therapie." Stuttgart, 1893.

LEHMANN, Dr. ALFRED. "Die Hypnose und die damit verwandten normalen Zustände." Leipzig, 1890.

MOLL, Dr. ALBERT. "Der Hypnotismus." Berlin, 1889. "Der Rapport in der Hypnose." Leipzig, 1892.

PREYER, Dr. W. "Die Entdeckung des Hypnotismus." Berlin, 1881. "Der Hypnotismus." Ausgewählte Schriften von J. Braid. Deutsch herausgegeben von W. Preyer. Berlin, 1892.

"Der Hypnotismus." Vorlesungen gehalten an der K. Friedrich-Wilhelms-Universität zu Berlin. Vienna and Leipzig, 1890.

RIEGER, Dr. CONRAD. "Der Hypnotismus." Jena, 1884.

RINGIER, Dr. GEORG. "Erfolge des therapeutischen Hypnotismus in der Landpraxis." Munich, 1891.

SCHRENCK-NOTZING, Dr. VON. "Suggestion, Suggestivtherapie, Psychische Behandlung." Real-Encyclopedia.

"Ein Beitrag zur therapeutischen Verwerthung des Hypnotismus." Leipzig, 1888.

"Ueber Hypnotismus und Suggestion." Munich, 1889.

"Die gerichtliche Bedeutung und missbräuchliche Anwendung des Hypnotismus." Munich, 1889.

"Die Bedeutung narcotischer Mittel für den Hypnotismus." Schriften der Gesellschaft für psychologische Forschung. Leipzig, 1891.

"Die Suggestions-Therapie bei krankhaften Erscheinungen des Geschlechtsinnes." Stuttgart, 1892.

"Über Suggestion und suggestive Zustände." Munich, 1893.

STADELMANN, Dr. "Der Psychotherapeut." Würzburg, 1896.

VERWORN, Dr. MAX. "Erregung und Lähmung." Leipzig, 1896.

"Die sogenannte Hypnose der Thiere." Jena, 1898.

WETTERSTRAND, Dr. OTTO G. "Der Hypnotismus und seine Anwendung in der praktischen Medicin." Vienna and Leipzig, 1891.

"Ueber den künstlich verlängerten Schlaf, besonders bei der Behandlung von Hysterie." Dritter Internationaler Congress für Psychologie in München, 1896, p. 361.

Dritter Internationaler Congress für Psychologie in München von 4 bis 7 August 1896. Munich, 1897.

ENGLISH REFERENCES.

BARRETT, Prof. W. F., F.R.S.E., M.R.I.A. "Appendix to the Report on Thought-Reading." Proceedings of the Society for Psychical Research, vol. i. 1882-83, p. 47. Also "Second Report," vol. i. p. 70, and "Third Report," vol. i. p. 161.

BASTIAN, Dr. H. CHARLTON. "Braidism," vol. i. p. 131. "Mesmerism," vol. ii. p. 972. A Dictionary of Medicine. Edited by Richard Quain, M.D. London, 1882.

BENNETT, Prof. JOHN HUGHES, M.D., F.R.S.E. "The Mesmeric Mania of 1851." A Lecture. Edinburgh, 1851.

"Text-book of Physiology," part ii. pp. 357-361. Edinburgh, 1871.

BERNHEIM, Prof., M.D. "Suggestive Therapeutics: A Treatise on the Nature and Uses of Hypnotism." (Translated from the second and revised edition by Christian A. Herter, M.D.) Second edition. Edinburgh and London, 1890.

BINET and FÉRÉ, Profs. "Animal Magnetism." London, 1888.

BJÖRNSTRÖM, FREDERICK. "Hypnotism, its History and Present Development." New York, 1889.

BOOTH, Dr. T. ARTHUR. "Hysterical Amblyopia and Amaurosis." Report of five cases treated by hypnotism. *Medical Record*, August 24th, 1895. New York.

BRAMWELL, J. MILNE, M.B. "On Imperative Ideas." *Brain*, parts lxx. and lxxi. 1895.

"James Braid, Surgeon and Hypnotist." *Ibid.* part lxxiii. 1896.

"On the Evolution of Hypnotic Theory." *Ibid.* part lxxvi. 1896.

"Hypnotism: A Reply to Recent Criticisms." *Ibid.* part lxxxv. 1899.

"Hypnotic and Post-Hypnotic Appreciation of Time : Double and Multiple Personalities." *Ibid.* 1890.

"James Braid : his Work and Writings." *Proceedings of the Society for Psychical Research*, 1896.

"Personally observed Hypnotic Phenomena; and What is Hypnotism?" *Ibid.* 1896.

"On the so-called Automatism of the Hypnotised Subject." *Dritter Internationaler Congress für Psychologie.* München, 1896.

"On the Appreciation of Time by Somnambules." *Ibid.*

"The Phenomena of Hypnotism, and the Theories as to its Nature." *British Medical Journal*, 1898.

"Hypnotic Anæsthesia." *Practitioner*, 1896.

"On the Treatment of Dipsomania and Chronic Alcoholism by Hypnotic Suggestion." *Ibid.* 1902.

"Hypnotism in the Treatment of Insanity and Allied Disorders." Allbutt's *System of Medicine*, vol. viii.

"Dipsomania and its Treatment by Suggestion." *Proceedings of the Society for the Study of Inebriety*, 1900.

"Suggestion : its Place in Medicine and Scientific Research." Being a Lecture delivered on behalf of the Leigh Browne Trust. February, 1897.

"Hypnotism : An Outline Sketch." Being a Lecture delivered before the King's College Medical Society. *Clinical Journal*, May 7th and 14th, 1902.

BRITISH MEDICAL JOURNAL. "Hypnotism as an Anæsthetic." April 5th, 1890, p. 801.

"Report of the Hypnotic Committee, 1892." July 29th, 1893.

BRUCE, LEWIS C., M.B. "Notes of a Case of Dual Brain Action." *Brain*, vol. xviii. (1895), p. 54.

CARPENTER, Prof. WILLIAM B., M.D. "Mesmerism, Spiritualism, etc." London, 1877.

"Principles of Mental Physiology." Second edition, London, 1881.

"Electro-Biology and Mesmerism." *The Quarterly Review*, vol. xciii. 1853, Article VI. p. 501 (supposed to be by Carpenter).

CHARCOT, Prof., and TOURETTE, Dr. GILLES DE LA. "Hypnotism in the Hysterical." *A Dictionary of Psychological Medicine.* Edited by D. Hack Tuke, M.D. London, 1892. Vol. i. p. 606.

CLIFFORD, HUGH. "Studies in Brown Humanity." London, 1898.

CRUISE, Sir FRANCIS, M.D. "Hypnotism." *Dublin Journal of Mental Science*, 1891.

"DAGONET" (SIMS, G. R.). "Mustard and Cress." *The Referee*, January 31st, 1897.

DAVEY, S. J., and HODGSON, RICHARD. "The Possibilities of Mal-Observation
    and Lapse of Memory from a Practical Point of View." *Proceedings
    of the Society for Psychical Research*, vol. iv. pp. 381, 405.
DELBŒUF, Prof. J. "On Criminal Suggestion." *The Monist*, April, 1892,
    p. 383.
DERCUM, FRANCIS X., M.D. "Saltatoric Spasm." *Text-book of Nervous
    Diseases by American Authors*, p. 262.
DESSOIR, Dr. MAX. · "Experiments in Muscle-Reading and Thought-Trans-
    ference." *Proceedings of the Society for Psychical Research*, vol. iv. p. 111.
    " Experiments in Thought-Transference." *Ibid.* vol. v. p. 355.
DICTIONARY OF NATIONAL BIOGRAPHY. "John Elliotson." By the late
    Robert Hunt, F.R.S. Vol. xvii. p. 264. (Edited by Leslie Stephen.)
ELLIOTSON, Dr. JOHN. Numerous articles in *The Zoist*, a Journal of Cerebral
    Physiology and Mesmerism, 1844-56.
    " Pencillings of Eminent Men." *The Medical Times*, February 1st, 1845,
    p. 392.
ENCYCLOPÆDIA BRITANNICA. " Animal Magnetism." Ninth edition, part lviii.
    p. 277.
ESDAILE, Dr. JAMES. 1. "Letters from the Red Sea, Egypt, and the
    Continent." Calcutta, 1839.
    2. "Mesmeric Feats." Reported by James Esdaile, M.D., Civil
    Assistant-Surgeon, Hooghly, 1845. (Reprinted from the *India
    Journal of Medical and Physical Science*, vol. iii. Nos. 5, 6, 1845.)
    3. " Mesmerism in India, and its Practical Application in Surgery and
    Medicine." London, 1846.
    4. " A Record of Cases treated in the Mesmeric Hospital, from
    November, 1846, to December, 1847, with Reports of the Official
    Visitors. Printed by Order of the Government." Calcutta,
    1847.
    5. " Review of my Reviewers." Calcutta, 1848. (Reprinted from the
    India Register of Medical Science, vol. i.)
    6. " The Introduction of Mesmerism as an Anæsthetic and Curative
    Agent into the Hospitals of India." Perth, 1852.
    7. " Natural and Mesmeric Clairvoyance, with the Practical Application
    of Mesmerism in Surgery and Medicine." London, 1852.
    All, unfortunately, have long been out of print, and only Nos. 1, 3, 6,
    and 7 are to be found in the Library of the British Museum.
FELKIN, R. W., M.D. "Hypnotism or Psycho-Therapeutics." Edinburgh
    and London, 1890.
FÉRÉ and BINET, Profs. *See* BINET.
GREGORY, WILLIAM, M.D., F.R.S.E. " Animal Magnetism: or Mesmerism
    and its Phenomena." London, 1877.
GURNEY, EDMUND. " Second Report on Thought-Transference." *Proceedings
    of the Society for Psychical Research*, vol. i. p. 70.
    " Third Report on Thought-Transference." *Ibid.* vol i. p. 161.
    " The Stages of Hypnotism." *Ibid.* vol. ii. p. 61.
    " An Account of some Experiments in Mesmerism." *Ibid.* vol. ii.
    p. 201.
    " The Problems of Hypnotism." *Ibid.* vol. ii. 1884, p. 265.
    " Hallucinations." *Ibid.* vol. iii. p. 151.

(and MYERS, F. W. H.). "Some Higher Aspects of Mesmerism." *Ibid.* vol. iii. p. 401.

"Peculiarities of Certain Post-Hypnotic States." *Ibid.* vol. iv. 1887, p. 268.

"Stages of Hypnotic Memory." *Ibid.* vol. iv. p. 515.

"Recent Experiments in Hypnotism." *Ibid.* vol. v. 1888, p. 3.

"Hypnotism and Telepathy." *Ibid.* vol. v. p. 216.

(and MYERS, F. W. H.). "On Apparitions occurring soon after Death." *Ibid.* vol. v. p. 403.

HART, ERNEST. "Hypnotism and Humbug." *Nineteenth Century.* January, 1892.

"The Revival of Witchcraft." *Ibid.* February, 1893, p. 347.

"Hypnotism, Mesmerism, and the New Witchcraft." London, 1893.

"The Eternal Gullible." *The Century Illustrated Magazine.* October, 1894, p. 835.

HEIDENHAIN, RUDOLF, M.D. "Hypnotism or Animal Magnetism." Translated from the German by L. C. Wooldridge, M.D., D.Sc. London, 1888.

HODGSON, Dr. RICHARD. "A Case of Double Consciousness." *Proceedings of the Society for Psychical Research,* vol. vii. p. 221.

See DAVEY, S. J.

HOLLAND, Sir HENRY, M.D. "Effects of Mental Attention on Bodily Organs." *Medical Notes and Reflections* (London, 1839), p. 64.

"Chapters on Mental Physiology." Second edition, revised and enlarged. London, 1858.

HUDSON, T. J. "The Law of Psychic Phenomena." London, 1893.

HULST, HENRY, A.M., M.D. "Artificial Multiple Personality." *Bulletin of the Psychological Section of the Medico-Legal Society.* June, 1894, p. 1. (Grand Rapids, Mich., U.S.A.)

HYSLOP, T. B., M.D. "Mental Physiology" (London, 1895), pp. 349-353, 423-424, 440.

JAMES, Prof. WILLIAM, LL.D., etc. "The Principles of Psychology." London, 1890.

"The Varieties of Religious Experience : A Study in Human Nature." London, New York, and Bombay, 1903.

JOURNAL OF MENTAL SCIENCE. "Hypnotism" and "Hypnotism in Court." July and October, 1898.

KINGSBURY, Dr. G. C. "Dupuytren's Contraction of the Palmia fascia treated by Hypnotism." *British Medical Journal,* 1890.

"Should we give Hypnotism a Trial ?" *Dublin Journal of Mental Science,* 1891.

"The Practice of Hypnotic Suggestion." Bristol, 1891.

KRAFFT-EBING, Dr. R. VON. "An Experimental Study in the Domain of Hypnotism." Translated from the German by Charles G. Chaddock, M.D. New York and London, 1889.

LANCET, THE. "Demonstration of Hypnotism as an Anæsthetic during the Performance of Dental and Surgical Operations." April 5th, 1890.

LANGLEY, J. N., M.A., F.R.S. "Details of a Series of Valuable Investigations carried out by Mr. J. N. Langley, M.A., F.R.S., in conjunction with Mr. Wingfield, B.A." In "Report of the Committee appointed to investigate the Nature and Phenomena of Hypnotism, its Value as a Therapeutic Agent, and the Propriety of using it." *British Medical Journal*, July 29th, 1893.

MAYO, THOMAS, M.D., F.R.C.S. "Case of Double Consciousness." *London Medical Gazette*, New Series, vol. i. 1845, p. 1202.

MITCHELL, Dr. WEIR. "Case of Mary Reynolds." *Trans. of the College of Physicians of Philadelphia*, April 4th, 1888.

MOLL, Dr. ALBERT. "Hypnotism." Fourth edition, revised and enlarged. London, 1897.

MYERS, A. T., M.D. "The Life History of a Case of Double or Multiple Personality." (Reprinted from the *Journal of Mental Science*, January, 1886.) London, 1886.

"Hypnotism at Home and Abroad." (Reprinted from the *Practitioner*, March, 1890.) London, 1890.

(and SMITH, R. PERCY, M.D.). "On the Treatment of Insanity by Hypnotism." (Reprinted from the *Journal of Mental Science*, April, 1890.) London, 1890.

MYERS, F. W. H. "Second Report on Thought-Transference." *Proceedings of the Society for Psychical Research*, vol. i. p. 70.

"Third Report." *Ibid.* vol. i. p. 161.

"On a Telepathic Explanation of some so - called Spiritualistic Phenomena." *Ibid.* vol. ii. p. 217, part i.

(and GURNEY, EDMUND). "Some Higher Aspects of Mesmerism." *Ibid.* vol. iii. p. 401.

"Human Personality in the Light of Hypnotic Suggestion." *Ibid.* vol. iv. p. 1.

"On Telepathic Hypnotism, and its Relation to other Forms of Hypnotic Suggestion." *Ibid.* vol. iv. p. 127.

"Automatic Writing." III. *Ibid.* vol. iv. p. 209.

"Multiplex Personality." *Ibid.* vol. iv. p. 496.

"Note on Certain Reported Cases of Hypnotic Hyperæsthesia." *Ibid.* vol. iv. p. 532.

"Critical Notices." *Ibid.* vol. v. pp. 260, 263.

"Edmund Gurney's Work in Experimental Psychology." *Ibid.* vol. v. p. 359.

"French Experiments on Strata of Personality." *Ibid.* vol. v. p. 374.

"Automatic Writing. IV. The Dæmon of Socrates." *Ibid.* vol. v. p. 522.

"A Defence of Phantasms of the Dead." *Ibid.* vol. vi. p. 314.

Introduction to "A Record of Observations of Certain Phenomena of Trance." *Ibid.* vol. vi. p. 436.

"Review of A. Aksakof's *Animismus and Spiritismus*." *Ibid.* vol. vi. p. 665.

"Professor William James' *The Principles of Psychology*." *Ibid.* vol. vii. p. 111.

"On Alleged Movements of Objects, without Contact, occurring not in the Presence of a Paid Medium." *Ibid.* vol. vii. p. 146.

"The Subliminal Consciousness." *Ibid.* vol. vii. p. 298.

"The Subliminal Consciousness. Chap. v. Sensory Automatism and Induced Hallucinations." *Ibid.* vol. viii. p. 436.

" The Subliminal Consciousness." Chaps. vi. and vii. *Ibid.* vol. ix. pp. 3, 26.

(and MYERS, Dr. A. T.). "Mind-Cure, Faith-Cure, and the Miracles of Lourdes." *Ibid.* vol. ix. p. 160.

"The Experiments of W. Stainton Moses." I. *Ibid.* vol. ix. p. 245, and vol. xi. p. 24.

" Resolute Credulity." *Ibid.* vol. xi. p. 213.

" The Subliminal Self." *Ibid.* vol. xi. p. 334.

" Glossary of Terms used in Psychical Research." *Ibid.* vol. xii. p. 166.

" Recent Experiments in Normal Motor Automatism." *Ibid.* vol. xii. p. 316.

"The Psychology of Hypnotism." *Ibid.* vol. xiv. p. 100.

" Human Personality and its Survival of Bodily Death." (Longmans, Green and Co.) London, New York, and Bombay, 1903.

OSGOOD, HAMILTON, M.D. "Outcome of Personal Experience in the Application of Hypnotism and Hypnotic Suggestion." Boston, U.S.A., 1891.

"The Treatment of Sclerosis, various forms of Paralysis, and other Nervous Derangements by Suggestion." Boston, 1895.

PALL MALL GAZETTE, April 4th, 1895. "To inculcate contempt of others."

PEREIRA, JONATHAN, M.D., F.R.S. "The Elements of Materia Medica and Therapeutica." Second edition. Vol. ii. p. 1097. London, 1842.

PETERSON, FREDERICK, M.D., and KENNELLY, A. E., Chief Electrician, Edison Laboratory, Vice-President, American Institute of Electrical Engineers. "Some Physiological Experiments with Magnets at the Edison Laboratory." Read before the Section in Neurology of the New York Academy of Medicine, October 14th, 1892.

PRINCE, MORTON, M.D. "An Experimental Study of Visions." *Brain*, 1898, p. 528.

PROCEEDINGS OF THE SOCIETY FOR PSYCHICAL RESEARCH. "Report of the Hypnotic Committee for 1894-95." Vol. xi. p. 594.

RIBOT, Prof. TH. "The Psychology of Attention." London, 1890.

ROBERTSON, Dr. GEORGE M. "Hypnotism at Paris and Nancy: Notes of a Visit." *Journal of Mental Science*, 1892.

"The Use of Hypnotism among the Insane." *Ibid.* 1893.

ROMANES, G. J. "Hypnotism." *Nineteenth Century*, September, 1880, p. 474.

SMITH, Dr. R. PERCY, and MYERS, Dr. A. T. *See* MYERS, Dr. A. T.

SIDIS, BORIS, M.A., Ph.D. "The Psychology of Suggestion." New York, 1898.

STURGIS, RUSSELL, M.D. "The Use of Suggestion of the First Degree as a Means of modifying or of completely eliminating a Fixed Idea." *Medical Record*, New York, February 17th, 1894.

SULLY, Prof. JAMES. "Illusions: A Psychological Study." London, 1887.

SUTTON, C. W. "James Braid." *Dictionary of National Biography*, vol. vi p. 198. London, 1886.

TUCKEY, Dr. C. LLOYD. "Psycho-Therapeutics; or Treatment by Hypnotism." London, 1891.

"The Value of Hypnotism in Chronic Alcoholism." London, 1892.

"The Use of Hypnotism in Chronic Alcoholism." London, 1896.

"Case of Mischievous Morbid Impulse in a Child treated by Hypnotism." *Edinburgh Medical Journal*, June, 1897.

TUKE, D. HACK, M.D., LL.D. "Sleep - walking and Hypnotism." London, 1884.

"Imperative Ideas." *Brain*, part. ii., 1894, p. 179.

"A Dictionary of Psychological Medicine." Edited by. London, 1892.

TURNER, W. ARTHUR, L.D.S.ENG. "Extractions under Hypnotism." *Journal of the British Dental Association*, March 15th, 1890.

VINCENT, RALPH HARRY. "The Elements of Hypnotism." London, 1897.

WALLER, AUGUSTUS D., M.D., F.R.S. "An Introduction to Human Physiology." London, 1893.

WILKS, Sir SAMUEL, M.D., F.R.S. "Stray Thoughts on Some Medical Subjects." *The Lancet*, November 24th, 1894, p. 1197.

WILLIAMSON, WILLIAM CRAWFORD, LL.D., F.R.S. "Reminiscences of a Yorkshire Naturalist." London, 1896.

WOODS, JOHN F., M.D. "The Treatment by Suggestion with or without Hypnosis." *Journal of Mental Science*, April, 1897.

International Congress of Experimental Psychology. Second session, London, 1892.

'*The Zoist.* A Journal of Cerebral Physiology and Mesmerism." Thirteen volumes published from 1844 to 1856.

JAMES BRAID.

The following are all the books and articles by BRAID I have been able to trace :—

1. "Satanic Agency and Mesmerism reviewed, in a letter to the Rev. H. M'Neile, M.A., in Reply to a Sermon preached by him" (1842, 12mo).

2. "Neurypnology, or the Rationale of Nervous Sleep, considered in Relation to Animal Magnetism, illustrated by numerous cases of successful application in the Relief and Cure of Disease" (1843, 12mo, p. 381).

3. "The Power of the Mind over the Body : an Experimental Inquiry into the Nature and Cause of the Phenomena attributed by Baron Reichenbach and others to a 'New Imponderable'" (1846).

4. "Observations on Trance or Human Hybernation" (1850).

5. "Electro - Biological Phenomena, considered physiologically and psychologically," from the *Monthly Journal of Medical Science* for June, 1851, with Appendix.

6. "Magic, Witchcraft, Animal Magnetism, Hypnotism and Electro-Biology : being a Digest of the latest Views of the Author on these Subjects." Third edition, greatly enlarged, embracing observations on J. C. Colquhoun's *History of Magnetism* (1852).

7. "Hypnotic Therapeutics, illustrated by Cases, with an Appendix on Table-turning and Spirit-rapping." Reprinted from the *Monthly Journal of Medical Science* for July, 1853.

8. "The Physiology of Fascination and the Critics criticised" (1855). The second part is a reply to the attacks made in *The Zoist.*
9. "Observations on the Nature and Treatment of Certain Forms of Paralysis (1855).

Articles in the *Medical Times* :—

10. "Animal Magnetism." Vol. v. 1841-42, p. 283.
11. "Animal Magnetism." Vol. v. p. 308.
12. "Neuro-Hypnotism." Vol. vi. 1842, p. 230.
13. "Phreno-Mesmerism." Vol. ix. 1843-44, p. 74.
14. "Mr. Braid on Mesmerism." Vol. ix. p. 203.
15. "Observations on some Mesmeric Phenomena." Vol. ix. p. 225.
16. "Observations on Mesmeric and Hypnotic Phenomena." Vol. x. 1844, pp. 31 and 47.
17. "Cases of Natural Somnambulism and Catalepsy, treated by Hypnotism : with Remarks on the Phenomena presented during Spontaneous Somnambulism, as well as that produced by various Artificial Processes." Vol. xi. 1844-45, pp. 77, 95, and 134.
18. "Experimental Inquiry whether Hypnotic and Mesmeric Manifestations can be adduced in Proof of Phrenology." Vol. xi. p. 181.
19. "Magic, Mesmerism, Hypnotism, etc., historically and physiologically considered." Vol. xi. pp. 201, 224, 270, 296, 399, and 439.
20. "Case of Natural Somnambulism, etc." Vol. xii. 1845, p. 117 (article giving further history of case already reported).
21. "The Fakirs of India." Vol. xii. 1845, p. 437.
22. "Dr. Elliotson and Mr. Braid." Vol. xiii. 1845-46, pp. 99, 120, and 141.
23. "On the Power of the Mind over the Body : an Experimental Inquiry into the Nature and Cause of the Phenomena attributed by Baron Reichenbach and others to a 'New Imponderable.'" Vol. xiv. 1846, pp. 214, 252, and 273.
24. "Facts and Observations as to the Relative Value of Mesmeric and Hypnotic Coma and Ethereal Narcotism, for the Mitigation or entire Prevention of Pain during Surgical Operations." Vol. xv. 1846-47, p. 381 ; continued, vol. xvi. 1847, p. 10.
25. "Observations on the Use of Ether for preventing Pain during Surgical Operations, and the Moral Abuse it is capable of being converted to." Vol. xvi. p. 130.
26. "Mr. Braid and Dr. Elliotson." Vol. xvii. 1847-48, p. 106.
27. "Mr. Braid and Mr. Wakley." Vol. xvii. p. 163.
28. "Observations on Trance or Human Hybernation." Vol. xxi. 1850, pp. 351, 401, and 416.

In *The Lancet* :—

29. "Queries respecting the alleged Voluntary Trance of Fakirs in India." Vol. ii. 1845, p. 325.

In the *Monthly Journal of Medical Science* :—

30. "Hypnotic Therapeutics, illustrated by Cases." Vol. viii. Third Series, 1853, p. 14.

In the *Edinburgh Medical and Surgical Journal :—*

31. "The Power of the Mind over the Body: an Experimental Inquiry into the Nature and Cause of the Phenomena attributed by Baron Reichenbach and others to a 'New Imponderable.'" Vol. lxvi. 1846, p. 286.

32. "Facts and Observations as to the Relative Value of Mesmeric and Hypnotic Coma, and Ethereal Narcotism, for the Mitigation or entire Prevention of Pain during Surgical Operations." Vol. lxvii. 1847, p. 588.

33. "On the Use and Abuse of Anæsthetic Agents, and the best Modes of rousing Patients who have been too intensely affected by them." Vol. lxx. 1848, p. 486.

34. "On the Distinctive Conditions of Natural and Nervous Sleep." Manchester, December 17th, 1845. A manuscript first published in a German translation in Preyer's book, *Der Hypnotismus*, 1890.

35. *Manchester Times*, September 1st, 1842. Account of case of total deafness successfully treated by hypnotism.

36. "Abstract Report of a Course of Six Lectures on the Physiology of the Nervous System—with particular reference to the States of Sleep, Somnambulism (natural and induced), and other conditions allied to these—delivered at the Royal Manchester Institution, in March and April, 1853, by William B. Carpenter." *Manchester Examiner and Times* of April 30th, 1853. By James Braid.

37. "On Table-moving: a Letter to the Editor of the *Manchester Examiner and Times.*" This letter appeared on June 22nd, 1853, and was afterwards published as a pamphlet.

38. A Manuscript on Hypnotism by James Braid. January, 1860. Translated into French by Dr. Jules Simon as an appendix to *Neurypnologie*, and into German by Preyer in *Die Entdeckung des Hypnotismus.*

39. "Talipes." *The Lancet*, vol. i. 1841-42, p. 202.

40. "Entire Absence of Vagina, with Rudimentary State of Uterus, and Remarkable Displacement of Rudimentary Ovaries and their Appendages, in a married female, 74 years of age." *Monthly Journal of Medical Science*, vol. xvi. (Third Series, vol. vii.) 1853, p. 230.

41. "Observations on Talipes, Strabismus, Stammering, and Spinal Contortion, and the best Methods of removing them." *Edinburgh Medical and Surgical Journal*, vol. lvi. 1841, p. 338.

In the *London Medical Gazette*, New Series :—

42. "Lateral Curvature of the Spine—Strabismus." Vol. i. 1840-41, p. 445.

43. "Stammering." Vol. i. p. 445.

44. "Cure of Stammering." Vol. ii. 1840-41, p. 116.

45. "On the Operation of Talipes." Vol. ii. p. 186.

46. "Case of Congenital Talipes varus of a Foot with Ten Toes." With illustration. 1848.

47. "Arsenic as a Remedy for the Bite of the Tsetse, etc." *British Medical Journal*, March 13th, 1858.

48. The Manchester and Salford Sanitary Association. A letter (on the means of improving the air of Manchester and upon the connection between cholera and sewers) of November 15th, 1853, in the *Examiner and Times.*
49. The Manchester Geological and Natural History Societies. A controversial letter in the *Manchester Courier* of November 26th, 1859.

The following are the principal references to BRAID'S work that I have been able to trace :—

In the *Medical Times* :—

1. "The New Theory of Animal Magnetism." Vol. v. 1841-42, p. 175. Editorial account of a lecture given by Mr. Duncan on Animal Magnetism, at the Hanover Square Rooms, on December 31st, 1841. The lecturer, who had adopted Braid's views, explained them.
2. "Animal Magnetism." Vol. v. 1841-42, p. 283. Editorial account of two lectures by Braid, one on March 1st, 1842, at Hanover Square, and the other next day at the London Tavern.
3. "On Mr. Braid's Experiments." By Dr. Herbert Mayo. Vol. vi. 1842, p. 11.
4. "Mesmerism." Vol. vi. 1842, p. 47. Editorial account of two lectures delivered by Braid.
5. "Hypnotism, or Mr. Braid's Mesmerism." Vol. x. 1844, p. 98. Letter to Editor from "S." in praise of Braid's researches and of the open-mindedness of the *Medical Times.*
6. "Conversazione on Hypnotism." Vol. x. 1844, p. 137. Editorial account of the Conversazione held by James Braid, at the Royal Manchester Institution, on April 22nd, 1844, by invitation of the Committee.
7. "Jenny Lind and Hypnotism." Vol. xvi. 1847, p. 602. An interesting account of Braid's experiments to show the power of somnambulists in imitating languages and song.
8. "Operations under Hypnotism in Paris." Vol. xix. 1859, p. 646. Account of Azam, with reference to Braid.
9. "Mr. Braid of Manchester." Vol. i. 1860 (new series), p. 355. Obituary notice.
10. "The Late Mr. Braid." Vol. i. 1860 (new series), p. 396. Letter to Editor from A. W. Close, F.R.C.S., exposing the absurdity of certain statements in the above account of Mr. Braid's death.

In *The Lancet* :—

11. "Mr. Braid's new Operation for Club Foot." Vol. i. 1841-42, p. 326.
12. "Hypnotism in Paris." Vol. ii. 1859, p. 650. Article referring to Azam, Velpeau, Broca, etc., and stating that they had copied the methods of Braid and Esdaile.
13. "Sudden Death of Mr. James Braid, Surgeon, of Manchester." Vol. i. 1860, p. 335.

In the *Edinburgh Medical and Surgical Journal*:—

14. Critical article on Braid's "Observations on Trance or Human Hybernation." Vol. lxxiv. 1850, p. 421.
15. "Abstract of a Lecture on Electro-Biology," delivered at the Royal Institution, Manchester, on March 26th, 1851, by James Braid. Vol. lxxvi. 1851, p. 239.
16. "Death of Mr. James Braid, Surgeon, of Manchester." Vol. v. 1859-60, p. 1068.
17. "Case of Contracted Foot with Severe Pain, cured by Mesmerism." *The Zoist*, vol. iii. 1845-46, p. 339. Article by Elliotson, referring to Braid.
18. "Researches in Magnetism, Electricity, Heat, Light, Crystallisation, and Chemical Attraction in their Relations to Vital Force." By Karl, Baron von Reichenbach, Ph.D. Translated by William Gregory, M.D. London, 1850.
19. Article V. *The British and Foreign Medico-Chirurgical Review*, vol. viii., July to October, 1851, p. 378. An article on Mesmerism, Magnetism, and Hypnotism, with favourable reference to Braid and his views.
20. "Death of Mr. Braid, Surgeon." *The Manchester Courier*, Saturday March 31st, 1860. This article gives an account of Braid's life and writings.
21. "Observations on Animal Magnetism." By M. Andral. *London Medical Gazette*, vol. i. 1832-33, p. 792.
22. "Electrical Psychology; or the Electrical Philosophy of Mental Impressions, including a New Philosophy of Sleep and of Consciousness." From the works of the Rev. John Bovee Dods and Prof. J. S. Grimes. Revised and edited by H. G. Darling, etc. London, Glasgow. Printed 1851.
23. "Spirit Manifestations examined and explained: Judge Edwards refuted; or an Exposition of the Involuntary Powers and Instincts of the Human Mind." By J. B. Dods. New York, 1854.
24. "The Philosophy of Mesmerism and Electrical Psychology . . . comprised in two Courses of Lectures, by J. B. Dods." Edited by J. Burns. London, 1876.
25. "Mystères des sciences occultes." Par un Initié. Paris (no date). A short account of Braid is given, pp. 296-300, and at p. 289 is to be found a portrait of Braid. (Facsimile d'une lithographie d'après nature, imprimée à Liverpool, en 1854.)
26. "Ephémérides de l'hypnotisme." This contains an account of Braid, without reference to his later works. *Revue de l'Hypnotisme*, vol. ii. 1888, p. 276.
27. "Neurypnology, or The Rationale of Nervous Sleep." By James Braid, M.R.C.S., etc. A New Edition, edited, with an Introduction, Biographical and Bibliographical, embodying the Author's Views, and further Evidence on the Subject, by Arthur Edward Waite. London, 1899.

Note.—Numerous other works and articles containing accounts of Braid are included in the general references.

APPENDIX.

(A) JAMES BRAID.

SINCE writing the historical chapter of this book, my attention has been drawn to the following independent account of the origin of Braid's researches, from the pen of the late Dr. Williamson, formerly Professor of Natural History at Owens College, Manchester. This I think of sufficient interest to quote in detail :—

"During the fourth decade of this century the subject of clairvoyance had been much discussed in social circles, and in the early days of my professional life two men who lectured on the subject visited Manchester. The first of these was a Frenchman, who illustrated his lecture by experiments on a young woman. At one of his lectures the girl was declared to be in a state of sound sleep. A considerable number of medical men were present, including our leading ophthalmist, Mr. Wilson, and one Mr. Braid. The latter gentleman was loud in his denunciation of the whole affair. The audience then called upon Mr. Wilson for his opinion of the exhibition. Of course the question was, 'Is this exhibition an honest one or is it a sham?' 'Is the girl really asleep, or is she only pretending to be so?' In reply to the call of the audience, Mr. Wilson stood up and said : 'The whole affair is as complete a piece of humbug as I ever witnessed.' The indignant lecturer, not familiar with English slang phrases, excitedly replied : 'The gentleman says it is all *Bog;* I say it is not *Bog;* there is no *Bog* in it at all.' By this time several of us, including Mr. Wilson, had gone upon the platform to examine the girl. I at once raised her eyelids, and found the pupils contracted to two small points. I called Wilson's attention to this evidence of sound sleep, and he at once gave me a look and a low whistle, conscious that he was in a mess. Braid then tested the girl by forcing a pin between one of her nails and the end of her finger. She did not exhibit the slightest indication of feeling pain, and Braid soon arrived at the conclusion that it was not all 'Bog.'

"He subsequently commenced a long series of elaborate experiments, which ended in his placing the subject on a more philosophical basis than had been done by any of his predecessors. For the term

2 H

'Animal Magnetism' and other popular phrases, Braid substituted
'Hypnotism' and 'Monoideism.'

"The hypothesis which he adopted was that the subjects of these
experiments required to have their mental faculties concentrated upon
one idea; this accomplished, two effects will be produced in a few
moments. The first is a state of sound sleep, which he succeeded in
obtaining through either of the several senses, sight, hearing, or touch;
but his favourite plan was to seat the individual operated upon in an
arm-chair, whilst he held a bright silver object, usually his lancet case,
a few inches above the person's eyebrows, and required him to raise
his eyes upwards until he saw the shining metal, soon after doing
which, the patient went off into a sound sleep. But a still more remarkable result followed, indicating a condition of mind not so easily
explained as illustrated.

"On one occasion I called Braid in to see a young lad who had
been suffering fearfully from a succession of epileptic attacks, which
had failed to yield to medical treatment. So far as the epilepsy was
concerned the hypnotic treatment was a perfect success; the boy, after
having long endured numerous daily attacks, was perfectly relieved
after the third day's hypnotic operation. For five subsequent years,
during which the youth remained under my observation, the epilepsy
did not return.

"Braid always awoke his subjects from their hypnotic condition by
sharply clapping his hands close to the sleepers' ears, which at once
aroused them. One day, before doing this, Braid said to me, 'I will now
show you another effect of hypnotism. Lend me your pocket-book and
pencil.' I did so. He then placed the book in the boy's left hand,
which he raised into a convenient position in front of the lad's breast.
My pencil was placed in his right hand, which was lifted into such a
position that the point of the pencil rested upon one of the pages of
the book. This attitude was rigidly maintained until Braid whispered
in his ear: 'Write your name and address.' The lad did so: 'John
Ellis, Lloyd Street, Manchester.' This done, the book and pencil were
restored to my pocket. Braid then awoke the boy and asked, 'John,
what were you doing just now?' He looked about rather wildly for
a moment, and persistently answered, 'Nothing.' Braid then sent him
off to sleep again. The question was again asked: 'John, what were
you doing just now?' The lad answered promptly, but in a low voice:
'Writing my name and address.' A succession of similar experiments
clearly indicated two things: first, that a mesmerised individual would
do what he was told to do; second, that things done when in that
state were remembered only when the same condition was resumed;
otherwise they were forgotten, indicating a *dual state of mind*, which, so
far as I know, has not yet been satisfactorily explained. I cannot
learn that Braid's method of experimental inquiry and of philosophical
induction has been continued by any person since he died.

"The second visitor to Manchester was of a different type. He appeared to be a man of some financial position in the world, since he had a gentlemanly demeanour and kept a yacht, of which the lad whom he brought with him to Manchester was said to be cabin-boy. It was affirmed that this lad was a clairvoyant, who could see to read, however much his eyes were plastered up. Some persons were invited out of the audience to apply this plastering, and after they had done so, the lad certainly read as easily as before. I at once expressed myself dissatisfied with the test, and was requested by some of the audience to undertake the closing of the eyes with these plasters. I tried to do so, but careful watching convinced me that by vigorous movements of the muscles acting upon the eyelids, the lad contrived to loosen a minute fold of the plaster close to his eye; through this fold he managed to read the books. I saw at once that this could be stopped by cutting a long strip of plaster which should cover the eyebrows, and at the same time binding down the edges of all the plasters with which the eyes were closed. In order to prevent any muscular action from disturbing this additional bandage, I stretched it tightly round the temples and fastened the two ends firmly together at the back of his head. I had no sooner done this with one of his eyes, than he prevented me from adopting the same plan with the other; he began to yell and declared I was killing him with pain. His master instantly turned upon me, and affirmed that I had covered that part of the lad's forehead with which he did see. Then the credulous fools in the audience fell foul of me for being so cruel. Of course I threw the thing up and resumed my seat. The next day a few medical friends met the two fellows at their hotel and plugged each of the boy's eyes with small balls of cobbler's wax; the clairvoyant's vision at once terminated, they left, and no more was afterwards heard of them."

(B) SPIRITUALISM, CLAIRVOYANCE, TELEPATHY

A certain section of the general public believe that there is a connection between hypnotism and spiritualism, and that those who practise the former must be in sympathy with the latter. Any connection with the Society for Psychical Research is also regarded as affording still stronger evidence of spiritualistic belief. I wish, therefore, to supplement what I have already said as to spiritualistic and other so-called occult phenomena. On pages 146-7, I called attention to some alleged spiritualistic manifestations which were said to have occurred during hypnotic trance. In the case referred to, the medium's condition was obviously not one of hypnosis. Further, I have never seen a single instance in which hypnotic phenomena could with justice be claimed to be of spiritualistic origin.

Although undoubtedly certain members of the Society for

Psychical Research are believers in spiritualism, the main work of that body has been destructive. Thus, the late Professor Henry Sidgwick said : "We have continually combated and exposed the frauds of professional mediums, and have never yet published in our *Proceedings* any report in favour of any of them." The following are examples of this destructive work :—

(1) A report of an investigation by Sir William Crookes, Sir Victor Horsley, and the late Dr. A. T. Myers, of an alleged supernatural phenomenon to which the spiritualists attached great importance, and the investigators none at all.

(2) The complete destruction by Dr. Hodgson of the Theosophical claim to miraculous powers, and of the existence of Mahatmas.

(3) A series of experiments contrived to illustrate the " Possibilities of Mal-observation and Lapse of Memory." These practically refuted the assertions that certain phenomena must be due to spirits, because they could not have been produced by mortals. Mr. S. J. Davey, a member of the Society, since deceased, gave several years to the assiduous practice of certain tricks of sleight of hand; these he so successfully supplemented by ingenious psychological artifices as to render them inexplicable. It would be difficult to find any piece of laboratory work on attention comparable in subtlety and skill with Mr. Davey's demonstrations; while, if we wish to protect ourselves and our fellow-creatures against fraud and imposture, this kind of reply is more effective (though more difficult to obtain) than any mere denial or attempt at ridicule can be.

Although I have seen nothing to convince me of the genuineness of alleged spiritualistic phenomena, the subject is not without interest to the physician. From time to time I see patients whose health has undoubtedly suffered from their taking part in spiritualistic *séances*. One of these, a young lady now under my care, was supposed to be what is termed a "sensitive," and underwent training with a view of developing this quality. She informed me that during the *séances* she was frequently conscious of the presence of a spirit. Her hands then became lifeless and fell from the table, and she experienced a peculiar sensation of suffocation. She is now ill both mentally and physically, and fears that she is losing her reason.

Although I know of no genuine case of clairvoyance, many persons believe in its existence. The latter may be divided into two groups :—

(1) *Those who are the victims of self-deception.* I have been assured by several persons, whose honesty and good faith were undoubted, that they had succeeded in making hypnotic somnambules see what was taking place at a distance. When the experiment was repeated in my presence, the source of fallacy was at once obvious. The operator gave the necessary information to the subject by leading questions and the like.

In some instances it is the ignorance of the spectators which causes belief in the so-called occult powers. For example, an unqualified man, who practised "mesmeric healing," informed me that he had a somnambule in his pay who possessed the power of clairvoyance. She could, he said, diagnose in this way the diseases of his patients, and also give important suggestions as to their treatment. The man obviously believed his own statements. I pointed out to him, however, that he took no steps to confirm his clairvoyant's diagnosis, and that this might possibly be a wrong one. As he was quite willing to put the matter to the test, I offered myself for experiment. The clairvoyant, after holding my hand for some time, informed me that I had disease of the liver. Although I doubtless possess this organ, it has certainly never forced itself on my notice through disordered function. I was, however, suffering from a poisoned wound of the finger, and the axillary glands and lymphatics of my arm were inflamed. My hand was swollen and enveloped in a poultice, and my arm was in a sling. These obvious outward indications of disease the clairvoyant failed to notice.

(2) *Cases where the alleged clairvoyant power is assumed for purposes of deception.* Of this the following is a typical example :—

I was asked one day by a young woman to buy tickets for a lecture on clairvoyance. She assured me that not only could she see what was taking place at a distance, but also that she was able to foretell future events. She could, for example, predict the rise and fall of stocks, or name the winner of the next Derby. I pointed out that if this were true, she might easily have saved herself the trouble of calling : her clairvoyant powers ought to have informed her that I had no intention of purchasing tickets for her lecture.

As already stated, although successful telepathic experiments were formerly reported by several members of the Society for Psychical Research, these have not been confirmed by later observers. Despite this, the belief in telepathy is widespread. A typical example is cited by William James, not, however, as evidence in favour of telepathy (*The Varieties of Religious Experience*, p. 125). The patient sat quietly with a Christian Science healer for half an hour each day, and attributed the result of the treatment to telepathy, although he admitted that verbal suggestions were given. The messages were received, he said, in a mental stratum quite below the level of his immediate consciousness, and reached him from a corresponding mental stratum of the healer's mind. As we have seen, many of the errors of the mesmerists and of the Salpêtrière school arose through unconscious suggestion. In the case just cited, suggestion was obviously present, and in others, where the telepathic healing was said to be done from a distance, suggestion was not excluded. The patients knew that an attempt was being made to influence them, and thus self-suggestion came into play.

The idea that one may be influenced from a distance, against one's will and without one's knowledge, is startling enough, even when the supposed influence is asserted to be for one's good. What must one think, however, of the mystic who was an anti-vivisectionist as well as a telepathist, and who claimed to have killed Pasteur by means of malign telepathic influences? With a few exceptions, *i.e.* the more or less rigorously conducted experiments already referred to, the so-called telepathy of the present day is simply an attempt to represent in pseudo-scientific language the superstitions and practices of the dark ages. The occultist who claims to kill telepathically differs little, if at all, from the witch who was willing to do an enemy to death by the slow melting of his waxen counterfeit and the like.

INDEX.

---

[1] In all instances where "cases" are cited, it is to be understood that these have been treated by *suggestion*, associated with *hypnotic methods*.

AUTHORS AND AUTHORITIES REFERRED TO.

Albrecht, 86
Alcock, 81, 90, 92
Allbutt, Clifford, 164
Allden, 224
Arndt, 209
Artigalas, 82
Ashburner, 10
Audiffrent, 172
Avenbrugger, 5
Azam, 26, 29, 30, 386

Babinski, 365
Backman, 266
Bagnold, Col., 277
Baillarger, 247
Baillif, 48, 68
Balfour, A. J., 35
Balfour, G. W., 35
Ball, 246
Bamberger, 356
Barclay, 129, 135
Barkworth, 129, 135
Barrett, W. F., 35
Bartrum, 138
Bauer, 232, 238
Beach, Fletcher, 236
Beard, 209
Beaunis, 33, 34, 35, 42, 48, 55, 60, 68, 82, 83, 87, 89, 93, 105, 113, 115, 307, 329, 348, 370, 377, 398, 400, 402, 403, 409
Bechterew, 225, 238
Benedikt, 357
Bennett, John Hughes, 30, 38, 294, 303, 304, 307, 308, 375, 483
Berger, 48 68, 76
Bergson, 89
Bérillon, 57, 62, 181, 199, 207, 209, 232, 237, 238, 251, 252, 260, 263, 266, 299
Bertrand, 68, 280

Berry, Mrs. Dickinson, 197
Bernheim, 28, 31, 33, 34, 35, 42, 47, 48, 53, 55, 57, 62, 63, 65, 66, 68, 69, 70, 73, 75, 83, 94, 97, 104, 105, 106, 108, 153, 154, 181, 191, 198, 208, 225, 245, 274, 275, 296, 298, 307, 309, 311, 314, 325, 328, 330, 337, 338, 339, 340, 342, 343, 344, 345, 348, 350, 366, 376, 398, 401, 409, 425, 426, 427
Billinger, 86
Binet, 32, 75, 94
Bingswanger, 209
Boismont, Brierre de, 246
Bouchut, 306
Bouffé, 238
Boulting, 195, 201, 203, 235, 243
Bourdon, 173, 207, 208, 225, 238, 245
Bourru, 82, 208
Bouveret, 209
Bowditch, 35
Braid, James, 1, 4, 21, 29, 30, 38, 39, 40, 45, 52, 55, 61, 64, 73, 75, 78, 79, 87, 88, 90, 91, 92, 97, 106, 107, 141, 144, 145, 148, 150, 152, 161, 198, 212, 244, 258, 275, 278, 283, 286, 287, 290, 293, 300, 301, 304, 310, 311, 328, 338, 340, 342, 344, 345, 348, 354, 425, 433, 437, 438, 465
Braithwaite, 164
Bramwell, J. P., 38
Brémaud, 214
Briand, 199
Broca, 27

Brochin, 251
Brouardel, 329
Brown, W. H., 164
Brown-Séquard, 305
Bruce, Lewis C., 164, 380
Brügelmann, 207, 208
Brunnberg, Tyko, 199
Bugney, 199
Burckhardt, 208, 216
Burot, 82, 189, 199, 208, 215, 245
Bushnell, 225

Caddy, 164
Calonder, 429
Carpenter, W. B., 30, 75, 294, 306, 343, 370, 388, 390, 438
Carter, T., 164, 166
Chambers, 211
Charcot, 34, 39, 77, 85, 297, 300, 301, 366, 425
Charpentier, 266
Charpignon, 329
Chenevix, 6
Churton, 164, 264
Clausner, 86
Clifford, 356
Cobbe, 371, 373
Conrad, 358
Copland, 10, 355
Corval, von, 208, 262
Crawfurd, Raymond, 196, 209
Crocq, 55, 329
Crookes, Sir William, 468
Cruise, Sir Francis, 36
Cullerre, 238

"Dagonet," 382
Davidson, 277
Debove, 95
Dècle, 199

475

THE END

Printed by R. & R. CLARK, LIMITED, *Edinburgh.*

PRESS NOTICES

self or patients to hypnotic treatment. The first is the erroneous belief that a capacity for being hypnotised is a sign of weakness of mind or even of actual mental defect. The exact opposite appears to be the case. . . . The second great prejudice lies in the fear that the subject may become so subservient to the will of the operator that he or she will be placed wholly in the latter's power. . . . It is clear from Dr. Bramwell's book that in at least the great majority of instances the subject possesses, while hypnotised, plenty of will power to resist unpleasant or immoral suggestions. . . .

". . . In conclusion, we would cordially recommend Dr. Bramwell's book to all who are interested in the subject of hypnotism either professionally or merely scientifically. It is written in a strictly scientific spirit; no exaggerated claims are made for his specialty, nor are facts put forward in a startling manner to attract the curious reader. It constitutes a valuable account of a branch of psychology possessing a distinct medical interest, apart from the light which it may one day shed upon difficult problems in mental activity."

THE LIVERPOOL MEDICO-CHIRURGICAL JOURNAL, July 1903.

"The time has gone by when the phenomena of hypnotism can be dismissed as partaking merely of quackery and deception, and the genuineness of many of its manifestations is now generally recognised. . . . A work on the subject, therefore, from Dr. Milne Bramwell, whose name is well known in connection with the revived interest in hypnotism which took place a few years ago, is to be welcomed, and the more so since there is a deficiency of authoritative expositions on the subject in this country."

THE LIVERPOOL MEDICO-CHIRURGICAL JOURNAL, January 1904.

". . . Although we are far from looking on hypnotism as such a valuable curative agent as it is represented to be by Dr. Bramwell, yet we can cordially recommend his book to all those who take an interest in psychological subjects. It is pleasantly and clearly written, contains the results of much research, and the writer evidently endeavours to avoid exaggeration of every kind, and to put his case forward as fairly as he can. . . . We can only repeat, in conclusion, that, while there is much in this book concerning which we have grave doubts, the work is one of great merit and full of interest. . . ."

MEDICAL CHRONICLE, December 1903.

". . . Dr. Milne Bramwell has produced in this interesting volume a valuable contribution to the English literature of the subject. Well written and clear in style, moderate in tone, while not disguising the author's sincere conviction of the therapeutic value of hypnotic suggestion, and presenting in moderate compass a fairly complete account of the phenomena of the hypnotic state, this book will be welcomed by many medical and scientific readers. . . . The extensive bibliography and copious index largely increase its value for purposes of reference."

THE SCOTTISH MEDICAL AND SURGICAL JOURNAL.

"Dr. Bramwell's book ought to be welcomed by a great number of readers, for it appeals to several different sections of the thinking public. Students of the history of medicine, moralists, psychologists, physiologists, as well as physicians and surgeons, may all learn much to their advantage from it, and we imagine a class of sensational novelists will seek for ideas and guidance in these pages. . . . While we have here a handbook for those who desire to study or practise hypnotism, no practitioner can peruse the work without learning much, were it only as a fresh demonstration of the immense value of the force of the mind."

MIND. New Series, No. 53, January 1905.

"The author of this work is well known as one of the very few English physicians who, at the present time, apply hypnotism regularly and successfully to the cure of disease. In this volume he presents a summary of the more important observations made by himself during the twelve years that he has actively practised hypnotism; and gives also a clear and very readable sketch of the history, facts, theories, and methods of hypnotism. . . . Amongst the most interesting and carefully made experiments are those of Dr. Bramwell on the post-hypnotic measurement of time, here fully reported and discussed. The results of these experiments are among the most remarkable of all the many astonishing and puzzling achievements of hypnotised persons. . . . In two chapters on hypnotic treatment of disease, Dr. Bramwell reviews the many types of cases that have been successfully treated, and illustrates them, for the most part, from his own practice. He concludes this section with some admirable maxims, which are summed up in the one weighty sentence: 'The central factor in all hypnotic treatment ought to be the development of the patient's control of his own organism.' A fact of great theoretical interest is that Dr. Bramwell obtains in many cases marked therapeutic effects by simple suggestions repeated to patients who sit with closed eyes in a drowsy state, but in whom no symptoms of hypnosis are discoverable. So good are the results thus obtained, that he relies in an increasing degree upon this method, deeming it unnecessary to induce a distinctly hypnotic state. . . . In conclusion, it may be said that the book is especially well suited to introduce medical men to the study and practice of hypnotism, and to prove to them that in it we have an aid to the treatment of disease that is of great power and value in many cases, and devoid of danger in all, when practised on the sound lines laid down by the author; and it must be added that it contains much matter of the deepest interest to every student of the mind."

PROCEEDINGS OF THE SOCIETY FOR PSYCHICAL RESEARCH.

"This is a remarkable book—remarkable not only for what it says, but even more for what it abstains from saying. Dr. Bramwell is best known perhaps as a distinguished practitioner, who has had no small share in raising hypnotism to the recognised and almost orthodox position which, after many decades of calumny, is now accorded to it by the medical profession in Great Britain. This alone would entitle him to our attention. But he is more than this; he is an active and acute inquirer. He has made himself the historian of hypnotism, and has been the first to bring fully to light the splendid work of his countryman and predecessor, James Braid: work which has been too long ignored, and must now take its place among the most original and illuminating contributions of Great Britain to mental and medical science. And he is besides a keen and trenchant psychologist—not merely a critic of the theories of others, but the author of a remarkable series of experiments which have done much to throw fresh light on the theory of his craft. . . . It is no small gain that the question should at length, and perhaps for the first time in its history, be removed from the heated atmosphere of rash assertion, blind prejudice, and more than theological persecution in which it has passed its stormy and none too healthy infancy. It is one of the hardest of scientific lessons to learn to state mere facts uncoloured by preconceived ideas, and it is at least a proof of courage that Dr. Bramwell, in spite of all temptations, should have held fast to this attitude of detachment. . . . The average medical man, no less than the average patient, needs to have the whole subject stripped of the supernatural and abnormal, and put before him in the driest light of dispassionate science; and perhaps for the benefit of sufferers at least, Bramwell's chief service is that he should so resolutely have struck out of his book anything that has the least savour of the uncanny or abnormal or sensational, and given us a treatise which offers little for the paragraphist of the halfpenny press, but infinite interest, not only to the scientific thinker, but to every one who desires to know more of the workings of that extraordinary complex which we call Self."

REVUE PHILOSOPHIQUE.

"Ce volume constitue une monographe aussi complète que possible sur l'hypnotisme, d'une utilité incontestable, aujourd'hui surtout, où l'hypnotisme, après avoir subi tant d'attaques et avoir été traité avec tant de mépris, a fini par s'imposer par l'évidence de ses résultats et des services qu'il rend journellement, soit comme procédé thérapeutique, soit comme moyen d'expérimentation psychologique. Réunir ces résultats, en discuter la valeur, analyser et comparer les différents procédés d'hypnotisation, employés par les expérimentations, poser enfin autant que possible des règles précises concernant les indications et les contre-indications de l'hypnotisme, et cela en se basant sur douze années d'expérience personnelle, tel a été le but de M. Bramwell en écrivant ce volume. . . ."

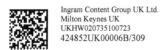

Ingram Content Group UK Ltd.
Milton Keynes UK
UKHW020735100723
424852UK00006B/309